Handbook
of Clinical
Nutrition

Provided as an educational service by

THIRD EDITION

Handbook
of Clinical
Nutrition

Douglas C. Heimburger, MD, MS
Associate Professor and Director,
Division of Clinical Nutrition
Departments of Nutrition Sciences and Medicine

Roland L. Weinsier, MD, DrPH
Professor and Chairman,
Department of Nutrition Sciences
Professor, Department of Medicine

University of Alabama at Birmingham
Schools of Medicine, Health-Related Professions,
and Dentistry

with 29 illustrations

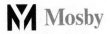

St. Louis Baltimore Boston Carlsbad Chicago Naples New York
Philadelphia Portland London Madrid Mexico City Singapore
Sydney Tokyo Toronto Wiesbaden

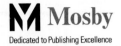

M Mosby

Dedicated to Publishing Excellence

A Times Mirror Company

Vice President and Publisher: Anne S. Patterson
Executive Editor: James Shanahan
Developmental Editors: Carolyn Malik Kruse,
Laura Berendson
Project Manager: Linda McKinley
Production Editor: Catherine Bricker
Design Manager: Elizabeth Fett
Book Designer: Tenenbaum Design,
Jane Tenenbaum

THIRD EDITION

Printed in the United States of America
Composition by Clarinda Company
Printing/binding by RR Donnelley & Sons Company

Mosby-Year Book, Inc.
11830 Westline Industrial Drive
St. Louis, Missouri 63146

Library of Congress Cataloging in Publication Data
Heimburger, Douglas C.
    Handbook of clinical nutrition. — 3rd ed. / Douglas C.
Heimburger, Roland L. Weinsier.
        p.   cm.
    Rev. ed. of: Handbook of clinical nutrition / Roland L. Weinsier,
Douglas C. Heimburger, Charles E. Butterworth, Jr. 2nd ed. 1989.
    Includes bibliographical references and index.
    ISBN 0-8151-9274-6
    1. Diet therapy—Handbooks, manuals, etc. I. Weinsier, Roland L.
Handbook of clinical nutrition.   II. Weinsier, Roland L.   III. Title.
    [DNLM: 1. Diet Therapy—handbooks.   2. Nutrition—handbooks.
WB 39 H467h 1996]
RM217.2.H45 1996
615.8'54—dc20
DNLM/DLC
for Library of Congress   96-20199
                                                              CIP

96 97 98 99 00 / 9 8 7 6 5 4 3 2 1

Contributors

Reinaldo Figueroa-Colon, MD
Assistant Professor,
Division of Pediatric
  Gastroenterology and
  Nutrition,
Departments of Pediatrics and
  Nutrition Sciences,
University of Alabama at
  Birmingham,
Birmingham, Alabama

Frank A. Franklin, Jr, MD, PhD
Professor and Director,
Division of Pediatric
  Gastroenterology and
  Nutrition,
Departments of Pediatrics and
  Nutrition Sciences,
University of Alabama at
  Birmingham,
Birmingham, Alabama

Douglas C. Heimburger, MD, MS
Associate Professor and Director,
Division of Clinical Nutrition,
Departments of Nutrition
  Sciences and Medicine,
University of Alabama at
  Birmingham,
Birmingham, Alabama

Adrian F. Heini, MD
Associate/Fellow,
Division of Clinical Nutrition,
Departments of Nutrition
  Sciences and Medicine,
University of Alabama at
  Birmingham,
Birmingham, Alabama

Donald D. Hensrud, MD, MPH, MS
Assistant Professor of Preventive
  Medicine and Nutrition,
Mayo Clinic,
Rochester, Minnesota

Cora E. Lewis, MD, MSPH
Assistant Professor,
Division of Preventive Medicine,
Department of Medicine,
University of Alabama at
  Birmingham,
Birmingham, Alabama

Sarah L. Morgan, MD, MS, RD
Associate Professor,
Division of Clinical Nutrition,
Departments of Nutrition
  Sciences and Medicine,
University of Alabama at
  Birmingham,
Birmingham, Alabama

Lisa L. Mullins, MA, RD
Clinical Dietetic Specialist,
Division of Human Nutrition and
    Dietetics,
Department of Nutrition Sciences,
University of Alabama at
    Birmingham,
Birmingham, Alabama

Christopher M. Reinold,
    MPH, RD
Senior Nutrition Consultant,
Jefferson County Department of
    Health

Christine S. Ritchie, MD
Assistant Professor,
Division of Gerontology and
    Geriatric Medicine,
Department of Medicine,
University of Alabama at
    Birmingham,
Birmingham, Alabama

Delia Smith, PhD
Assistant Professor,
Division of Preventive Medicine,
Department of Medicine,
University of Alabama at
    Birmingham,
Birmingham, Alabama

Charles B. Stephensen, PhD
Associate Professor,
Division of International Health,
Department of Public Health
    Sciences,
Division of Public Health
    Nutrition,
Department of Nutrition Sciences,
University of Alabama at
    Birmingham,
Birmingham, Alabama

David R. Thomas, MD
Assistant Professor,
Division of Gerontology and
    Geriatric Medicine,
Department of Medicine,
University of Alabama at
    Birmingham,
Birmingham, Alabama

Glen Thompson, PharmD
Division Director,
Department of Pharmacy,
University of Alabama Hospital,
University of Alabama at
    Birmingham,
Birmingham, Alabama

Roland L. Weinsier, MD, DrPH
Professor and Chairman,
Department of Nutrition
    Sciences;
Professor,
Department of Medicine,
University of Alabama at
    Birmingham,
Birmingham, Alabama

Nancy H. Wooldridge, MS, RD
Assistant Professor,
Pediatric Pulmonary Center,
Departments of Pediatrics and
    Nutrition Sciences,
University of Alabama at
    Birmingham,
Birmingham, Alabama

James A. Wright, Jr, MD
Associate Professor,
Division of Gastroenterology and
    Nutrition,
Departments of Pediatrics and
    Nutrition Sciences,
University of Alabama at
    Birmingham,
Birmingham, Alabama

Preface

In 1977, we wrote the first version of the *Handbook of Clinical Nutrition*. This version was published locally in response to the demand of our medical students, residents, and ward dietitians for a pocket-sized nutrition manual in a ready-reference format. It came at a time when nutrition support services were just beginning to appear and little practical information or guidance was available for members of the health care team who were interested in providing nutritional support for hospitalized patients.

In 1981, Mosby published the first edition of our *Handbook*. However, with the rapid expansion of information on nutritional support of the acutely ill patient, a second edition became necessary almost immediately. Now we have been asked to prepare the third edition to better inform clinicians of the many medical-nutrition advances that have appeared in the last few years and expand the sections dealing with health promotion and preventive nutrition services. Thus not only have all sections been updated to incorporate new concepts and references, but this edition also contains important new information on the role of nutrition in the following areas:

- Childhood and adolescence
- Aging
- Obesity
- Gastrointestinal disorders
- Bone disease
- AIDS
- Transplantation

We hope once again that you as physicians, nurses, dietitians, pharmacists, and other health care providers will find valuable information in our *Handbook of Clinical Nutrition* that will strengthen your role in the team approach to providing effective health care and disease prevention through nutrition.

Douglas C. Heimburger, MD, MS
Roland L. Weinsier, MD, DrPH

Acknowledgments

This book is a publication of the Departments of Nutrition Sciences and Medicine of the University of Alabama at Birmingham. It was supported in part by PHS Grant # 1-R25-CA47888, awarded by the National Cancer Institute, DHHS.

We deeply appreciate the assistance of Garland W. Scott in attending to many details without which this book would not have been possible.

Introduction

For some time now the American public has shown a significant interest in the relationships between nutrition and health. The media continually fuel this interest, overwhelming consumers with books, articles, testimonials, and advertisements proclaiming the health advantages of certain food and diets while denouncing others as life-threatening. The scientific community and media have often reversed advice previously given on health issues, prompting many persons to become either wary or cynical of their suggestions. Time-honored associations between what is consumed and a person's physical health, such as the association of certain food with a stomachache or of a hearty meal with a sense of well-being, have made many individuals susceptible to questionable health claims, whereas increasing scientific sophistication and rising skepticism have led others to justify maintaining unhealthy habits. The upward spiral in health care expenditures has made the public increasingly hopeful that an ounce of nutritional prevention may be worth well more than a pound of cure.

Unfortunately, physicians are all too often unprepared or ill-equipped to provide guidance to their patients. The stock phrase, "Before going on this or any other diet, seek the advice of your physician," is often little more than a device to protect commercial interests rather than the public. Nevertheless, many individuals prefer to receive information about nutrition from their doctors and tend to trust its validity more than if it were to come from other sources.

We live in a time during which remarkable scientific progress is being made in our understanding of nutrient requirements and the interactions between diet and health. With the development of new laboratory methods, electronic devices, computers, and radioisotopes for medical use, a person's nutritional status can be assessed more rapidly and accurately than ever before. There have been equally important advances in clinical nutrition. Methods have been developed that can sustain a satisfactory nutritional status in a patient for indefinite periods, even when that patient has lost virtually the entire gastrointestinal tract. Thus intestinal failure is now often less life-threatening than failure of organs such as the kidneys, heart, and lungs that can be replaced with transplants; intestinal transplantation holds additional promise for these patients. Considerable progress is also being made in understanding nutrient metabolism in specific disease states. The role of nutrition in the etiology and management of heart disease, cancer, and other leading causes of death is being intensively studied. Nutrition promises to be an increasingly important component of the physician's armamentarium in the years ahead.

Public demand coupled with rapid advances in nutrition science and biomedical technology has increased the pressure on medical professionals to learn about and incorporate nutrition into their practice. Therefore there must be a well-informed community of nutrition professionals who can perform nutritional assessments and provide nutritional support and counseling. To be effective, these professionals must have essential information and practical references at their fingertips and even the bedside in well-organized and indexed formats—this compact volume is intended to meet this need. It is our hope that by equipping health care professionals with the tools needed to deliver nutritional care, this book will contribute to the welfare of healthy persons and patients alike.

Contents

PART II
Nutritional Support in Patient Management, *167*

27 AIDS, 520

28 Organ Transplantation, 529

Appendixes, 539

PART I

Nutrition for Health Maintenance

1

Health Promotion and Disease Prevention

NUTRITION AND DISEASE PREVENTION

It has been argued that it is more reasonable to identify individuals who are at risk for disease and need intervention strategies than to modify the health behaviors of the general public. However, dietary recommendations aimed at reducing the general population's risk for disease can have a major benefit for the nation's health. A relatively small risk reduction for a disease that occurs in many moderate-risk people could lead to a larger risk reduction for the total population than a large risk reduction for a smaller number of high-risk people. For example, modifying diets to reduce coronary artery disease in the general population is considered worthwhile because most deaths occur in people who have only moderate elevations in serum cholesterol (200 to 240 mg/dl) and not in those at high risk due to high serum cholesterol levels. Similarly, decreasing salt and fat intake may substantially reduce the risk of hypertension and certain cancers, but the effects on many individuals may be small or absent. Although genetic factors can affect individual susceptibility, they appear to account for only a small part of the observed variation in disease incidence among populations as exemplified by the tendency of migrants to acquire the disease rates of their adoptive countries. With future advances in understanding genetic variability and its interaction with the environment, we will be increasingly able to supplement recommendations for the general population with more sophisticated, individually based dietary intervention.

TRENDS IN DIET AND DISEASE

At the turn of the century the leading causes of death were infectious diseases, and curing them would have reduced death rates. Today most of the leading causes of death in Western countries are strongly influenced by how people live, and medical resources are mainly invested in treating diseases associated with specific lifestyles. Heart disease, cancer, and stroke account for two thirds of all deaths in the United States; one third of us will die of coronary artery disease (CAD) before age 65. Many others will be disabled by these illnesses and their complications.

Changes in eating patterns parallel history's disease trends. In lieu of the high-fiber, low-fat foods once used, refined starches, sweets, saturated fats, and salt comprise a major share of today's typical American diet. Table 1-1 lists eight of the ten current leading causes of death. Of these, five are strongly linked with unhealthy dietary habits, and three are associated with alcohol abuse. The table also details the many dietary factors related to significant causes of morbidity, such as obesity, hypertension, osteoporosis, diverticular disease, and neural tube defects.

Traditionally, our health care system's goal and measure of success have been related to an increase in life expectancy, regardless of well-being or quality of life. However, reducing morbidity—improving quality of life and maximizing the period of good health—may be more important. If prevention guidelines like the ones in this chapter are followed, there should be a resulting decrease in morbidity.

CURRENT DIETARY HABITS IN THE UNITED STATES

Surveys suggest that people in higher educational and income brackets have been more responsive to public health recommendations, yet most Americans do not follow published dietary guidelines. Although the percentage of calories from fat has fallen from about 41% to 36%,

TABLE 1-1 Dietary influences on the major causes of death and morbidity in the United States[1]

Cause of death or morbidity	Factors associated with a decrease in risk	Factors associated with an increase in risk
Death		
Coronary heart disease	Intake of complex carbohydrates, particular fatty acids (e.g., monounsaturated, polyunsaturated, and ω-3 fatty acids from fish), soluble fiber, antioxidants (vitamins E and C, β-carotene, selenium), folic acid, soy protein, alcohol in moderation.	Intake of saturated fat, *trans* fatty acids, and cholesterol; excess of calories, sodium, animal protein; abdominal distribution of body fat
Cancer	Intake of fruits, vegetables (for β-carotene—vitamins A, C, D, and E; folic acid; calcium; selenium; phytochemicals), fiber	Intake of excess calories, fat, alcohol, red meat, salt- and nitrite-preserved meats, possibly grilled meats; abdominal distribution of body fat
Stroke	Intake of potassium, calcium, ω-3 fatty acids	Sodium, alcohol consumption (as with hypertension)
Accidents	—	Alcohol consumption
Diabetes mellitus	Fiber intake	Intake of excess calories, fat, alcohol; abdominal distribution of body fat

Continued

TABLE 1-1 Dietary influences on the major causes of death and morbidity in the United States[1]—cont'd

Cause of death or morbidity	Factors associated with a decrease in risk	Factors associated with an increase in risk
Death—cont'd		
Suicide	—	Alcohol consumption
Chronic liver disease	—	Alcohol consumption
Atherosclerosis (peripheral)	Intake of particular fatty acids (e.g., monounsaturated, ω-3 fatty acids), soluble fiber, antioxidant vitamins	Saturated fat, cholesterol consumption
Morbidity		
Obesity	—	Excess calories, fat consumption
Hypertension	Intake of potassium, calcium, ω-3 fatty acids	Intake of sodium, alcohol, excess calories; abdominal distribution of body fat
Osteoporosis	Calcium, vitamin D intake	Excess of sodium, phosphorus, protein consumption
Diverticular disease, constipation	Fiber intake	—
Neural tube defects	Folic acid intake	—

and Americans are more likely to choose low-fat than whole milk, the use of high-fat cheeses has more than doubled and cream intake is rising. Fruits and vegetables, specifically cruciferous (e.g., broccoli, cauliflower) and carotenoid-containing (most green and yellow) vegetables that are thought to play a role in reducing cancer risk, are still consumed in relatively small amounts. According to the latest USDA Nationwide Food Consumption Survey (1987 to 1988)[2] of more than 10,000 Americans, only a small proportion reported daily consumption of any food thought to reduce the risk of cancer; a mere 18% ate dark-green and yellow vegetables high in carotene. By contrast the proportion of Americans consuming foods that have the potential to increase cancer risk was high; 74% ate red meat and 25% ate sausage and luncheon meats.

As of 1995 substantial progress has been made with certain diet-related disorders relative to the goals of the 1990 U.S. Public Health Service report *Healthy People 2000.* Heart disease and stroke, blood-pressure control, and cancer deaths have all improved. By contrast, no progress has been made in reducing diabetes-related deaths, and the prevalence of obesity has risen by an astounding 33% despite a reduction in total fat intake.

EATING FOR OPTIMUM HEALTH

There have been at least five reports of dietary guidelines for Americans published in recent years, and at least 19 reports of national dietary guidelines outside of the United States. It is noteworthy that there is close agreement on the general recommendations made in these reports, which enhances their credibility. The most widely publicized guidelines are those in the USDA/DHHS food guide pyramid (Figure 1-1), which pictorially prioritizes food groups in terms of their importance to health. The guidelines discussed are distilled from various recent publications, although there is not total agreement on every aspect.

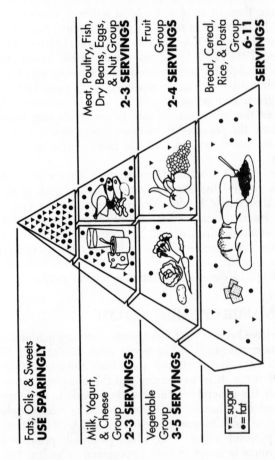

**Fats, Oils, & Sweets
USE SPARINGLY**

**Milk, Yogurt,
& Cheese
Group
2-3 SERVINGS**

**Meat, Poultry, Fish,
Dry Beans, Eggs,
& Nut Group
2-3 SERVINGS**

**Vegetable
Group
3-5 SERVINGS**

**Fruit
Group
2-4 SERVINGS**

**Bread, Cereal,
Rice, & Pasta
Group
6-11
SERVINGS**

▼ = sugar
● = fat

FIGURE 1-1 USDA/DHHS food guide pyramid.

Dietary Guidelines
1. Eat Less Fat, Particularly Saturated Fat

Aim: Consume less than 25% of calories as total fat, less than 7% of calories as saturated fat, and less than 300 mg/day of dietary cholesterol. Because there is no risk and great potential benefit, some experts suggest reducing total fat intake to as low as 10% of calories. Eat less than three 3-oz servings (roughly the size of a deck of playing cards) of red meat a week.

Comments: Fats, whether in the form of oils, margarine, or butter, provide two times more calories (9 kcal/g) than carbohydrates and protein (each 4 kcal/g), so reducing all fats is an important method for reducing energy intake and the risk of obesity (and therefore diabetes). Decreasing total fat intake may also reduce the risk of cancers such as cancer of the colon, prostate, and breast; reducing saturated fat specifically lowers the risk of CAD.

Saturated fats are solid at room temperature and found primarily in meat and dairy products (butter, cream, cheese, red meat) and some vegetable products (solid margarine made from coconut oil, palm oil, cocoa butter, and vegetable oil that have been hydrogenated). Dietary cholesterol comes solely from animal products. As a substitute for saturated fats, complex carbohydrates (i.e., fruit, vegetables, whole-grain products) have the advantage over polyunsaturated fats (i.e., oil, margarine) of being lower in energy content and higher in many essential nutrients and fiber. Intake of saturated fat and cholesterol can be reduced by substituting fish, poultry without skin, lean meats, and low-fat dairy products for fatty meats and whole-milk dairy products.

Liberal use of polyunsaturated fat is not advised, as high intakes have promoted tumors in animals. In addition, *trans* fatty acids, which are formed by the partial hydrogenation of liquid vegetable oil in the production of margarine and vegetable shortening, do not increase high-density lipoprotein (HDL) or reduce low-density lipoprotein (LDL) levels in serum as do polyunsaturated fats, and they have also been associated with CAD. By contrast, the largely monounsaturated olive oil appears to be beneficial except for its high energy content. The apparent CAD risk reduction that is associated with olive oil may be related in part to the fact that LDL particles formed in a diet high in monounsaturated fat are relatively resistant to oxidation, an important step in the atherosclerotic process.

An additional benefit of decreasing total fat intake, especially animal fat, is an anticipated reduction in cancers of the breast, colon, and prostate. Although a reduced fat intake should help diminish the prevalence of obesity, the recent U.S. trend in which people use low-fat products must be viewed with skepticism. The fat is often substituted with sugar and diglycerides (which are not classified as fat on food labels), so calorie intake does not necessarily decline.

2. Adjust Energy Intake for Weight Control

Aim: Achieve and/or maintain ideal body weight.

Comments: Shakespeare admonished, *"Leave gourmandizing. Know the grave doth gape for thee thrice wider than for other men."* The following statements, found printed on Egyptian papyrus, are even earlier warnings about the adverse effects of excess energy intake: *"Most of what we eat is superfluous. Hence, we only live off a quarter of all we swallow; doctors live off the other three quarters."* These statements summarize well the health risks of obesity or excessive weight; weight control entails an understanding of how to match average daily energy intake to actual daily requirements. Recommendations on diet modification for weight control are discussed in Chapter 15.

3. Eat More Vegetables, Fruit, and Whole-Grain Food

Aim: Consume at least 55% of calories as carbohydrates. Eat at least 7 servings of a combination of vegetables and fruit and at least 6 servings of a combination of unrefined starch and legumes.

Comments: Preferred carbohydrates include fresh fruit, green and yellow vegetables, whole-grain bread and cereal, beans, baked potatoes, and other unrefined starch. Recommendations to eat liberal amounts of vegetables and fruit are supported by a wealth of research data indicating they are associated with a reduced risk of developing cancer, especially cancers of the lung, breast, colon, and stomach. The reasons these foods are beneficial are not completely clear but may relate to the fact that they are good sources of fiber, folic acid, and antioxidants such as B-carotene and vitamin C. Vegetables, fruit, and unrefined starch are all low in calorie content and help displace foods with higher energy densities, such as fats and simple sugars, that are conducive to obesity. Because of their natural high nutrient content, when sufficient quantities of complex carbohydrates are eaten, vitamin supplements are not necessary or recommended.

4. Reduce Salt Intake

Aim: Consume less than 6 g/day.

Comments: The taste for salt is acquired and can be modified. On average, Americans consume about 10 to 12 g of salt per day, about 20 times the requirement (less than 0.5g/day, equivalent to less than 200 mg of sodium). Because susceptibility to salt-induced hypertension (i.e., salt-sensitive individuals) cannot be identified easily, and reducing salt intake has no detrimental effects, the reduced salt intake recommendation is reasonable for the entire population and specifically beneficial for hypertension-prone individuals. It entails refraining from adding salt to foods in preparation or at the table; infrequently using sodium-rich items such as steak and soy sauce, bouillon cubes, soups, chips, and crackers; and reading labels to avoid packaged and canned foods that have high sodium contents (i.e., greater than 150 mg/serving).

5. Consume Protein-Rich Food in Moderation

Aim: Consume less than 2 to 3 servings/day of high-protein foods (i.e., meat, poultry, fish, eggs, nuts).

Comments: The average protein intake in this country, about 100 to 140 g/day, is well in excess of need, which is closer to 40 to 60 g/day for the average adult. Most adults can consume an adequate amount of protein without the use of animal products by following a diet that contains a variety of vegetables and starch. In fact, animal protein causes increased calcium loss in the urine and in excessive amounts can contribute to osteoporosis.

6. Consume Dairy Products in Moderation

Aim: Consume 2 to 3 servings/day of low-fat dairy products such as milk, yogurt, and cheese.

Comments: The optimal calcium intake remains uncertain; recommendations have varied from 800 mg to 1500 mg/day. To achieve these levels by using an appropriate diet would necessitate the use of dairy products because they are relatively high in calcium content. For example, 8 oz of milk provides 250 to 300 mg of calcium. However, there are reasons to be cautious about the liberal use of dairy products: (1) Adult populations in other countries with low bone-fracture rates generally consume few dairy products and actually have low calcium intakes by our standards. (2) Using dairy products to achieve high calcium-intake levels may not equate to taking calcium supplements, which have been shown to reduce the number of fractures in older adults. (3) Dairy products contain substantial amounts of protein (which increases calcium loss), they may increase the intake of saturated fat, and their lactose content is not tolerated by a large segment of the population. (4) Milk consumption can decrease iron absorption by as much as 50% which may induce iron deficiency in individuals with marginal iron status. (5) Dairy products are not the only source of calcium; greens, spinach, broccoli, and beans also contain substantial amounts. Rather than relying heavily on dairy foods or even calcium supplements, it may be possible to reduce the incidence of bone fractures by following an active exercise program, reducing animal-protein intake, consuming significant amounts of vegetables, and when appropriate using estrogen replacement therapy.

7. Drink Alcohol in Moderation, If at All

Aim: Consume less than 1 oz of pure alcohol per day (2 cans of beer, 2 small glasses of wine, or 2 average cocktails). Pregnant women should avoid alcoholic beverages.

Comments: Although some studies suggest that a moderate alcohol intake is associated with a lower risk of CAD, it is not recommended that nondrinkers actually start consuming alcohol; drinking poses other health risks that may offset any potential advantages. In addition, because alcohol is high in energy density (7 kcal/g or 200 kcal/oz of ethanol), alcoholic beverages may contribute significantly to total calorie intake.

Summary of Dietary Guidelines

Experimental data and lessons derived from populations with low rates of chronic diseases, such as atherosclerosis, obesity, diabetes, and cancer, commonly reveal several components that should form the dietary foundation for our daily eating patterns. These data indicate that our meals should be based mainly on whole grains, legumes (beans, peas) and other vegetables, and generous amounts of fruit. Poultry and fish should be used in moderation, and red meat and eggs should be used infrequently or completely excluded. Although less certain, it is likely that a healthy diet may also include moderate consumption of low-fat dairy products and little or no alcohol consumption.

Food Labels

In 1994 the U.S. government published regulations for food labels so that the public could receive reliable information to help them follow the recommended dietary patterns. The objective was to standardize the nutrient contents, terminology, and serving sizes that are printed on labels to prevent the food industry from confusing consumers with misleading terms and varying serving sizes. In addition, standard guidelines were issued regarding health

TABLE 1-2 Definitions of terms used on food labels

Term	Definition
Low fat	≤3 g per serving
Low saturated fat	≤1 g per serving, ≤15% of calories
Low calorie	≤40 calories per serving
High	≥20% of desired daily value per serving
Light	Half the fat or one third the calories of the regular product
Reduced	≤75% of the content of the regular product
Free	None or an insignificant amount (e.g., <1 g fat or <0.5 g sugar per serving)
Healthy	Low total and saturated fat, sodium, and cholesterol; ≥10% daily value for vitamin A, vitamin C, iron, calcium, protein, or fiber

Modified from U.S. DHHS, FDA, USDA.

claims because food manufacturers wanted to make health-positive claims on their labels. The guidelines are summarized in Tables 1-2 and 1-3.

Dietary Supplements

Approximately one half of the adults in the United States report using nutritional supplements. In many cases they are self-prescribed. Accumulating evidence suggests that for some persons, supplementation with certain vitamins may be beneficial (e.g., folic acid for women with child-bearing potential and vitamin E for persons with CAD). However, the most desirable dietary approach for the general public to take is to obtain the recommended levels of nutrients by eating a variety of whole foods as described previously. When the diet is optimal, routine use of nutritional supplements may be of little benefit to most people, and unprescribed daily use of vitamin B_6, selenium, and

TABLE 1-3	Permissible health claims for food labels
Items on label	**Permissible claim**
Calcium	May lower the risk for osteoporosis
Fat	May increase the risk for cancer
Saturated fat and cholesterol	Increase the risk for CAD
Fiber-containing grain products, fruits and vegetables	May reduce the risk for CAD and cancer
Sodium	May increase the risk for high blood pressure
Folic acid supplementation	Reduces the risk for neural tube defects

Modified from U.S. DHHS, FDA, USDA.

fat-soluble vitamin supplements in amounts exceeding the Recommended Dietary Allowances (RDA) should be avoided.

Dietary Guidelines for Vegetarians

Because of the recognized health advantages of a vegetarian diet, more and more people are selecting meatless diet patterns as a way of life. Many choose simply to eliminate red meat. Others also avoid poultry, fish, and perhaps even eggs, and some avoid dairy products as well (vegans). The benefits of these diets are that they are generally low in saturated fat and cholesterol and high in complex carbohydrates such as fruit, vegetables, and unrefined starch. Vegetarians usually have lower rates of CAD, obesity, hypertension, and cancer.

All of the described variations of a vegetarian diet can provide adequate nutrition, although a little extra planning may be necessary for those who are vegans, especially children and pregnant or nursing women. The protein content of vegetarian diets is generally adequate for adults, and no special adjustments need to be made or supplements taken. Although consuming complementary plant proteins was stressed in the past, it is now believed that an adequate mix of amino acids will be consumed by simply eating a variety of plant foods. Children and pregnant women who are vegans and do not use any animal products are at greater risk of protein deficiency because of their increased requirements. In such cases it is wise to combine specific food groups at each meal to be certain that the specific essential amino acid that is deficient in one food source is available in another. For example, either nuts and seeds can be combined with legumes (beans and peas), legumes can be combined with cereal grains, or cereal grains can be combined with leafy vegetables to ensure that the appropriate complement of all amino acids is consumed.

The individuals at greatest risk for nutrient deficiency are those who rely on a single plant food source rather than a variety of foods in their diets. Legumes are rich in protein, B vitamins, and iron. Unrefined grain is a good source of protein, thiamin, iron, and trace minerals. Nuts and seeds contribute essential fats, protein, B vitamins, and iron. Dark green, leafy vegetables contribute calcium, riboflavin, and carotene (a precursor of vitamin A). By contrast, plant foods provide no vitamin B_{12}, and although milk and eggs are satisfactory sources of this vitamin, vegans should consume fortified soybean milk or vitamin B_{12} supplements.

Nutrition and Athletic Performance

With the increasing interest in sports and fitness has come an increase in research on the role of diet in athletic performance. Unfortunately, there has also been a dramatic rise in misinformation and advertisements touting the benefits of a variety of nutrient supplements. Although anecdotal information has exceeded scientific data, there is sound information on several aspects of diet and performance that warrants consideration.

Protein Requirements

Protein metabolism may change during endurance exercise or rigorous weight training, increasing skeletal muscle catabolism and the need for amino acids. However, the amount required is small and is expected to be met by a daily intake of only about 12 g of protein (supplied by approximately 1.5 oz of a protein-rich food). Sweating during vigorous physical activity also increases nitrogen loss but only to a very small extent. Approximately 4 hours of strenuous exercise results in a loss of about 7.5 g of protein. During weight training muscle mass will increase; to add 1 oz of muscle mass a day, an adult male would require an additional 7.5 g of protein/day. Theoretically, if the described conditions were combined (strenuous exercise and adding muscle mass), requirements may increase to 27 g of additional protein per day at most. This need is likely to be met by protein consumption in the average American diet, which generally exceeds requirements by 40 to 50 g/day. In addition, there is no evidence performance is enhanced by taking amino acid supplements. Thus supplementary amino acids and high-protein foods are not necessary for either endurance- or weight-trained athletes.

Electrolyte Requirements

The major source of loss of electrolytes during exercise is sweat. Each liter of sweat contains about 10 to 30 mEq (230 to 690 mg) of sodium and 3 to 10 mEq (120 to 390 mg) of potassium. For the conditioned and acclimated athlete, sweating does not usually cause electrolyte imbalances and salt tablets are unnecessary. For the unacclimated individual who is exposed to extreme conditions with heavy fluid losses, diluted, commercially-available, electrolyte-containing fluids may be needed.

Vitamin/Mineral Requirements

The need for some vitamins increases with physical activity in proportion to the increase in energy requirements.

However, this increased requirement is small and easily met by a balanced, unsupplemented diet. A number of studies have been performed on athletes to test the potential benefits of additional vitamin intake of a variety of vitamins, including riboflavin, vitamin C, and vitamin E. None of the studies demonstrated any measurable improvement in the athletic performance of athletes who took vitamin supplements as compared with those who took placebos.

Sports anemia or runner's anemia has been reported as a transient phenomenon during the early stages of strenuous physical training, especially among females. Although iron deficiency is not usually present, it must be ruled out as the cause of the anemia. If iron status is normal, iron supplements are not indicated and are unlikely to increase red blood cell production.

Precompetition Meals and Glycogen Loading

Preparation for competition requires attention to dietary intake patterns. Although practices vary, many athletes have found that performance is enhanced by adhering to a few basic dietary principles on the day of the event. The goal is generally to avoid foods that delay gastric emptying, produce flatulence, leave a heavy residue, and suppress fatty acid mobilization. These goals can be accomplished by choosing low-fat, low-bulk, high-carbohydrate foods. The carbohydrates should not be in a form that is too concentrated such as candy, honey, or concentrated sugar drinks because they tend to increase movement of fluid into the intestinal tract and may also impair performance by inhibiting the release of free fatty acids from adipose tissue for use by the muscle. Instead, a dilute sugar solution can be comfortably consumed periodically (even during the athletic event); this practice is encouraged during prolonged endurance exercise. Caffeine-containing drinks have variable effects on exercise performance and may be disadvantageous because their diuretic effect increases the risk of dehydration and need to urinate during the event.

There is a positive relationship among dietary carbohydrate content, muscle-glycogen concentration, and endurance exercise performance. On the basis of this information, various glycogen-loading techniques have been used by athletes to increase performance during long-distance events. One commonly used approach involves following a low-carbohydrate, glycogen-depletion diet and then switching to a high-carbohydrate, glycogen-repletion regimen before the event. Some researchers have found that similarly high levels of glycogen stores can simply be achieved with a precompetition, high-carbohydrate diet and rest. Because of the uncertainty of the safety of the depletion/repletion diet, it may be wiser to use the simpler carbohydrate-loading approach.

References

1. Heimburger DC: *Nutrition's interface with health and disease.* In Bennett JC, Plum F, eds: *Cecil textbook of medicine,* ed 20, Philadelphia, 1996, WB Saunders.
2. US Department of Agriculture—Human Nutrition Information Service: *Food and nutrient intakes by individuals in the United States, 1 day, 1987-1988,* Nationwide Food Consumption Survey, 1987-1988, Report No 87-I-1, Washington, DC, 1993.

Suggested Readings

Are you eating right? *Consumer Reports,* October, 1992.
McArdle WD, Katch FI, Katch VL: *Exercise physiology: energy, nutrition, and human performance,* ed 3, Philadelphia, 1991, Lea & Febiger.
National Heart, Lung, and Blood Institute: *Report of the task force on research in epidemiology and prevention of cardiovascular diseases,* Washington, DC, 1994, US DHHS.
U.S. DHHS, Public Health Service: *Promoting health/preventing disease: year 2000 objectives for the nation,* Washington, DC, 1989, US DHHS.
Willett WC: Diet and health: what should we eat?, *Science* 264:532-537, 1994.

2

Nutrients: Metabolism, Requirements, and Sources

This chapter comprises tables of basic information about nutrients. Although the tables are far from exhaustive, they can serve as quick references for important facts about each of the major nutrients. Information on human nutrient requirements from the Recommended Dietary Allowances (RDA) is listed in Tables 2-1, 2-2, and 2-3. Table 2-4 details the functions, body stores, deficiencies, assessments, treatments, and potential toxicities of the nutrients, and Table 2-5 gives additional information about dose ranges for prevention and treatment of vitamin deficiencies. The food sources of most of the nutrients are listed in the remaining tables (Tables 2-6 to 2-27).

VITAMIN SUPPLEMENTS

With billions of dollars being spent annually on vitamin and mineral supplements in the United States, appropriate usage is an important issue. Reasons cited for supplement use include health enhancement, disease prevention, prophylaxis against the stresses of daily living, restoration of vigor and energy, and prevention or cure of a variety of conditions, including the common cold, arthritis, cancer, depression, and premenstrual syndrome. Many of these reasons are unfounded. Although vitamin deficiencies cause a variety of signs and symptoms (see Table 2-4), the deficiencies may not be a frequent cause of these symptoms in the United States; nutrient supplements may not improve symptoms caused by other factors. (See

Chapter 1 for guidelines and indications for use of nutrient supplements.)

VITAMIN TOXICITIES

Most vitamins act as cofactors in biochemical reactions and are required in the minute quantities that are supplied by a varied diet. The minimum daily requirement (formerly referred to as the "MDR") is the smallest amount of a vitamin needed to prevent the signs and symptoms of a deficiency from occurring. The RDAs outline the levels of daily nutrient intake that are estimated to cover the nutritional requirements of 97% of the population; these are generally 2 to 6 times the minimum daily requirement. In dose levels far in excess of the requirements, vitamins act not only as cofactors but as pharmacologic agents as well. In some cases these two actions are very different. Therefore it cannot be assumed that high doses simply amplify the effects of lower doses.

Because they are stored in the body, an excess intake of certain fat-soluble vitamins can result in an accumulation of toxic quantities. For example, vitamin A taken by an adult in daily doses greater than 50,000 IU for several months can precipitate liver abnormalities, bone and joint pain, hypercalcemia, scaling of the skin, and headaches (from increased intracranial pressure [pseudotumor cerebri]).

When present in excess amounts most water-soluble vitamins are excreted in the urine, so it is often assumed that water-soluble vitamins are less likely to cause toxicity. Although this is generally true, water-soluble vitamins can be toxic. A prolonged intake of large doses of vitamin B_6 (pyridoxine) can cause peripheral neuropathy with numbness and paresthesia, especially in the lower extremities. Because these symptoms have been caused by dosages as low as 200 mg/day for several months and do not always completely resolve after discontinuation, using pyridoxine in this manner should be discouraged.

See Table 2-4 for the known toxicities of other vitamins and minerals; clinical findings in some vitamin toxicities are also shown in Table 8-2.

Text continued on p. 82.

TABLE 2-1 Recommended dietary allowances[a]

Category	Age (yr) or condition	Weight[b] (kg)	Weight[b] (lb)	Height[b] (cm)	Height[b] (in)	Protein (g)	Fat-soluble vitamins Vitamin A (µg RE)[c]	Vitamin D (µg)[d]	Vitamin E (mg α-TE)[e]	Vitamin K (µg)
Infants	0.0-0.5	6	13	60	24	13	375	7.5	3	5
	0.5-1.0	9	20	71	28	14	375	10	4	10
Children	1-3	13	29	90	35	16	400	10	6	15
	4-6	20	44	112	44	24	500	10	7	20
	7-10	28	62	132	52	28	700	10	7	30
Males	11-14	45	99	157	62	45	1000	10	10	45
	15-18	66	145	176	69	59	1000	10	10	65
	19-24	72	160	177	70	58	1000	10	10	70
	25-20	79	174	176	70	63	1000	5	10	80
	51+	77	170	173	68	63	1000	5	10	80

Females									
11-14	46	101	157	62	46	800	10	8	45
15-18	55	120	163	64	44	800	10	8	55
19-24	58	128	164	65	46	800	10	8	60
25-50	63	138	163	64	50	800	5	8	65
51+	65	143	160	63	50	800	5	8	65
Pregnant	—	—	—	—	60	800	10	10	65
Lactating First 6 mo	—	—	—	—	65	1300	10	12	65
Second 6 mo	—	—	—	—	62	1200	10	11	65

From National Research Council, Food and Nutrition Board: Recommended dietary allowances, ed 10, Washington, DC, 1989, National Academy Press.

[a]Designed for the maintenance of good nutrition of practically all healthy people in the United States; the allowances, expressed as average daily intakes over time, are intended to provide for individual variations among most normal persons as they live in the United States under usual environmental stresses. Diets should be based on a variety of common foods in order to provide other nutrients for which human requirements have been less well defined.

[b]Weights and heights of reference adults are actual medians for the U.S. population of the designated age, as reported by NHANES II. The median weights and heights of those under 19 years of age were taken from Hamill et al (1979). The use of these figures does not imply that the height-to-weight ratios are ideal.

[c]Retinol equivalents. 1 retinol equivalent = 1 μg retinol or 6 μg β-carotene.

[d]As cholecalciferol. 10 μg cholecalciferol = 400 IU vitamin D.

[e]α-Tocopherol equivalents. 1 mg d-α tocopherol = 1 α-TE.

Continued

TABLE 2-1   Recommended dietary allowances[a] —cont'd

Category	Age (yr) or condition	Weight (kg)	Weight (lb)	Height (cm)	Height (in)	Protein (g)	Vitamin C (mg)	Thiamin (mg)	Riboflavin (mg)	Niacin (mg NE[f])	Vitamin B6 (mg)	Folate (µg)	Vitamin B12 (µg)
Infants	0.0-0.5	6	13	60	24	13	30	0.3	0.4	5	0.3	25	0.3
	0.5-1	9	20	71	28	14	35	0.4	0.5	6	0.6	35	0.5
Children	1-3	13	29	90	35	16	40	0.7	0.8	9	1	50	0.7
	4-6	20	44	112	44	24	45	0.9	1.1	12	1.1	75	1
	7-10	28	62	132	52	28	45	1.0	1.2	13	1.4	100	1.4
Males	11-14	45	99	157	62	45	50	1.3	1.5	17	1.7	150	2
	15-18	66	145	176	69	59	60	1.5	1.8	20	2	200	2
	19-24	72	160	177	70	58	60	1.5	1.7	19	2	200	2
	25-50	79	174	176	70	63	60	1.5	1.7	19	2	200	2
	51+	77	170	173	68	63	60	1.2	1.4	15	2	200	2
Females	11-14	46	101	157	62	46	50	1.1	1.3	15	1.4	150	2
	15-18	55	120	163	64	44	60	1.1	1.3	15	1.5	180	2
	19-24	58	128	164	65	46	60	1.1	1.3	15	1.6	180	2
	25-50	63	138	163	64	50	60	1.0	1.2	13	1.6	180	2
	51+	65	143	160	63	50	60	1.0	1.2	13	1.6	180	2
Pregnant	—	—	—	—	—	60	70	1.5	1.6	17	2.2	400	2.2
Lactating	First 6 mo	—	—	—	—	65	95	1.6	1.8	20	2.2	280	2.6
	Second 6 mo	—	—	—	—	62	90	1.6	1.7	20	2.1	260	2.6

[f] 1 NE (niacin equivalent) = 1 mg niacin or 60 mg dietary tryptophan.

TABLE 2-1 Recommended dietary allowances[a] —cont'd

Category	Age (yr) or condition	Weight[b] (kg)	(lb)	Height[b] (cm)	(in)	Protein (g)	Minerals Calcium (mg)	Phosphorus (mg)	Magnesium (mg)	Iron (mg)	Zinc (mg)	Iodine (µg)	Selenium (µg)
Infants	0.0-0.5	6	13	60	24	13	400	300	40	6	5	40	10
	0.5-1	9	20	71	28	14	600	500	60	10	5	50	15
Children	1-3	13	29	90	35	16	800	800	80	10	10	70	20
	4-6	20	44	112	44	24	800	800	120	10	10	90	20
	7-10	28	62	132	52	28	800	800	170	10	10	120	30
Males	11-14	45	99	157	62	45	1200	1200	270	12	15	150	40
	15-18	66	145	176	69	59	1200	1200	400	12	15	150	50
	19-24	72	160	177	70	58	1200	1200	350	10	15	150	70
	25-20	79	174	176	70	63	800	800	350	10	15	150	70
	51+	77	170	173	68	63	800	800	350	10	15	150	70
Females	11-14	46	101	157	62	46	1200	1200	280	15	12	150	45
	15-18	55	120	163	64	44	1200	1200	300	15	12	150	50
	19-24	58	128	164	65	46	1200	1200	280	15	12	150	55
	25-50	63	138	163	64	50	800	800	280	15	12	150	55
	51+	65	143	160	63	50	800	800	280	10	12	150	55
Pregnant	—	—	—	—	—	60	1200	1200	320	30	15	175	65
Lactating	First 6 mo	—	—	—	—	65	1200	1200	355	15	19	200	75
	Second 6 mo	—	—	—	—	62	1200	1200	340	15	16	200	75

26

TABLE 2-2 Summary table: estimated safe and adequate daily dietary intakes of selected vitamins and minerals[a]

		Vitamins		Trace Elements[b]				
Category	Age (yr)	Biotin (µg)	Pantothenic acid (mg)	Copper (mg)	Man-ganese (mg)	Fluoride (mg)	Chromium (µg)	Molybdenum (µg)
Infants	0-0.5	10	2	0.4-0.6	0.3-0.6	0.1-0.5	10-40	15-30
	0.5-1	15	3	0.6-0.7	0.6-1	0.2-1	20-60	20-40
Children and adolescents	1-3	20	3	0.7-1	1-1.5	0.5-1.5	20-80	25-50
	4-6	25	3-4	1-1.5	1.5-2	1-2.5	30-120	30-75
	7-10	30	4-5	1-2	2-3	1.5-2.5	50-200	50-150
	11+	30-100	4-7	1.5-2.5	2-5	1.5-2.5	50-200	75-250
Adults	—	30-100	4-7	1.5-3	2-5	1.5-4	50-200	75-250

National Research Council, Food and Nutrition Board: Recommended dietary allowances, ed 10, Washington, DC, 1989, National Academy Press.

[a]Because there is less information on which to base allowances, these figures are not given in the main table of the RDA and are provided here in the form of ranges of recommended intakes.

[b]Since the toxic levels for many trace elements may be only several times usual intakes, the upper levels for the trace elements given in this table should not be habitually exceeded.

TABLE 2-3 Median heights and weights and recommended energy intake

Category	Age (yr) or condition	Weight (kg)	Weight (lb)	Height (cm)	Height (in)	REE[a] (kcal/day)	Average energy allowance (kcal)[b] Multiples of REE	Average energy allowance (kcal)[b] Per kg	Average energy allowance (kcal)[b] Per day[c]
Infants	0.0-0.5	6	13	60	24	320	—	108	650
	0.5-1	9	20	71	28	500	—	98	850
Children	1-3	13	29	90	35	740	—	102	1300
	4-6	20	44	112	44	950	—	90	1800
	7-10	28	62	132	52	1130	—	70	2000
Males	11-14	45	99	157	62	1440	1.70	55	2500
	15-18	66	145	176	69	1760	1.67	45	3000
	19-24	72	160	177	70	1780	1.67	40	2900
	25-50	79	174	176	70	1800	1.60	37	2900
	51+	77	170	173	68	1530	1.50	30	2300

From National Research Council, Food and Nutrition Board: Recommended dietary allowances, ed 10, Washington, DC, 1989, National Academy Press.
[a]Calculation based on FAO equations, then rounded.
[b]In the range of light to moderate activity, the coefficient of variation is ± 20%.
[c]Figure is rounded.

Continued

TABLE 2-3 Median heights and weights and recommended energy intake—cont'd

Category	Age (yr) or condition	Weight (kg)	Weight (lb)	Height (cm)	Height (in)	REE[a] (kcal/day)	Average energy allowance (kcal)[b] Multiples of REE	Average energy allowance (kcal)[b] Per kg	Average energy allowance (kcal)[b] Per day[c]
Females	11-14	46	101	157	62	1310	1.67	47	2200
	15-18	55	120	163	64	1370	1.60	40	2200
	19-24	58	128	164	65	1350	1.60	38	2200
	25-50	63	138	163	64	1380	1.55	36	2200
	51+	65	143	160	63	1280	1.50	30	1900
Pregnant	First trimester	—		—	—	—	—	—	+0
	Second trimester	—		—	—	—	—	—	+300
	Third trimester	—		—	—	—	—	—	+300
Lactating	First 6 months	—		—	—	—	—	—	+500
	Second 6 months	—		—	—	—	—	—	+500

From National Research Council, Food and Nutrition Board: Recommended dietary allowances, ed 10, Washington, DC, 1989, National Academy Press.

[a]Calculation based on FAO equations, then rounded.

[b]In the range of light to moderate activity, the coefficient of variation is ± 20%.

[c]Figure is rounded.

TABLE 2-4 Nutrients: functions, stores, deficiencies,
             assessments, treatments, and toxicities

Proteins and amino acids

Functions

Constituents of structural proteins (e.g., muscle), enzymes,
  antibodies, hormones, neurotransmitters, nucleic acids;
  transport other substances in the blood; perform many
  other vital functions; diet must provide some (essential),
  body can synthesize others (nonessential); provide 4 kcal/g

Stores, longevity with minimal intake

All lean tissues, months (depends on total energy intake)

Conditions predisposing to deficiency°

Acute, critical illness (see Chapters 7 and 21); monotonous
  low-protein diet

Clinical signs, symptoms, syndromes of deficiency

Hypoproteinemia, edema, easy hair pluckability, skin
  changes, poor wound healing, lymphopenia, impaired
  immune function, many others; many signs due to
  functional metabolic impairment and not just dietary
  deficiency (see Chapter 7)

Treatment of deficiency

1.5-4 g/kg/day orally, enterally, or parenterally

Lab tests (normal values†)

Serum albumin (3.5-5.5 g/dl)

Serum total iron binding capacity [TIBC] (270-400 µg/dl)

Serum transferrin (212-415 mg/dl)

Indications for therapeutic doses/megadoses‡

—

Toxicity/side effects

Azotemia possible at high doses, especially in patients with
  impaired renal function

Carbohydrates

Functions

Source of energy (provides 4 kcal/g, 3.4 kcal/g for IV
  dextrose), stored as glycogen mainly in liver and muscle,
  main source of dietary fiber

Continued

TABLE 2-4   Nutrients: functions, stores, deficiencies,
assessments, treatments, and toxicities—cont'd

Carbohydrates—cont'd

Stores, longevity with minimal intake
Liver, muscle (glycogen); hours (see Chapter 7)

Conditions predisposing to deficiency°
Diet limited to refined and/or simple carbohydrates (fiber)

Clinical signs, symptoms, syndromes of deficiency
Ketosis, constipation from inadequate fiber

Treatment of deficiency
Adequate amount to prevent ketosis (usually 60 g/day for
adults)

Lab tests (normal values†)
—

Indications for therapeutic doses/megadoses‡
—

Toxicity/side effects
Obesity (calories), dental caries (simple sugars), flatulence
and bulky stools (fiber)

Fat

Functions
Source of energy (provides 9 kcal/g); precursors or
constituents of cell membranes and steroid hormones;
essential fatty acids (EFA)—precursors of prostaglandins,
thromboxanes, prostacyclins, leukotrienes

Stores, longevity with minimal intake
Adipose tissue, months (depends on total energy intake)

Conditions predisposing to deficiency°
Anorexia from various causes (energy), prolonged fat-free
parenteral nutrition (EFA, rare)

Clinical signs, symptoms, syndromes of deficiency
Weight loss if total energy intake is inadequate (see
Chapter 7); EFA deficiency—dry, scaling skin and poor
wound healing

TABLE 2-4 Nutrients: functions, stores, deficiencies, assessments, treatments, and toxicities—cont'd

Fat—cont'd

Treatment of deficiency

EFA—250-500 ml lipid intravenously (IV) 2-3 times/week; EFA deficiency prevention in TPN patients by daily application of 15-30 ml vegetable oil to skin (but not a reliable treatment)

Lab tests (normal values†)

EFA (plasma lipid triene/tetraene ratio <0.4)
Lipoproteins (see Chapter 18)

Indications for therapeutic doses/megadoses‡
—

Toxicity/side effects

Obesity; high-fat diets associated with increased risk of coronary artery disease, several cancers (Chapters 18 and 19)

Vitamin A (fat soluble)

Functions

Ocular rod and cone formation, embryonic development and bone growth, sperm formation; necessary for growth and differentiation of epithelial tissue

Stores, longevity with minimal intake

Liver (not exclusively); > 1 year

Conditions predisposing to deficiency°

Chronic fat malabsorption, insufficient intake (children); inadequate diet (common in developing countries), smoking (β-carotene)

Clinical signs, symptoms, syndromes of deficiency

Follicular hyperkeratosis, scaling skin, night blindness, male sterility, growth retardation, xerophthalmia, keratomalacia, Bitot's spots, blindness

Treatment of deficiency

5,000-30,000 IU/day orally; single 100,000 IU injection intramuscularly (IM), possibly repeated after 1-4 weeks

Continued

TABLE 2-4 Nutrients: functions, stores, deficiencies, assessments, treatments, and toxicities—cont'd

---

Vitamin A (fat soluble)—cont'd

Lab tests (normal values†)
Plasma retinol (25-70 µg/dl)
Plasma carotene (79-233 µg/dl)

Indications for therapeutic doses/megadoses‡
Measles, Darier's disease

Toxicity/side effects
>50,000 IU/day—dry and itching skin, desquamation, erythematous dermatitis, hair loss, headaches, bone and joint pain, liver injury, hypercalcemia, anorexia, fatigue
>10,000 IU/day during pregnancy—increased risk of birth defects

---

Thiamin (vitamin B₁ [water soluble])

Functions
Coenzyme in decarboxylation of α-keto acids and in transketolation in the hexose-monophosphate shunt

Stores, longevity with minimal intake
None appreciable, weeks

Conditions predisposing to deficiency°
Alcoholism; inadequate diet, especially with superimposed glucose load (e.g., IV fluids)

Clinical signs, symptoms, syndromes of deficiency
Precipitated by carbohydrate loading (e.g., IV glucose)
Wet beriberi—cardiomegaly, tachycardia, high output congestive heart failure
Dry beriberi—peripheral polyneuropathy with paresthesia, hypesthesia, anesthesia
Alcoholic polyneuropathy—myelopathy, cerebellar signs, anorexia, hypothermia
Wernicke-Korsakoff syndrome—confabulation, disorientation, ophthalmoplegia, cerebellar ataxia

Treatment of deficiency
At least 10-15 mg/day, up to 100 mg/day p.o. or IM (parenteral route preferable in alcoholics because of decreased absorption)

TABLE 2-4 Nutrients: functions, stores, deficiencies, assessments, treatments, and toxicities—cont'd

Thiamin (vitamin B₁ [water soluble])—cont'd

Lab tests (normal values†)
Erythrocyte thiamin (1.6-4 μg/dl)
Erythrocyte transketolase activity coefficient (1-1.23 [deficiency indicated by high level])
Urinary thiamin (270-780 μg/24 hr)

Indications for therapeutic doses/megadoses‡
Transketolase defect (Wernicke-Korsakoff), branched-chain keto acid dehydrogenase and/or decarboxylase deficiency (maple syrup urine disease), pyruvate dehydrogenase deficiency (subacute necrotizing encephalopathy), pyruvate kinase deficiency, thiamine-responsive megaloblastic anemia (in diabetes mellitus)

Toxicity/side effects
None documented up to 200 times RDA

Riboflavin (vitamin B₂ [water soluble])

Functions
Coenzyme (FAD, FMN) of active prosthetic group of flavoproteins involved with tissue oxidation and respiration

Stores, longevity with minimal intake
None appreciable, weeks

Conditions predisposing to deficiency°
Inadequate diet (uncommon)

Clinical signs, symptoms, syndromes of deficiency
Soreness and burning of lips, mouth, tongue; depapillation of tongue; tearing, burning, itching of eyes; desquamation and seborrhea (especially nasolabial folds and scrotum)

Treatment of deficiency
10-15 mg/day p.o. for 1 week

Lab tests (normal values†)
Erythrocyte glutathione reductase (EGR) activity coefficient (1-1.67 [deficiency indicated by high level])
Urine riboflavin (children: (270 μg/g creatinine, adults: (80 μg/g creatinine)

Continued

TABLE 2-4   Nutrients: functions, stores, deficiencies, assessments, treatments, and toxicities—cont'd

---

Riboflavin (vitamin B_2 [water soluble])—cont'd

Indications for therapeutic doses/megadoses ‡
Carnitine synthetase deficiency with lipid myopathy, acyl-coenzyme A (acyl-CoA) dehydrogenase deficiency, ethyl-adipic aciduria

Toxicity/side effects
None documented at dosages far above RDA

Niacin (vitamin B_3 [water soluble])

Functions
Component of coenzymes NAD and NADP involved in glycolysis and tissue respiration

Stores, longevity with minimal intake
None appreciable, weeks

Conditions predisposing to deficiency°
Inadequate dietary niacin and tryptophan (uncommon)

Clinical signs, symptoms, syndromes of deficiency
Pellagra—diarrhea, dermatitis, dementia; tongue can be scarlet, raw, depapillated, and fissured
Hartnup disease—aminoaciduria, pellagra-like rash, cerebellar ataxia

Treatment of deficiency
50-500 mg/day p.o. or IV

Lab tests (normal values†)
Urine N-methyl nicotinamide, adults (>0.5 mg/g creatinine)

Indications for therapeutic doses/megadoses ‡
Hartnup disease (nicotinamide or nicotinic acid), elevated low-density lipoprotein (LDL) and/or very low-density lipoprotein (VLDL) cholesterol (nicotinic acid)

Toxicity/side effects
<1 g/day—flushing (usually manageable) and possible nausea, vomiting, diarrhea, liver injury (the latter especially with sustained-release forms)

TABLE 2-4 Nutrients: functions, stores, deficiencies, assessments, treatments, and toxicities—cont'd

Pyridoxine (vitamin B₆ [water soluble])

Functions
Cofactor in numerous reactions, mostly associated with amino acid metabolism

Stores, longevity with minimal intake
None appreciable, weeks (inversely related to protein intake)

Conditions predisposing to deficiency°
Inadequate diet, especially with high-protein intake (clinically uncommon)

Clinical signs, symptoms, syndromes of deficiency
Polyneuropathy, oxalate stone formation, seborrheic dermatitis, microcytic anemia, glossitis, cheilosis, muscular twitching, convulsions

Treatment of deficiency
At least 2 mg/day, up to 50 mg/day

Lab tests (normal values†)
Erythrocyte aspartate aminotransferase—AST or GOT—activity coefficient (1.15-1.89 [deficiency indicated by high level])
Urine pyridoxine (children: ≥50 µg/g creatinine, adults: ≥20 µg/g creatinine)

Indications for therapeutic doses/megadoses‡
Infantile convulsive disorders, cystathioninuria, homo-cystinuria, kynureninase deficiency, ornithine (γ-amino transferase deficiency, sideroblastic anemia, oxaluria

Toxicity/side effects
Ataxia and sensory neuropathy with dosages as low as 200 mg/day for several months

Folic acid (folacin, folate [water soluble])

Functions
Formyl group transfer; biosynthesis of purine bases, histidine, choline, and serine

Stores, longevity with minimal intake
Liver, weeks

Continued

TABLE 2-4 Nutrients: functions, stores, deficiencies, assessments, treatments, and toxicities—cont'd

Folic acid (folacin, folate [water soluble])—cont'd

Conditions predisposing to deficiency°
Inadequate diet, pregnancy, smoking, antifolate medications

Clinical signs, symptoms, syndromes of deficiency
Macrocytic anemia, leukopenia, thrombocytopenia, glossitis, stomatitis, diarrhea, malabsorption (see Chapter 24); neural tube defects in babies born to genetically susceptible mothers with less than optimal diets.

Treatment of deficiency
1 mg/day p.o. or IV

Lab tests (normal values†)
Plasma folate (3-10 ng/ml)
RBC folate (160-369 ng/ml)

Indications for therapeutic doses/megadoses‡
Formiminotransferase deficiency, folate reductase deficiency, homocystinuria; to reverse effects of antifolates such as methotrexate; lower-dose supplementation advisable in planned or suspected pregnancy

Toxicity/side effects
Mask B_{12} deficiency (methyl-folate trap), convulsion in one seizure patient after 14 mg IV

Vitamin B_{12} (water soluble)

Functions
Isomerization of methylmalonyl CoA to succinyl CoA; interacts with folic acid in methionine synthetase, homocysteine/methionine conversion, methylation reactions, and synthesis of proteins, purines, and pyrimidines

Stores, longevity with minimal intake
Liver, several years

Conditions predisposing to deficiency°
Pernicious anemia, resection or disease (e.g., Crohn's) of terminal ileum, strict vegetarianism (uncommon cause of deficiency)

TABLE 2-4 Nutrients: functions, stores, deficiencies, assessments, treatments, and toxicities—cont'd

Vitamin B$_{12}$ (water soluble)—cont'd

Clinical signs, symptoms, syndromes of deficiency
Macrocytic anemia (mainly pernicious anemia), leukopenia, thrombocytopenia, stomatitis, glossitis (see Chapter 24); includes peripheral and central neuropathy with decreased vibratory and position senses, paresthesia, unsteady gait, delusions, even psychosis

Treatment of deficiency
100 μg/day IM for several days; 100 μg/month IM for maintenance

Lab tests (normal values†)
Plasma B$_{12}$ (200-700 pg/ml)
Schilling test (see Chapter 24)

Indications for therapeutic doses/megadoses‡
Rare congenital B$_{12}$ metabolism defect (e.g., B$_{12}$-responsive methylmalonic acidemia), homocystinuria

Toxicity/side effects
None documented

Vitamin C (ascorbic acid [water soluble])

Functions
Affects growth of developing cartilage and bone (fibroblasts, osteoblasts, and odontoblasts), hydroxylation of proline and lysine, formation of neurotransmitters (dopamine to norepinephrine, tryptophan to 5-hydroxytryptophan), enhances GI iron absorption and inhibits copper absorption

Stores, longevity with minimal intake
None, about 6 weeks

Conditions predisposing to deficiency°
Inadequate diet with or without physiologic stress from illness; smoking

Clinical signs, symptoms, syndromes of deficiency
Scurvy—follicular hyperkeratosis, corkscrew hairs, perifollicular petechiae, ecchymoses, bleeding gums (in

Continued

TABLE 2-4   Nutrients: functions, stores, deficiencies,
                assessments, treatments, and toxicities—cont'd

---

Vitamin C (ascorbic acid [water soluble])—cont'd

Clinical signs, symptoms, syndromes of deficiency—cont'd
patients with teeth), dry skin, dry mouth, scorbutic
arthritis, impaired wound healing

Treatment of deficiency
Up to 1-2 g/day

Lab tests (normal values†)
Plasma vitamin C (0.5-1.5 mg/dl), scurvy indicated when
  level < 0.2

Indications for therapeutic doses/megadoses‡
Chédiak-Higashi syndrome; 1-2 g/day to enhance
  compromised wound healing; rheumatoid arthritis

Toxicity/side effects
Occasional diarrhea; increased uric acid excretion; possible
  interference with tests for urine glucose (false positive with
  copper reagents, false negative with glucose-oxidase
  method); possible false-negative result in test for stool
  occult blood; possible interference with anticoagulant
  therapy

Biotin (water soluble)

Functions
Cofactor for carboxylase enzymes involved in fatty acid,
  carbohydrate, protein, and cholesterol metabolism

Stores, longevity with minimal intake
Unknown, influenced by intestinal flora synthesis and avidin
  intake

Conditions predisposing to deficiency°
Substantial consumption of avidin (raw egg whites); biotin-
  free parenteral nutrition (rare)

Clinical signs, symptoms, syndromes of deficiency
Biotin deficiency—dermatitis, atrophic lingual papillae,
  graying of mucous membranes, hypercholesterolemia,
  electrocardiographic abnormalities

TABLE 2-4 Nutrients: functions, stores, deficiencies,
assessments, treatments, and toxicities—cont'd

Biotin (water soluble)—cont'd

Clinical signs, symptoms, syndromes of deficiency—cont'd
Holoenzyme synthetase deficiency—erythematous rash,
  persistent vomiting, impaired immune function
Biotinidase deficiency—delayed neuromotor development,
  nystagmus, hypotonia, impaired immune function, ketosis,
  accumulation of lactate in tissues

Treatment of deficiency
300 µg/day for several days

Lab tests (normal values†)
Whole blood biotin (200-500 pg/ml)
Urinary biotin (6-100 µg/24 hr)

Indications for therapeutic doses/megadoses‡
Holoenzyme synthetase deficiency, biotinidase deficiency,
  propionicacidemia, β-methylcrotonyl glycinuria

Toxicity/side effects
None documented

Pantothenic acid (water soluble)

Functions
Integral component of coenzyme A; involved in fatty acid
  and cholesterol synthesis and lipid, carbohydrate, and
  amino acid metabolism

Stores, longevity with minimal intake
Unknown; weeks (intestinal flora synthesis suspected)

Conditions predisposing to deficiency°
—

Clinical signs, symptoms, syndromes of deficiency
Demonstrated only in experimental circumstances—
  vomiting, malaise, abdominal distress, burning feet,
  cramps, fatigue, insomnia, paresthesia of the hands and
  feet

Treatment of deficiency
Uncertain because of unclear existence of deficiency

Continued

TABLE 2-4   Nutrients: functions, stores, deficiencies,
                assessments, treatments, and toxicities—cont'd

---

Pantothenic acid (water soluble)—cont'd

Lab tests (normal values†)
Whole blood pantothenic acid (100-300 µg/dl)

Indications for therapeutic doses/megadoses‡
—

Toxicity/side effects
Occasional diarrhea with 10-20 g/day

Vitamin D (fat soluble)

Functions
Facilitates calcium and phosphorus absorption and
  utilization, maintenance of skeletal integrity

Stores, longevity with minimal intake
Liver, skin; months to years (depends on sun exposure)

Conditions predisposing to deficiency°
Chronic fat malabsorption, inadequate sun exposure, breast-
  feeding without supplemental vitamin D

Clinical signs, symptoms, syndromes of deficiency
Rickets (children)—bony deformities due to enlargement of
  epiphyseal growth plates, stunted growth
Osteomalacia (adults)—pathologic fractures, possibly
  hypocalcemia and hypophosphatemia (see Chapter 26)

Treatment of deficiency
Rickets—1000 IU/day
Osteomalacia—50,000 IU/day vitamin D_3 or 50 µg/day
  calcifediol

Lab tests (normal values†)
Serum 25-OH vitamin D (9-52 ng/ml)
Serum 1,25-$(OH)_2$ vitamin D (30-75 pg/ml)

Indications for therapeutic doses/megadoses‡
Vitamin D dependency, familial hypophosphatemia

Toxicity/side effects
Serum 25-OH vitamin D level > 400 ng/ml associated with
  weakness, fatigue, headache, nausea, vomiting,
  hypercalcemia, impaired renal function; can cause growth
  arrest in children

TABLE 2-4 Nutrients: functions, stores, deficiencies, assessments, treatments, and toxicities—cont'd

---

Vitamin E (fat soluble)

Functions
Antioxidant, free-radical scavenger (primarily in membranes)

Stores, longevity with minimal intake
Liver, cell membranes, all lipid-rich tissues; years

Conditions predisposing to deficiency°
Very long-term fat malabsorption, prematurity

Clinical signs, symptoms, syndromes of deficiency
Hemolytic anemia, retinopathy, bronchopulmonary dysplasia in premature newborns; neuropathy, myopathy with creatinuria in adults with severe, longstanding malabsorption

Treatment of deficiency
0.2-2 g/day (200-2000 IU) p.o.

Lab tests (normal values†)
Serum tocopherol (0.6-1.4 mg/dl), lower in patients with low blood lipids, higher in patients with hyperlipidemia

Indications for therapeutic doses/megadoses‡
Premature birth; chronic cholestasis; pancreatic insufficiency; uncontrolled celiac disease; inborn errors such as glucose-6-phosphate dehydrogenase deficiency, glutathione peroxidase deficiency, glutathione synthetase deficiency, thalassemia major, sickle cell anemia; coronary artery disease, intermittent claudication (peripheral atherosclerosis)

Toxicity/side effects
None documented

Vitamin K (fat soluble)

Functions
Carboxylation of glutamic acid residues in formation of clotting factors II, VII, IX, X

Continued

TABLE 2-4   Nutrients: functions, stores, deficiencies, assessments, treatments, and toxicities—cont'd

Vitamin K (fat soluble)—cont'd

Stores, longevity with minimal intake
Liver, cell membranes; weeks (despite synthesis by intestinal flora, shortened by antibiotic use)

Conditions predisposing to deficiency°
Inadequate diet plus antibiotic use (uncommon except in hospitalized patients)

Clinical signs, symptoms, syndromes of deficiency
Increased prothrombin time, ecchymoses, bleeding

Treatment of deficiency
5-10 mg IV or IM to restore prothrombin time to normal
Newborn infants: routine single dose of 0.5 to 1.0 mg IM at birth

Lab tests (normal values†)
Prothrombin time (≤1-2 sec beyond control, 70%-100% of normal activity)

Indications for therapeutic doses/megadoses‡
Parenchymal liver disease with hypoprothrombinemia

Toxicity/side effects
None documented

Calcium

Functions
Forms structure of bones and teeth; integral to neurotransmission, muscle contraction, blood clotting

Stores, longevity with minimal intake
Bones, years

Conditions predisposing to deficiency°
Inadequate diet, malabsorption

Clinical signs, symptoms, syndromes of deficiency
Hypoparathyroidism—paresthesia, neuromuscular excitability, muscle cramps, tetany, convulsions
Osteoporosis, osteomalacia—bone fractures, bone pain, height loss (see Chapter 26)

TABLE 2-4 Nutrients: functions, stores, deficiencies,
assessments, treatments, and toxicities—cont'd

Calcium—cont'd

Treatment of deficiency
Hypoparathyroidism—calcium and vitamin D replacement
Osteoporosis—calcium, vitamin D, potentially estrogen
   therapy
Osteomalacia—vitamin D (see vitamin D entry), calcium
   therapy (1-1.5 g/day)

Lab tests (normal values†)
Serum calcium (8.5-10.5 mg/dl)
Urine calcium (30-250 mg/24 hr)

Indications for therapeutic doses/megadoses‡
—

Toxicity/side effects
Constipation, rarely kidney stones

Chloride

Functions
Principal extracellular anion, plays a key role in fluid and
   electrolyte balance; acidifies gastric juice

Stores, longevity with minimal intake
None, days (very unusual without sodium depletion)

Conditions predisposing to deficiency*
Chloride-free parenteral fluids, sodium depletion (e.g.,
   heavy sweating); gastric suction or prolonged vomiting

Clinical signs, symptoms, syndromes of deficiency
Volume depletion

Treatment of deficiency
About 60 mEq/day NaCl p.o. or IV

Lab tests (normal values†)
Serum chloride (95-108 mEq/L)

Indications for therapeutic doses/megadoses‡
—

Toxicity/side effects
Possible elevated blood pressure

Continued

TABLE 2-4 Nutrients: functions, stores, deficiencies,
assessments, treatments, and toxicities—cont'd

Chromium

Functions
Cofactor for insulin in glucose metabolism

Stores, longevity with minimal intake
Unknown

Conditions predisposing to deficiency°
Chromium-free parenteral nutrition (rare)

Clinical signs, symptoms, syndromes of deficiency
Glucose intolerance, peripheral neuropathy, weight loss

Treatment of deficiency
200 μg/day chromium chloride or 10 g/day brewers' yeast

Lab tests (normal values†)
None reliable

Indications for therapeutic doses/megadoses‡
—

Toxicity/side effects
None documented at 50-200 μg/day

Copper

Functions
Influences iron absorption and mobilization, a component of
a number of metalloenzymes (e.g., ceruloplasmin,
lysyloxidase, cytochrome C, superoxide dismutase)

Stores, longevity with minimal intake
Unknown

Conditions predisposing to deficiency
Copper-free parenteral nutrition (rare)

Clinical signs, symptoms, syndromes of deficiency
Menkes'syndrome—mental deterioration, hypothermia,
defective keratinization of hair, metaphyseal lesions,
degeneration of aortic elastin, depigmentation of hair
Microcytic anemia—indistinguishable from iron deficiency
anemia (see Chapter 26)

Treatment of deficiency
2-3 mg/day copper sulfate

| TABLE 2-4 | Nutrients: functions, stores, deficiencies, assessments, treatments, and toxicities—cont'd |

Copper—cont'd

Lab tests (normal values†)
Serum copper (80-120 µg/dl [adults])
Urine copper (15-30 µg/24 hr)

Indications for therapeutic doses/megadoses‡
—

Toxicity/side effects
Doses > 15 mg—possible nausea, vomiting, headache, diarrhea, abdominal cramps
Wilson's disease (genetic)—possible chronic copper toxicity (accumulation in liver, kidney, brain)

Fluoride (Fluorine)

Functions
Protects against dental caries

Stores, longevity with minimal intake
Unknown

Conditions predisposing to deficiency°
—

Clinical signs, symptoms, syndromes of deficiency
Dental caries (true requirement in humans is debatable)

Treatment of deficiency
1-2 mg/day sodium fluoride for persons living in a nonfluoridated area

Lab tests (normal values†)
—

Indications for therapeutic doses/megadoses‡
—

Toxicity/side effects
Mottling of teeth

Iodine

Functions
Component of thyroid hormones

Stores, longevity with minimal intake
Thyroid gland, unknown

Continued

TABLE 2-4   Nutrients: functions, stores, deficiencies,
                 assessments, treatments, and toxicities—cont'd

---

Iodine—cont'd

Conditions predisposing to deficiency°
— (Inadequate diet common in developing countries)

Clinical signs, symptoms, syndromes of deficiency
Goiter, hypothyroidism

Treatment of deficiency
2 g/day iodized salt

Lab tests (normal values†)
Serum thyroxine [T4] (5-12.3 µg/dl)
Serum triiodothyronine [T3] (80-240 ng/dl)
Serum thyroid-stimulating hormone [TSH] (0-5 µIU/ml)

Indications for therapeutic doses/megadoses‡
—

Toxicity/side effects
Possible goiter from >2 mg/day

Iron

Functions
Oxygen transport (hemoglobin, myoglobin), electron
  transport (cytochromes)

Stores, longevity with minimal intake
Bone marrow, liver, spleen (ferritin, hemosiderin); months

Conditions predisposing to deficiency°
Blood loss, especially menstrual or gastrointestinal;
  inadequate diet, especially in infancy and adolescence;
  pregnancy

Clinical signs, symptoms, syndromes of deficiency
Microcytic anemia, pallor, fatigue, glossitis, tachycardia (see
  Chapter 24)

Treatment of deficiency
325 mg ferrous sulfate p.o. t.i.d. for 2-6 months to rebuild
  iron stores

Lab tests (normal values†)
Serum iron (42-135 µg/dl)
Total iron binding capacity (270-400 µg/dl)
Serum ferritin (10-300 ng/ml)

TABLE 2-4   Nutrients: functions, stores, deficiencies, assessments, treatments, and toxicities—cont'd

Iron—cont'd

Indications for therapeutic doses/megadoses‡

—

Toxicity/side effects
Hemochromatosis and/or hemosiderosis (iron overload)

Magnesium

Functions
Associated with more than 300 enzyme systems, especially in metabolism of ATP; therefore participates in glucose utilization, synthesis of proteins, fats, and nucleic acids, muscle contraction, membrane transport systems, and neurotransmission

Stores, longevity with minimal intake
Bones, muscles, soft tissues; about 3 weeks

Conditions predisposing to deficiency°
Malabsorption, alcoholism, protein-energy malnutrition

Clinical signs, symptoms, syndromes of deficiency
Paresthesia, neuromuscular excitability, muscle spasms progressing to tetany, seizures, coma; often hypocalcemia, hypokalemia

Treatment of deficiency
250-500 mg magnesium oxide p.o. b.i.d. to q.i.d., or 1-2 g/day IM or IV

Lab tests (normal values†)
Serum magnesium (1.8-2.4 mg/dl)
Urinary magnesium (17-19 mg/dl)

Indications for therapeutic doses/megadoses‡

—

Toxicity/side effects
Diarrhea, possible decreased neurotransmission and cardiorespiratory dysfunction if accumulates in patients with impaired renal function

Continued

TABLE 2-4 Nutrients: functions, stores, deficiencies, assessments, treatments, and toxicities—cont'd

Manganese

Functions
Cofactor in many enzymes; involved in glycosyl transferases, gluconeogenesis, lipid metabolism, and mucopolysaccharide metabolism

Stores, longevity with minimal intake
Unknown

Conditions predisposing to deficiency°
—

Clinical signs, symptoms, syndromes of deficiency
Uncertain but reported—weight loss, hypocholesterolemia, dermatitis, nausea and vomiting, changes in color and reduced growth rate of hair and beard

Treatment of deficiency
—

Lab tests (normal values†)
Serum manganese (4-14 ng/ml)

Indications for therapeutic doses/megadoses‡
—

Toxicity/side effects
Neuropsychiatric problems in miners who have inhaled manganese oxide

Molybdenum

Functions
Cofactor in oxidase enzymes

Stores, longevity with minimal intake
Unknown

Conditions predisposing to deficiency°
Prolonged molybdenum-free parenteral nutrition (rare)

Clinical signs, symptoms, syndromes of deficiency
Tachycardia, tachypnea, stupor, coma—reported in one long-term parenterally fed patient

Treatment of deficiency
300 µg/day IV

| TABLE 2-4 | Nutrients: functions, stores, deficiencies, assessments, treatments, and toxicities—cont'd |

Molybdenum—cont'd

Lab tests (normal values†)
Serum molybdenum (2.9-12 nmol/L)

Indications for therapeutic doses/megadoses‡
—

Toxicity/side effects
If high intakes, possible interference with copper
  metabolism

Phosphorus

Functions
Constituent of nucleic acids and cell membranes, essential
  in glycolysis and—as ATP—in all energy-producing
  reactions, involved in modification of tissue calcium
  concentrations and maintenance of acid/base equilibrium

Stores, longevity with minimal intake
Bones, years (although serum levels may fall within hours in
  starved patients given glucose loads)

Conditions predisposing to deficiency°
Glucose load (e.g., parenteral nutrition) in starved cachectic
  patients (see Chapter 9), phosphate-binding antacids

Clinical signs, symptoms, syndromes of deficiency
Serum and intracellular depletion resulting from renal
  tubular disease or parenteral nutrition without adequate
  phosphorus supplementation—weakness with
  cardiorespiratory failure, glucose intolerance, diminished
  red blood cell, leukocyte, and platelet function (see
  Chapter 9)
Children—growth retardation, skeletal deformities, bone
  pain

Treatment of deficiency
Serum phosphorus 1.0 to 2.5 mg/dl: 1 mmol/kg IV or p.o.
  over 24 hr
Serum phosphorus <1.0 mg/dl: 1.5 mmol/kg IV over 24 hr

Continued

TABLE 2-4 Nutrients: functions, stores, deficiencies, assessments, treatments, and toxicities—cont'd

Phosphorus—cont'd

Lab tests (normal values†)
Serum phosphorus (adults—2.5-4.8 mg/dl, children—4-7 mg/dl)
Urinary phosphorus (0.7-1.5 g/24 hr)

Indications for therapeutic doses/megadoses‡
—

Toxicity/side effects
Diarrhea resulting from oral phosphorus supplementation, secondary hyperparathyroidism from poor excretion in renal disease

Potassium

Functions
Principal intracellular cation, nerve impulse transmission, skeletal and autonomic muscle contraction, blood pressure maintenance

Stores, longevity with minimal intake
None, days

Conditions predisposing to deficiency°
Gastrointestinal fluid losses (e.g., gastric suctioning, vomiting, diarrhea), renal reabsorptive defects, diuretics, laxatives, potassium-free parenteral fluids

Clinical signs, symptoms, syndromes of deficiency
Muscle weakness, tetany, cardiac arrhythmias, hypotension, respiratory failure, ileus

Treatment of deficiency
20-60 mEq KCl p.o. or (gradually) IV

Lab tests (normal values†)
Serum potassium (3.5-5.2 mEq/L)

Indications for therapeutic doses/megadoses‡
—

Toxicity/side effects
Cardiac arrhythmias and arrest

| TABLE 2-4 | Nutrients: functions, stores, deficiencies, assessments, treatments, and toxicities—cont'd |

Selenium

Functions
A component of glutathione peroxidase and associated with vitamin E, scavenges free radicals and protects against lipid peroxidation

Stores, longevity with minimal intake
None appreciable, years

Conditions predisposing to deficiency°
Prolonged low-selenium parenteral nutrition (rare)

Clinical signs, symptoms, syndromes of deficiency
Cardiomyopathy (Keshan disease) and increased cancer rates (both mainly reported in China), nail changes

Treatment of deficiency
100-200 µg/day

Lab tests (normal values†)
Serum or whole blood selenium (6-20 µg/dl [require special tube])

Indications for therapeutic doses/megadoses‡
—

Toxicity/side effects
Major hair loss, brittle fingernails, fatigue, irritability

Sodium

Functions
Principal extracellular cation, primary regulator of fluid and electrolyte balance, blood pressure maintenance

Stores, longevity with minimal intake
None, days

Conditions predisposing to deficiency°
Sodium-free parenteral fluids, heavy sweating, gastrointestinal fluid losses (e.g., gastric suctioning, vomiting, diarrhea)

Clinical signs, symptoms, syndromes of deficiency
Volume depletion

Continued

TABLE 2-4 Nutrients: functions, stores, deficiencies, assessments, treatments, and toxicities—cont'd

Sodium—cont'd

Treatment of deficiency
About 60 mEq/day NaCl p.o. or IV

Lab tests (normal values†)
Serum sodium (135-145 mEq/L)

Indications for therapeutic doses/megadoses‡
—

Toxicity/side effects
Edema, hypertension

Zinc

Functions
Cofactor for over 70 enzymes involved in growth, sexual maturation, fertility and reproduction, night vision, taste activity, and immune function

Stores, longevity with minimal intake
Bone, muscle (small available pool); months (influenced by dietary protein, phosphorus, iron)

Conditions predisposing to deficiency°
Malabsorption, critical illness (e.g., trauma, surgery)

Clinical signs, symptoms, syndromes of deficiency
Growth retardation, hypogonadism, impaired taste and smell, poor wound healing, lethargy, poor appetite, dry, scaly skin, cellular immune deficiency, acrodermatitis enteropathica (hereditary)

Treatment of deficiency
60 mg elemental zinc (zinc sulfate 220 mg) p.o. 1 to 3 times daily or 5-10 mg/day elemental zinc IV

Lab tests (normal values†)
Serum zinc (80-120 µg/dl)
Urinary zinc (150-1200 µg/24 hr)

TABLE 2-4 Nutrients: functions, stores, deficiencies, assessments, treatments, and toxicities—cont'd

Zinc—cont'd

***Indications for therapeutic doses/megadoses*‡**

Therapeutic doses for possible enhancement of compromised wound healing in patients with increased requirements resulting from severe physiologic stress or with increased zinc losses; generally recommended dosages—220 mg 1-3 times/day p.o., or 5-10 mg/day IV (see Chapters 13 and 21)

Toxicity/side effects

Possible interference with iron or copper metabolism (sideroblastic anemia), possible immune function impairment

---

*These conditions are generally encountered in the United States. Many of these conditions can result in deficiency even when intake of the nutrient is consistent with the RDA. Specific (e.g., inherited) syndromes in which the nutrient deficiency is a central feature are considered under the heading clinical signs, symptoms, syndromes of deficiency.

†These values vary among laboratories and should be considered approximate. Activity coefficients, which are derived from a laboratory method to assess thiamin, riboflavin, and pyridoxine status, involve measuring the plasma or erythrocyte activity of an enzyme that requires the respective vitamin as a cofactor. The equation used to calculate activity coefficient follows:

$$\frac{\text{Enzyme activity with the vitamin added to the assay tube}}{\text{Enzyme activity without additional vitamin}}$$

When a vitamin deficiency is present, the enzyme activity increases with addition of the vitamin to the assay tube, making the ratio greater than 1; therefore high activity coefficients indicate deficiency.

‡The term *megadoses* is used to indicate established or widely accepted uses of nutrients at levels beyond those required to maintain nutritional sufficiency (RDA) or correct deficiency. Generally a megadose is greater than 10 times the RDA.

TABLE 2-5 Recommended daily dose ranges for prevention and treatment of various diseases[1]

Vitamin (units)	Prevention of vitamin deficiency	Treatment of vitamin deficiency	Treatment of deficiency in patients with malabsorption	Treatment of dependency syndromes
Vitamin A (IU)	250-2500	5000-10,000	10,000-25,000	—
Vitamin D (IU)	400[*]	400-5000	4000-20,000	50,000-200,000
Calcifediol (µg)	—	—	20-100	50-100
Calcitriol—1,25-dihydroxy-vitamin D (µg)	—	—	0.25-2	0.25-2
Vitamin E (IU)	6-30[†]	—	100-1000	—
Vitamin K (mg)	—	1[‡]	5-10[‡]	—
Ascorbic acid—vitamin C (mg)	50-100	250-500	500	25-500
Thiamine (mg)	1-2	5-25	5-25	—
Riboflavin (mg)	1-2	5-25	5-25	—
Niacin (mg)	10-20	25-50	25-50	50-250
Vitamin B$_6$ (mg)	1.5-2.5	5-25	2-25	10-250
Pantothenic acid (mg)	5-20[†]	5-20	5-20	—
Biotin (mg)	—	0.15-0.3	0.3-1	10
Folic acid (mg)	0.1-0.4	1.0	1.0	—[†]
Vitamin B$_{12}$ (µg)	3-10	—[‡]	—[‡]	1-40

[*]For infants and children; 200 IU/day for adults. [†]To be used only in conjunction with multivitamin mixtures.

[‡]To be used parenterally as needed.

TABLE 2-6 Energy content of selected foods

Food	Portion size	kcal/portion
Meat		
Beef, roast	3 oz	250
Chicken, roasted		
with skin	3 oz	250
without skin	3 oz	200
Egg	1 large	80
Haddock, broiled	3½ oz	140
Hamburger; lean, cooked	3 oz	160
Pork chop, no visible fat	3 oz	225
Sausage, pork	1 link	60
Shrimp	3½ oz	91
Tuna, light in water	3½ oz	127
Dairy products		
Cheese, cheddar	1 oz	114
Swiss	1 oz	107
cottage	4 oz	100-120
Ice cream, vanilla	½ cup	135
Milk, whole	1 cup	150
2%	1 cup	125
skim	1 cup	85
Yogurt; low-fat, plain	1 cup	140
Grain		
Bread, whole-wheat	1 slice	56
Corn flakes	1 cup	110
Oatmeal, cooked	½	70
Rice, cooked	½ cup	100

Continued

TABLE 2-6 Energy content of selected foods—cont'd

Food	Portion size	kcal/portion
Vegetables		
Beans; kidney, cooked	½ cup	110
green	½ cup	18
Carrots	1 medium	34
Corn on cob	5½-inch ear	160
Lettuce, iceberg	⅙ head	13
Peas, black-eyed	½ cup	86
Fruits		
Banana	1 medium	1
Orange	1 medium	1
Miscellaneous		
Peanuts	1 oz	8
Fruits		
Apple with skin	1 medium	80
Banana	1 medium	100
Orange	1 medium	65
Peach	1 medium	38
Pear with skin	1 medium	100
Miscellaneous		
Brownie, plain	1	130
Butter	1 tbsp	100
Candy bar, plain chocolate	1 oz	150
Peanuts	1 oz	172
Potato chips	10 chips	115

TABLE 2-7 Protein content of selected foods

Food	Portion size	Amount of protein (g/portion)
Meat		
Beef, roast	3 oz	19
Chicken, roasted	3 oz	24
Egg	1	6
Haddock, broiled	3½ oz	20
Pork chop	3 oz	24
Shrimp	3 ½ oz	19
Tuna; light in water	3½ oz	25
Dairy products		
Cheese, Swiss	1 oz	8
cheddar	1 oz	7
Cottage cheese	4 oz	14
Ice cream	½ cup	2
Milk, whole or 2%	1 cup	8
Yogurt; low-fat, plain	1 cup	12
Grain		
Bread, whole-wheat	1 slice	3
Cornflakes	1 cup	2
Oatmeal, cooked	½ cup	3
Rice, cooked	½ cup	2
Vegetables		
Beans; kidney, cooked	⅓ cup	6
green	½ cup	1
Carrots	1 medium	1
Corn on cob	5½-inch ear	4
Lettuce	⅙ head	1
Peas, black-eyed	⅓ cup	5
Fruits		
Banana	1 medium	1
Orange	1 medium	1
Miscellaneous		
Peanuts	1 oz	8

TABLE 2-8 Fat content of selected foods

Food	Portion size	Amount (g/portion)
Meat		
Bacon, crisp	3 slices	9
Beef, roast	3 oz	26
Chicken, baked		
with skin	3 oz	11
without skin	3 oz	6
Egg, boiled	1 large	6
Haddock, broiled	3½ oz	7
Pork chop	3 oz	19
Shrimp	3½ oz	1
Tuna, light in water	3½ oz	1
Dairy products		
Cheese, cheddar	1 oz	9
cottage, creamed	4 oz	5
mozzarella, part-skim	1 oz	5
Ice cream	½ cup	7
Milk, whole	1 cup	8
2%	1 cup	5
skim	1 cup	<1
Sour cream	1 tbsp	3
Yogurt, low-fat	1 cup	4

TABLE 2-8 Fat content of selected foods—cont'd

Food	Portion size	Amount (g/portion)
Grains		
Biscuit	1	4
Bread	1 slice	1
Cornbread	1 piece	7
Oatmeal, cooked	½ cup	1
Vegetables		
Starches, other vegetables	½ cup	<1
Fruit		
Most fruit	—	<1
Miscellaneous		
Avocado	⅛ medium	4
Butter	1 tsp	4
Margarine	1 tsp	4
Mayonnaise	1 tbsp	11
Mayonnaise, reduced fat	1 tbsp	5
Potato chips	10 chips	8
Peanut butter	1 tbsp	7
Sour cream	1 tbsp	3
Vegetable oil	1 tsp	5

TABLE 2-9 Cholesterol content of selected food

Food	Portion size	Amount of cholesterol (mg/portion)
Meat		
Beef, roast	3 oz	80
Chicken	3 oz	76
Egg	1 large	275
Haddock, broiled	3½ oz	60
Lamb	3 oz	83
Liver, beef	3 oz	370
Pork, roast	3 oz	80
Scallops, steamed	3½ oz	53
Shrimp	3½ oz	150
Tuna, light in water	3½ oz	60
Veal	3 oz	86
Dairy products		
Buttermilk, cultured	1 cup	9
Cheese, cheddar	1 oz	30
Swiss	1 oz	26
cottage, creamed	4 oz	17
Ice cream	½ cup	30
Milk, whole	1 cup	33
2%	1 cup	18
skim	1 cup	4
Yogurt, low-fat	1 cup	14
Grains		
Bread, cereal, oats	—	0
Vegetables		
All starches, other vegetables	—	0
Fruits		
All fruits	—	0
Miscellaneous		
Butter	1 tsp	11
Nuts, seeds	—	0
Vegetable oils	—	0

| TABLE 2-10 | Dietary fiber content of selected food | |

Food	Portion size	Amount of fiber (g/portion)
Meat		
Beef, pork, seafood, eggs	—	0
Dairy products		
Milk, yogurt, cheese/cottage cheese	—	0
Grain		
All Bran	½ cup	12.8
Bran muffin	1	4.2
Oatmeal, cooked	½ cup	1.1
Raisin bran	½ cup	3
Shredded wheat	1 biscuit	2.2
Special K cereal	½ cup	0.1
White bread	1 slice	0.8
Whole-wheat bread	1 slice	1.3
Vegetables		
Broccoli	½ cup	3.2
Carrots, cooked	½ cup	2.4
raw	1 medium	2.4
Corn	½ cup	4.6
Lettuce, iceberg	⅙ head	1.4
Fruit		
Apple with peel	1 medium	3
Applesauce	½ cup	2.4
Pear with peel	1 medium	3.8
Raspberries	½ cup	4.6

TABLE 2-11 Vitamin A content of selected foods

Food	Portion size	Amount of vitamin (RE/portion)*
Meat		
Beef liver, fried	3½ oz	10640
Calf liver, cooked	3½ oz	8116
Chicken liver, cooked	2 livers	7806
Egg	1 large	78
Vegetables		
Asparagus, cooked	5-6 medium	90
Broccoli, cooked	½ cup	110
Carrots, raw	1 large	2025
cooked	½ cup	800
Collard greens, cooked	½ cup	540
Lettuce, romaine	4 leaves	190
iceberg	¼ head	97
Mustard greens, cooked	½ cup	212
Potato, sweet, baked	1 medium	2488
Pumpkin, cooked	½ cup	800
Spinach, raw	3½ oz	810
cooked	½ cup	737
Squash, winter	½ squash	420
Tomatoes, raw	1 small	90
Turnip greens, cooked	½ cup	396

TABLE 2-11	Vitamin A content of selected foods—cont'd	
Food	**Portion size**	**Amount of vitamin (RE/portion)***
Fruit		
Apricots, raw	3 medium	277
dried	4 halves	101
Cantaloupe	¼ melon	430
Nectarine, raw	1 medium	165
Papaya, raw	⅓ medium	175
Watermelon	10- × 16-inch slice	531
Dairy products		
Cheese, cheddar	1 oz	86
cottage, 2% fat	1 cup	45
Milk, whole	1 cup	83
2%	1 cup	140
skim	1 cup	149
Grain		
Cereal; cold, fortified	1 oz	375
Miscellaneous		
Butter	1 tsp	38
Margarine	1 tsp	47

*One RE (retinol equivalent) = 3.33 IU from animal sources and 10 IU from plant sources.

TABLE 2-12 Thiamin (vitamin B_1) content of selected foods

Food	Portion size	Amount of vitamin (mg/portion)
Meat		
Beef liver, fried	3½ oz	0.26
Ham, fresh, cooked	3½ oz	0.96
Hamburger	1 patty	0.15
Hot dogs, pork	1 frank	0.08
Pork chops, cooked	3½ oz	0.98
Nuts		
Brazil	¼ cup	0.82
Cashew	¼ cup	0.11
Pecans	¼ cup	0.18
Grain		
Bread, white	1 slice	0.11
whole-wheat	1 slice	0.09
Cereal, cold	1 oz	0.40
barley cereal	½ cup	0.22
Oatmeal, cooked	½ cup	0.13
Wheat germ	1 tbsp	0.15
Vegetables		
Asparagus, cooked	5-6 medium	0.16
Beans, cooked		
Lima	½ cup	0.14
Kidney	½ cup	0.14
Corn on cob, cooked	4-inch ear	0.12
Green peas, cooked	½ cup	0.28
Soybeans, cooked	½ cup	0.21
Dairy products		
Milk; whole, 2%, skim	1 cup	0.09
Miscellaneous		
Brewers' yeast	1 tbsp	1.25

TABLE 2-13 Riboflavin (vitamin B_2) content of selected foods

Food	Portion size	Amount of vitamin (mg/ portion)
Meat		
Beef; ground, cooked	3½ oz	0.21
Beef liver, fried	3½ oz	4.10
Calf liver, fried	3½ oz	4.10
Chicken liver, cooked	3½ oz	1.75
Egg, boiled	1 large	0.14
Steak, cooked	3½ oz	0.16
Veal roast, cooked	3½ oz	0.44
Grain		
Bread, white	1 slice	0.07
whole-wheat	1 slice	0.05
Cereal, cold	1 oz	0.40
Barley cereal	½ cup	0.12
Dairy products		
Cheese; cottage, low-fat, 2%	⅓ cup	0.14
blue or Roquefort	1 oz	0.11
cheddar	1 oz	0.11
brick	1 oz	0.10
Ice cream (1 scoop)	½ cup	0.17
Milk, whole or 2%	1 cup	0.42
skim	1 cup	0.34
Vegetables		
Asparagus, cooked	5-6 medium	0.18
Broccoli, cooked	½ cup	0.20
Brussels sprouts, cooked	½ cup	0.14
Collard greens, cooked	½ cup	0.20
Mustard greens, cooked	½ cup	0.14
Spinach, cooked	½ cup	0.13
Spinach, raw	3½ oz	0.20
Miscellaneous		
Brewers' yeast	1 tbsp	0.43

TABLE 2-14   Niacin (vitamin B_3) content of selected foods

Food	Portion size	Amount of vitamin (mg/portion)
Meat		
Beef; ground, cooked	3½ oz	5.7
Beef liver, fried	3½ oz	14.4
Calf liver, fried	3½ oz	16.5
Chicken; battered, fried	3½ oz	9
Chicken, cooked	3½ oz	6.6
Chicken liver, cooked	3½ oz	4.5
Haddock, cooked	3½ oz	2.1
Hot dogs or luncheon meats	3½ oz	2.5
Pork chop	3½ oz	5.5
Steak, cooked	3½ oz	5
Turkey, roasted	3½ oz	5
Grain		
Bread, white	1 slice	0.9
whole-wheat	1 slice	1
Cereal; cold, fortified	1 oz	5
Nuts		
Peanut butter	2 tbsp	4.8
Peanuts, roasted	1 oz	5.6
Vegetables		
Asparagus, cooked	5-6 medium	1.4
Collard greens, cooked	½ cup	1.2
Corn on cob, cooked	4-inch ear	1.4
Green peas, cooked	½ cup	1.7
Lima beans, cooked	½ cup	1
Peas, black-eyed	½ cup	1.1
Potato; white, baked	1 medium	1.7
Miscellaneous		
Beer	12 oz	1.8
Brewers' yeast	1 tbsp	3.8
Coffee, brewed	6 oz	5

TABLE 2-15 Pyridoxine (vitamin B_6) content of selected foods

Food	Portion size	Amount of vitamin (mg/portion)
Meat		
Beef, ground	3½ oz	0.39
Beef liver, fried	3½ oz	0.35
Chicken, baked	3½ oz	0.52
Hot dogs or luncheon meats	3½ oz	0.22
Pork chop, broiled	3½ oz	0.35
Salmon, broiled	3½ oz	0.70
Tuna, canned	3 oz	0.34
Turkey, baked	3½ oz	0.27
Vegetables		
Asparagus	½ cup	0.13
Broccoli, cooked	½ cup	0.15
Potatoes, not fried	3½ oz	0.24
french-fried	3½ oz	0.19
Spinach, cooked	½ cup	0.22
Turnip greens	½ cup	0.13
Dairy products		
Milk; whole, 2%, or skim	1 cup	0.1
Grain		
Cereals; cold, regular	1 oz	0.5
superfortified	1 oz	1.5
Fruit		
Banana	1 medium	0.66
Cantaloupe	1 cup	0.18
Figs, dried	10	0.42
Orange	1 medium	0.08
Watermelon	1 cup	0.23
Miscellaneous		
Beer	12 oz	0.18
Brewers' yeast	1 tbsp	0.40

TABLE 2-16 Folic acid content of selected foods

Food	Portion size	Amount of vitamin (µg/portion)
Meat		
Beef liver, fried	3½ oz	175
Chicken liver	3½ oz	770
Egg	1 large	32
Vegetables		
Acorn squash, cooked	½ medium	17
Asparagus, cooked	5-6 medium	89-140
Beans; lima, canned; pinto, navy	⅓ cup	21
Broccoli, cooked	½ cup	26
Brussels sprouts, cooked	½ cup	20
Cauliflower, cooked	½ cup	16
Endive, raw	20 long leaves	27-63
Escarole, raw	4 large leaves	26
Kale, cooked	½ cup	34
Mustard greens, cooked	½ cup	17-38
Okra, cooked	8-9 pods	24
Peas, black-eyed		
frozen	⅓ cup	65
canned	⅓ cup	16
Spinach, cooked	½ cup	131
Turnip greens, cooked	½ cup	86
Fruit		
Orange juice from concentrate	8 oz	102
Grain		
Bread, white	1 slice	8
whole-wheat	1 slice	14
Cereals; cold, regular	1 oz	80
superfortified	1 oz	180

TABLE 2-16 Folic acid content of selected foods—cont'd

Food	Portion size	Amount of vitamin (µg/portion)
Nuts		
Almonds	12-15 nuts	7
Filberts	10-12 nuts	10
Peanuts	1 tbsp	9
Pecans	12 halves	4
Walnuts	8-10 halves	12
Miscellaneous		
Beer	12 oz	22
Tea, brewed	8 oz	13

TABLE 2-17 Vitamin B_{12} content of selected foods

Food	Portion size	Amount of vitamin (µg/portion)
Meat		
Beef liver, fried	3½ oz	21-120
Beef round	3½ oz	3.4-4.5
Egg, whole	1 large	0.6
Haddock	3½ oz	0.6
Ham	3½ oz	0.9-1.6
Dairy products		
Cheese, Swiss	1 oz	0.5
American	1 oz	0.2
Milk; whole, 2%, or skim	1 cup	1.3

TABLE 2-18 Vitamin C content of selected foods

Food	Portion size	Amount of vitamin (mg/portion)
Vegetables		
Broccoli, cooked	½ cup	90
Brussels sprouts, cooked	½ cup	87
Cabbage, raw	1 cup	33
Collard greens, cooked	½ cup	46
Green pepper, raw	1 large	128
Lettuce, iceberg	3½ oz	6
Mustard greens, cooked	½ cup	48
Parsley, raw	2 tbsp	34
Potato; white, baked	1 medium	20
Spinach, cooked	½ cup	25
Spinach, raw	3½ oz	51
Tomato, raw	1 small	23
Fruit		
Acerola	1 cup	1644
Cantaloupe	¼ medium	43
Fruit drinks, fortified	6 oz	60
Grapefruit	½ medium	39
Grapefruit juice from concentrate	8 oz	83
Honeydew melon	¼ small	23
Kumquats	5 medium	35
Lemon without skin	1 medium	31
Lime without skin	1 medium	20
Orange	1 medium	80
Orange juice from concentrate	8 oz	97
Papaya, raw	⅓ medium	63
Strawberries	1 cup	85
Tangerine	1 medium	26
Tomato juice, canned	8 oz	102

TABLE 2-19 Vitamin D content of selected foods

Food	Portion size	Amount of vitamin (IU/portion)*
Dairy products		
Cheese, Swiss	1 oz	30
cottage	1 cup	5
Milk, fortified	1 cup	100
Grain		
Cereal, cold; fortified	½ cup	20-25
superfortified	½ cup	50-100
Wheat germ	1 tbsp	3
Meat		
Egg	1 large	27
Liver, beef	3½ oz	45
Salmon, canned	3½ oz	500
Tuna	3½ oz	15
Miscellaneous		
Butter	1 tsp	1.5
Margarine	1 tsp	16
Mayonnaise	1 tbsp	2

*400 IU vitamin D = 10 µg cholecalciferol; limited data available.

TABLE 2-20 Vitamin E content of selected foods

Food	Portion size	Amount of vitamin (mg/portion)*
Grain		
Bread, white	1 slice	0.03
Cereal; cold, fortified	½ cup	20
Wheat germ	1 tbsp	2
Meat		
Egg	1 large	0.35
Salmon, broiled	3½ oz	1.35
Vegetables		
Greens, mustard, turnip	½ cup	1
Potatoes, baked	3½ oz	0.03
french-fried	3½ oz	0.19
sweet	3½ oz	4.56
Miscellaneous		
Butter	1 tsp	0.08
Cakes, doughnuts	3½ oz	0.8
Margarine	1 tsp	0.1
Mayonnaise and salad dressings	1 tbsp	2
Nuts	3½ oz	0.2-44
Oil; safflower, sunflower	1 tbsp	5.5
soybean, corn, peanut	1 tbsp	1.1

*1 mg = 1 IU; limited data available.

TABLE 2-21 Calcium content of selected foods

Food	Portion size	Amount of calcium (mg/portion)
Meat		
Egg	1 large	28
Dairy products		
Cheese, Swiss	1 oz	272
cheddar	1 oz	204
brick	1 oz	191
blue or Roquefort	1 oz	150
cottage, creamed	⅓ cup	42
Ice cream	½ cup	88
Milk, 2%, skim	1 cup	300
Milk, whole	1 cup	288
Grain		
Bread, white	1 slice	30
whole-wheat	1 slice	18
Vegetables		
Broccoli, cooked	½ cup	66
Cabbage, raw	1 cup	49
Carrot, raw	1 large	37
Collard greens, cooked	½ cup	152
Kidney beans, cooked	½ cup	48
Lima beans, cooked	½ cup	26
Mustard greens, cooked	½ cup	138
Spinach, cooked	½ cup	83
Turnip greens, cooked	½ cup	138
Fruit		
Orange	1 medium	56
Prunes	10	43
Tangerine	1 large	12
Miscellaneous		
Doughnuts, cookies, or cakes	1 oz	11
Spaghetti with tomato sauce	3½ oz	50

TABLE 2-22 Iron content of selected foods

Food	Portion size	Amount of iron (mg/portion)
Meat		
Beef; lean round, cooked	3½ oz	5.9
Beef liver, fried	3½ oz	8.8
Calf liver, fried	3½ oz	14.2
Chicken; cooked, no bone	3½ oz	1.3
Chicken liver, cooked	3½ oz	8.5
Egg, boiled	1	1
Hot dog	1 frank	0.5
Luncheon meats	2 slices	0.5
Pork	3½ oz	4
Grain		
Bread, white	1 slice	0.7
whole-wheat	1 slice	0.9
Cereal; cold, regular	1 oz	0.6-1
bran and superfortified	1 oz	4.5-8
Fruit		
Apricots, dried	4 halves	0.66
Dates, dried	10	0.96
Prunes	8 large	1.67
Raisins	¼ cup	0.78
Strawberries, raw	1 cup	0.57
Watermelon	1 cup	0.28
Vegetables		
Asparagus, canned	½ cup	0.6
Beans, cooked		
kidney	½ cup	3
lima	½ cup	2
Beans, dried	3½ oz	2.5
Cauliflower, raw	1 cup	1.1
Green peas, cooked	½ cup	1.4
Lettuce, iceberg	3½ oz	0.5
Mustard greens, cooked	½ cup	1.8

TABLE 2-22 Iron content of selected foods—cont'd

Food	Portion size	Amount of iron (mg/portion)
Spinach, raw	3½ oz	3.1
cooked	½ cup	2
Miscellaneous		
Coffee, brewed	6 oz	0.02
Doughnuts	1	0.4
Molasses, medium	1 tbsp	1.2
Tea, brewed	8 oz	0.1

TABLE 2-23 Magnesium content of selected foods

Food	Portion size	Amount of vitamin (mg/portion)
Meat		
Cheese, cheddar	1 oz	8
Chicken, cooked	3½ oz	25
Clams	3 oz	31
Shrimp, boiled	3½ oz	110
Fruit		
Apple	1 medium	6
Cantaloupe	1 cup	17
Figs, dried	5	56
Orange	1 medium	13
Peach, fresh	1 medium	6
Vegetables		
Broccoli, cooked	½ cup	47
Garbanzo beans	½ cup	57.5
Lima beans	½ cup	40
Peas, black-eyed	½ cup	58.5
Potato, baked	1 medium	55
Spinach, cooked	½ cup	78.5
Squash, cooked	½ cup	22
Miscellaneous		
Brewers' yeast	1 tbsp	18
Wheat germ	¼ cup	91

TABLE 2-24 Phosphorus content of selected foods

Food	Portion size	Amount of phosphorus (mg/portion)
Meat		
Beef; lean round, cooked	3½ oz	250
Calf liver, fried	3½ oz	537
Cod, broiled	3½ oz	260
Egg	1 large	90
Halibut, broiled	3½ oz	248
Pork; lean, cooked	3½ oz	249
Dairy products		
Cheese, swiss	1 oz	171
cheddar	1 oz	145
blue or Roquefort	1 oz	110
cottage, creamed	⅓ cup	92
Milk, whole	1 cup	227
Milk; whole, 2% or skim	1 cup	227
Grain		
Bread, white or whole-wheat	1 slice	25
Nuts		
Brazil	4 nuts	104
Peanut butter	1 tbsp	59
Peanuts, roasted	1 oz	124
Vegetables		
Artichoke, cooked	1 bud	69
Beans, cooked		
kidney	½ cup	175
lima	½ cup	97
Brussels sprouts, cooked	½ cup	55
Green peas; fresh, cooked	½ cup	74
Potato; white baked	1	65
Miscellaneous		
Beer	12 oz	50
Carbonated drinks	12 oz	1-94
Doughnut	1	55

TABLE 2-25 Potassium content of selected foods

Food	Portion size	Amount of potassium (mg/portion)
Meat		
Beef, lean round	3½ oz	508
Chicken, cooked	3½ oz	181
Pork, cooked	3½ oz	567
Salmon, pink	3½ oz	306
Fruit		
Apricots, dried	4 halves	193
Banana	1 medium	451
Cantaloupe	1 cup	494
Dates, dried	10	541
Figs, dried	10	1332
Orange	1 medium	250
Orange juice from concentrate	8 oz	474
Peach, raw	1 medium	171
Plums, raw	2 medium	226
Prunes	8 large	501
Raisins	½ cup	563
Grain		
Bread, white	1 slice	27
whole-wheat	1 slice	44
Dairy products		
Milk; whole or 2%	1 cup	370
skim	1 cup	400

Continued

TABLE 2-25 Potassium content of selected foods—cont'd

Food	Portion size	Amount of potassium (mg/portion)
Vegetables		
Artichoke, cooked	1 bud	301
Avocado	½ medium	645
Brussels sprouts, cooked	½ cup	206
Cabbage, raw	1 cup	233
Carrots, cooked	½ cup	168
Cauliflower, raw	1 cup	295
Collard greens, cooked	½ cup	234
Lettuce, iceberg	3½ oz	175
Lima beans, cooked	½ cup	338
Potatoes; french-fried, fast-food	3½ oz	530-830
Potato; white, boiled	1 medium	407
sweet, baked	1 small	300
Pumpkin, cooked	½ cup	274
Spinach, raw	3½ oz	470
cooked	½ cup	291
Tomato, raw	1 small	244
Miscellaneous		
Coffee, brewed	6 oz	117
Molasses, light	1 tbsp	300
Tea, brewed	8 oz	58

TABLE 2-26 Sodium content of selected foods

Food	Portion size	Amount of sodium (mg/portion)
Meat		
Beef; corned, canned	3 oz	800
roast	3 oz	40
Bologna	1 slice	230
Egg	1 large	70
Haddock	3½ oz	70
Ham	1 oz	370
Hot dog	1 frank	500
Sausage	1 link	640
Tuna, light in water	3½ oz	400
Dairy products		
Cheese, cottage	4 oz	460
cheddar	1 oz	175
Milk	1 cup	120
Grain		
Biscuit	1	350
Bread	1 slice	140
Corn bread	1 piece	230
Corn flakes	1 cup	260
Oatmeal; cooked, unsalted	½ cup	<1
Vegetables		
Carrots		
canned	½ cup	230
frozen	½ cup	38
fresh	½ cup	25

TABLE 2-26 Sodium content of selected foods—cont'd

Food	Portion size	Amount of sodium (mg/portion)
Vegetables—cont'd		
Corn		
canned	½ cup	240
frozen	½ cup	4
fresh	½ cup	<1
Peas		
canned	½ cup	240
frozen	½ cup	80
fresh	½ cup	<1
Potatoes, baked	3½ oz	4
french fried, fast-food	3½ oz	90-340
Fruit		
Most fresh fruit	1 medium	<10
Miscellaneous		
Catsup	1 tbsp	155
Doughnut	1	139
Peanuts, salted	1 oz	140
unsalted	1 oz	1
Pickle, dill	1 medium	925
Pizza, cheese	6 oz slice	925
Potato chips	10 chips	150
Soup, regular	1 cup	900-1100
low-sodium	1 cup	25-85
Spaghetti with tomato sauce	3½ oz	400
Table salt	1 tsp	2300

TABLE 2-27 Zinc content of selected foods

Food	Portion size	Amount of zinc (mg/portion)
Meat		
Beef, lean, round	3½ oz	2-5
Beef liver, fried	3½ oz	3-8.5
Clams	4 large/9 small	2
Eggs	1 large	0.7
Oysters	5-8 medium	160
Vegetables		
Beets, cooked	2 beets	2.8
Cabbage, cooked	½ cup	0.1-0.8
Carrots, cooked	½ cup	0.4-2.7
Corn, cooked	½ cup	0.43
Lettuce	¼ head	0.1-0.7
Peas, green, cooked	½ cup	2.3-3.8
Spinach, cooked	½ cup	0.3-0.8
Grain		
Barley	½ cup	0.6
Bread whole-wheat	1 slice	0.4-0.6
rye	1 slice	0.3
Fruit		
Cherries, canned	½ cup	0.08-0.13
Pear	1 medium	0.2

Tables 2-6 through 2-27 adapted from Pennington JAT, Church HN: *Bowes' and Church's food values of portions commonly used,* ed 16, Philadelphia, 1994, JB Lippincott.

References

1. American Medical Association, Council on Scientific Affairs: Vitamin preparations as dietary supplements and as therapeutic agents, *JAMA* 257:1929, 1987.

Suggested Readings

National Research Council, Food and Nutrition Board: *Recommended dietary allowances,* ed 10, Washington, DC, 1989, National Academy Press.

Shils ME, Olson JA, Shike M, eds: *Modern nutrition in health and disease,* ed 8, Philadelphia, 1994, Lea & Febiger.

Pregnancy and Lactation

Adequate maternal nutrition is very important during pregnancy and lactation; it affects the outcome of the pregnancy and determines the success of lactation. Ideally, the mother should have a good nutritional status prior to becoming pregnant.

There are many physiologic changes taking place during pregnancy that maintain the mother's health but still allow for the development of the fetus. These changes affect the mother's nutritional status by increasing her energy and nutrient needs. There is an increase in hormone levels. The plasma volume increases out of proportion to the expansion of red blood cells typically causing the hematocrit to drop during pregnancy. There is also an increase in cardiac output and resting metabolic rate.

Changes taking place in the gastrointestinal tract during pregnancy often result in symptoms that may affect the mother's nutritional intake. Heartburn results from the enlarging uterus pushing against the stomach and intestines, which causes an upward pressure. Progesterone decreases the integrity of the cardiac sphincter allowing reflux of food and acid. Constipation results from progesterone slowing the peristaltic action of smooth muscles in the bowel and the enlarging uterus displacing internal organs. In addition, nausea and vomiting frequently occur in the first trimester of pregnancy.

MATERNAL AND FETAL WEIGHT GAIN

Birth weight is the best indicator of a newborn's health. Low prepregnant weight and inadequate weight gain during pregnancy are the most significant contributors to intrauterine growth retardation and low birth weight. Prepregnancy body mass index (BMI) is used to establish a target for total weight gain in pregnancy, as shown in Table 3-1 is as follows:

$$BMI = \frac{Weight(kg)}{Height^2(m)}$$

TABLE 3-1   Recommended weight gain during pregnancy[1]

Prepregnancy BMI*	lb	kg
Low (BMI < 19.8)	28-40	12.5-18
Normal (BMI 19.8-26)	25-35	11.5-16
High (BMI > 26-29)	15-25	7-11.5
Obese (BMI > 29)	>15	>7

*Body mass index.

TABLE 3-2   Normal components of maternal weight gain during pregnancy[2]

Organ, tissue, or fluid	Weight (g)
Uterus	970
Breasts	405
Blood	1250
Water	1680
Fat	3345
MATERNAL COMPONENTS TOTAL	7650
Fetus	3400
Placenta	650
Amniotic fluid	800
NONMATERNAL COMPONENTS	4850
TOTAL (all components)	12500

The target weight gain for mothers with twin pregnancies is 35 to 45 lb (16 to 20 kg). Aside from the weight of the developing baby, the mother gains additional weight from the fat that is laid down between maternal organs. Expanded uterus and breast tissues also add to the weight gain of the mother as does a dramatic increase in fluid and blood volume. Table 3-2 details the components of maternal weight gain.

Although the mother should gain 3 to 8 lb during the first trimester, poor weight gain during this period is not usually a cause for concern. During the second and third trimesters, women with low BMIs (see Table 3-1) should gain just over 1 lb per week, those with normal BMIs should gain about 1 lb per week, and those with high BMIs should gain slightly less than 1 lb per week. Between the third month of gestation and term, fetal weight increases dramatically—as much as 3500 g—therefore appropriate maternal weight gain in the second and third trimesters is a major factor in the health of the newborn and should occur steadily.

Maternal characteristics associated with low gestational weight gain include age at time of conception (less than 18 or greater than 35 years of age); low socioeconomic status; history of previous pregnancy complications (spontaneous abortion, birth weight of less than 2750 g, or delivery prior to 37 weeks of gestation); maternal height of less than 62 inches; hypertension; use of alcohol, tobacco, or drugs; and restrictive eating habits from a desire to remain thin. Women with these characteristics should strive for gains at the upper end of the weight range. Although short women (less than 62 inches) should strive for an adequate weight gain, it should be at the lower end of the normal range.

SPECIFIC NUTRIENT NEEDS DURING PREGNANCY AND LACTATION
Pregnancy

A pregnant woman's energy needs do not increase during the first trimester of pregnancy. During the second and third trimesters the energy demands of pregnancy increase by only 300 kcal per day. The recommended daily allowance (RDA) for protein during pregnancy is an additional 10 g over the amount for a woman that is not pregnant.

The RDA for folic acid during pregnancy (published in 1989) is 400 µg, which is 220 µg more than the RDA for nonpregnant women but only half that recommended for pregnant women in the 1980 RDAs. In the early 1990s, supplementation with between 400 µg and 4 mg of folic acid in the first weeks of pregnancy was proved to reduce the incidence of neural tube defects such as spina bifida and myelomeningocele. Because the neural tube closes before most women even know they are pregnant, supplementation after this time is assumed to be ineffective. A debate has therefore ensued among scientists and public health officials as to the optimum level of folic acid intake and how it can be achieved by the entire population. At the present time the American College of Obstetricians and Gynecologists recommends that a woman who is planning a pregnancy and has previously had a child with a neural tube defect take 4 mg of folic acid daily beginning 1 month prior to conception and continuing through the first 3 months of pregnancy. To protect women with unplanned pregnancies the U.S. Public Health Service has recommended that all women of childbearing potential receive a daily supplement of 400 µg of folic acid, which is contained in many over-the-counter multivitamin preparations. Because not all women are likely to take a daily supplement or eat a diet high in folic acid, food fortification with folate is being discussed as another option.

The RDA for calcium during pregnancy is 1200 mg, 400 mg more than the RDA for nonpregnant women. Supplementation is necessary if the woman does not drink milk or eat dairy products. Vitamin D intake should be 10 µg, 5 µg more than the nonpregnant intake. Vitamin D deficiency during pregnancy can lead to hypocalcemia and poor tooth enamel development in the fetus. Conversely, pregnant women should avoid excess vitamin D intake because infantile hypercalcemia syndrome may result.

Iron requirements double during pregnancy; the RDA for pregnant women is 30 mg as compared with 15 mg for nonpregnant women. Because this amount is not often achieved from diet alone, supplementation with 30 mg of ferrous iron per day is recommended during the second and third trimesters. Unfortunately, supplementation can aggravate constipation.

Lactation

During lactation the energy needs of the infant must be met by the mother. This is accomplished in part by mobilizing the extra maternal fat stores deposited during pregnancy, but even so the mother must consume an additional 500 kcal per day more than a nonpregnant woman or 200 kcal more than during pregnancy. Lactating women typically lose 1 to 2 lb per month, and the loss of the extra body fat is usually complete by the time the infant is 6 months of age. Women who do not breast feed are more likely to have difficulty losing weight after delivery.

In addition to the requirements for pregnancy, lactating women on average need an extra 5 g of protein per day during the first 6 months of lactation and 2 g per day during the second 6 months of lactation. These recommendations reflect a decrease in the volume of milk produced during the second 6 months of the infant's life as solid food intake is established. Other important nutrients in the lactating woman's diet include calcium, magnesium, zinc, folate, and vitamin B_6. Adequate fluid intake, rest, and family support are also essential for successful lactation.

IMPLEMENTATION OF NUTRITION GUIDELINES

Women should eat enough food to gain weight at the recommended rate. Fruit and vegetables, grain, meat, and dairy products should be included daily in meals and snacks. Adequate dairy and overall energy intakes are particularly important. Women should be encouraged to eat or drink at least 3 servings of dairy products daily. Four to 5 servings per day are recommended for women less than 18 years of age. For better absorption of iron, meals should include poultry, fish, other meat, or a vitamin C source such as orange juice or other citrus fruits.

The USDA DHHS (see Figure 1-1) food guide pyramid recommends a range of servings for each major food group. The following revisions to the pyramid are appropriate for most pregnant women: 6 to 9 servings from the starch group, 2 to 3 servings of fruit, 3 to 5 servings of vegetables, 2 to 3 servings from the meat group, and at least 3 servings of dairy products per day.

The same dietary advice applies to lactating women. A well-balanced and varied diet should be encouraged, with special attention given to adequate intake of energy, calcium, zinc, and fluid. With an adequate diet and reasonable sun exposure, vitamin and mineral supplementation is not necessary during lactation.

Prenatal Vitamins

A well-planned diet can meet all the nutrient needs of pregnant women. Except for iron and folic acid as discussed previously, routine supplementation of other vitamins and minerals has not been associated with measurable health improvements in the general population of pregnant women.

There are specific groups of women at increased risk for having an inadequate nutrient intake who may benefit from vitamin and mineral supplementation. These groups include women who have low incomes or inadequate access to food, avoid certain types of foods because of intolerance, adhere to strict vegetarian diets, have a tightly scheduled lifestyle that is unlikely to support nutritional adequacy, restrict their diets in an attempt to control their weight, have pica, are unhappy about being pregnant, or have the previously mentioned demographic characteristics. Also at an elevated risk are those who are carrying

PRENATAL SUPPLEMENTATION GUIDELINES FOR WOMEN AT RISK FOR DEFICIENCY

Iron: 30-60 mg
Zinc: 15 mg
Copper: 2 mg
Calcium: 250 mg
Vitamin D: 400 IU
Vitamin C: 50 mg
Folate: 400 µg
Vitamin B_6: 2 mg
Vitamin B_{12}: 2 µg

more than one fetus or use cigarettes, alcohol, or illicit drugs. For these women a multiple-vitamin supplement that at least includes the nutrients listed in the prenatal supplementation box is usually recommended. Supplementation should begin by the twelfth week of gestation, with the exception of folic acid which preferably should begin prior to pregnancy. Patients should be cautioned that excessive doses of some vitamins can be toxic.

Additional iron may be required if the mother has anemia (other than sickle cell anemia). A supplement of 60 to 120 mg of iron should be taken if the hemoglobin level falls below 11 g/dl during the first or third trimester or below 10.5 g/dl during the second trimester. Iron supplements should be taken with juice and between meals if possible.

Other Recommendations
Sodium

Salt does not need to be restricted during pregnancy unless it is indicated for an underlying problem. Pregnant women may be advised to salt food to taste because the need for salt increases somewhat during pregnancy.

Caffeine

Evidence about the effects of caffeine on pregnancy is equivocal. Although one study suggested that moderate to heavy users of caffeine were more likely to have spontaneous abortions in the late first trimester and second trimester, there is no convincing evidence that caffeine affects embryonic development. It is best to advise pregnant women to limit coffee and other caffeinated beverages to no more than 2 to 3 servings per day.

Alcohol, Tobacco, and Drugs

It is best to avoid tobacco, alcohol, and illicit drugs entirely during pregnancy because of the potential for impaired fetal growth, fetal alcohol syndrome, and inadequate maternal food intake while using them. Cigarette smoking and alcohol use also increase requirements for some nutrients.

Artificial Sweeteners

Aspartame is safe for individuals who do not have phenylketonuria (PKU). Circulating phenylalanine, one of two amino acids contained in aspartame, is broken down by phenylalanine hydroxylase in normal individuals.

High-Risk Considerations
Pica

Pica is the ingestion of nonnutritive materials such as dirt, clay, laundry starch, cornstarch, ice, chalk, burnt matches, baking soda, hair, stone, gravel, charcoal, cigarette ashes, mothballs, coffee grounds, and even tire inner tubes. Groups with a higher prevalence of pica (up to 20%) include those living in rural areas and people with a positive childhood or family history of pica. Some reasons given for pica include the relief of nausea or nervous tension, having a pleasant sensation when chewing, an inherent craving for the substances, and encouragement by family members. Possible risks of pica include hematologic and gastrointestinal disorders and interference with nutrient ingestion and absorption.

Health professionals counseling patients who practice pica should remain nonjudgmental while simultaneously strongly discouraging continuation of the practice. The substance being ingested and the reason for ingestion should be determined and the dangers explained in a culturally appropriate way.

Gestational Diabetes Mellitus

Gestational diabetes mellitus appears in pregnant women who have no prior history of diabetes, and it generally resolves after delivery. It is associated with an increased incidence of prematurity, macrosomia, and perinatal mortality. Universal screening occurs at 24 to 28 weeks of gestation via a 1-hour, 50-g nonfasting oral glucose challenge. If the plasma glucose level is greater than 140 mg/dl (7.8 mM) at 1 hour, a 3-hour, 100-g oral glucose tolerance test (GTT) should be performed. Gestational diabetes is diagnosed if two or more of the levels in the box are found.

In patients with gestational diabetes, attempt to provide all required nutrients, prevent hyperglycemia and ketosis, and ensure appropriate weight gain. The composition of the diet should be 40% of energy from fat, 20% from protein, and 40% from carbohydrate; the distribution is as follows: breakfast—10% to 15%, snack—5% to 10%, lunch—20% to 30%, snack—5% to 10%, dinner—

GLUCOSE TOLERANCE CRITERIA FOR GESTATIONAL DIABETES MELLITUS

Fasting: >105 mg/dl (5.8 mM)
One hour: >190 mg/dl (10.6 mM)
Two hour: >165 mg/dl (9.2 mM)
Three hour: >145 mg/dl (8.1 mM)

30% to 40%, and snack—5% to 10%. The patient should avoid simple sugars and convenience foods and choose high-fiber foods instead.

Diabetes Mellitus

Patients with established diabetes are at increased risk for pregnancy complications and should be counseled before becoming pregnant. Those requiring insulin may need to monitor their blood glucose levels as often as 4 to 8 times daily during pregnancy and adjust insulin as necessary. The hemoglobin A_1C concentration, which reflects blood glucose levels during the previous 4 to 6 weeks, should be maintained at a level no higher than 5.5% to 6.5%. This is accomplished if blood glucose levels average between 110 and 150 mg/dl. Urine ketones should be checked whenever the blood glucose exceeds 200 mg/dl (11 mM). The diet should be individualized according to the patient's prepregnancy intake and adjusted to achieve the recommended weight gain. The meal pattern is similar to the pattern used for patients with gestational diabetes.

Preeclampsia (Pregnancy-Induced Hypertension [PIH])

Preeclampsia is characterized by hypertension, proteinuria, and edema developing after the twentieth week of pregnancy. It occurs most often in primiparas less than 20 or more than 35 years of age. Eclampsia ("toxemia") includes grand mal seizures or coma and is often fatal. When all the signs of preeclampsia are present, the baby must be delivered immediately. Patients with PIH should be counseled about maintaining a diet that is liberal in protein, energy, and fluids. Sodium restriction is not necessary.

Phenylketonuria

PKU is a genetic condition in which the liver cannot metabolize dietary phenylalanine because it lacks the enzyme phenylalanine hydroxylase. Spontaneous abortions, congenital heart disease, low birth weight, mental retardation, and facial dysmorphology may occur in babies born to women with PKU. The goal is to maintain very low maternal blood phenylalanine levels (between 2 and 6 mg/dl) both before and during pregnancy. This can only be accomplished by using specially designed foods that provide the major fraction (80% to 90%) of dietary protein.

Nutrition Counseling

Good prenatal care includes dietary assessment and nutrition education. A registered dietitian can be a valuable resource in assessing current dietary intake by identifying problems that may affect nutrient intake or absorption and educating the patient. A good diet history will indicate whether the mother is omitting a major food group from her diet. Nondietary factors that may influence a woman's nutritional requirements and/or intake, such as inadequate housing, poor access to food, and substance abuse should be identified and appropriate referrals made. The woman's attitude toward weight gain and concern about body size should also be assessed.

After the initial nutrition assessment the pregnant woman should be counseled about maintaining a diet that addresses her individual needs and takes into consideration her cultural food preferences and practices. As mentioned previously, the food guide pyramid and/or the U.S. dietary guidelines can be used as a good basis for nutrition education. Regular exercise during pregnancy and lactation should also be encouraged.

Strategies for managing common symptoms in pregnancy are listed in the boxes on the following page.

Food and Nutrition Resources

The Special Supplemental Nutrition Program for Women, Infants, and Children (WIC) is available in each county throughout the United States. Eligibility requirements are based on income level and a determined nutri-

RECOMMENDATIONS FOR NAUSEA AND VOMITING

Eat crackers, melba toast, or dry cereal before getting out
of bed in the morning.
Eat small, frequent meals.
Try to consume an adequate amount of fluids even if solid
foods are not tolerated.
Avoid drinking coffee and tea.
Avoid or limit intake of fatty and spicy foods.

RECOMMENDATIONS FOR HEARTBURN

Keep meals small and eat slowly.
Select low-fat foods.
Drink fluids mainly between meals.
Avoid spices.
Avoid lying down for 1 to 2 hours after eating or drinking.
Wear loose-fitting clothing.

RECOMMENDATIONS FOR CONSTIPATION

Drink 2 to 3 qt of fluids daily.
Eat high-fiber food including whole-grain bread and ce-
real, legumes, and fresh fruit and vegetables.
Be physically active to maintain abdominal muscle tone.
Avoid taking laxatives.

tional risk (e.g., anemia). Women who are pregnant, postpartum (up to 6 months) and breast-feeding (up to 1 year)
are eligible. The benefits include individualized food packages and nutrition education. On completion of certifica-
tion food vouchers are provided, in most cases on the day of
application. Health professionals who refer a client to the
WIC program need to provide the following information:
hemoglobin or hematocrit, medical risks if any, height and
weight, and special requirements if any. Local WIC agen-
cies should be able to provide standard referral forms.

The food stamps program is available for U.S. citizens from households with low income and other resources of less than $2000. Eligibility is determined after formal application to local public assistance or social service agencies.

References

1. National Academy of Sciences: *Nutrition during pregnancy and lactation: an implementation guide,* Washington, DC, 1992, National Academy Press.
2. American College of Obstetricians and Gynecologists: *Nutrition during pregnancy.* ACOG Technical Bulletin 179, Washington, DC, 1993, ACOG.

Suggested Readings

American College of Obstetricians and Gynecologists: *Nutrition during pregnancy,* ACOG Technical Bulletin 179, Washington, DC, 1993, ACOG.

American Diabetes Association Clinical Education Series: *Medical management of pregnancy complicated by diabetes,* ed 2, 1994.

National Research Council, Food and Nutrition Board, Institute of Medicine—Committee on Nutritional Status During Pregnancy and Lactation, Subcommittee for a Clinical Application Guide: *Nutrition during pregnancy and lactation: an implementation guide,* Washington, DC, 1992, National Academy Press.

National Research Council, Food and Nutrition Board: *Recommended dietary allowances,* ed 10, Washington, DC, 1989, National Academy Press.

Worthington-Roberts B, Williams SR: *Nutrition in pregnancy and lactation,* ed 5, St Louis, 1993, Mosby.

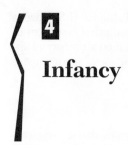

4

Infancy

THE FIRST YEAR OF LIFE

The first year of life is characterized by rapid growth and changes in body composition. Adequate infant nutrition is required to promote optimal growth and development, avoid illness, and allow infants to interact with and explore their environments. Infant nutritional requirements are different than those of adults. For example, protein, fat, and energy (which are important for growth) and iron, zinc, and calcium are required in greater proportions for infants.

Body Composition

Knowledge of the infant's body composition at various stages is of considerable importance. Characterizing changes in body composition is a means for understanding the process of growth and change in function that affect the nutritional needs of a growing infant. The body is composed of fat and fat-free body mass (FFBM), which includes water, protein, carbohydrates, and minerals. The percent of body weight that is fat increases throughout infancy from approximately 14% at birth to 23% by 1 year of age (Table 4-1). The accompanying decrease in the percentage of FFBM is principally the result of a decrease in water content. The contribution of protein, minerals, and carbohydrates remains relatively constant throughout infancy.

Body composition can be viewed in terms of its func-

TABLE 4-1 Body composition of reference infants (age 0-1 year; 50th percentile)[1,2]

Age (months)	Weight (kg)	Fat (kg)	Fat (%)	Fat-free body mass (kg)	Fat-free body mass (%)	Length (cm)	Head circumference (cm)
Boys							
Birth	3.5	0.5	14	3.1	86	50.5	34.8
3	6.4	1.5	23	4.9	77	61.1	40.6
6	8	2	25	6	75	67.8	43.8
9	9.2	2.2	24	7	76	72.3	45.8
12	10.2	2.3	23	7.9	77	76.1	47
Girls							
Birth	3.3	0.5	15	2.8	85	49.9	34.3
3	5.7	1.4	24	4.4	76	59.5	39.5
6	7.3	1.9	26	5.3	74	65.9	42.4
9	8.3	2.1	25	6.2	75	70.4	44.3
12	9.2	2.2	24	7	76	74.3	45.6

tional units, such as organs (brain, heart, liver, kidney), muscle mass, energy reserves (fat mass), extracellular fluid, and supporting structures (connective tissue, bone). The major organs and muscle mass account for most of the body protein, the fat mass is primarily used for energy when the diet is inadequate, and bone contains a reserve of calcium, phosphorus, and other minerals.

Growth

Growth increments in weight, length, and head circumference are extremely rapid before birth and during the first year of life (see Table 4-1). A normal 1-month-old infant grows approximately 1 cm per week and gains 20 to 30 g per day, gradually decreasing to 0.5 cm per week in length and 10 g per day in weight by 12 months of age. An average newborn weighs 3.5 kg, doubles its weight by 4 months, and triples it by 12 months of age. The energy cost of growth is the cost of depositing fat and protein. Fat deposition requires 10.8 kcal/g and protein deposition 13.4 kcal/g.

During early postnatal development, all organs appear to grow by cell division (hyperplasia) followed by a pattern of increasing cell size (hypertrophy). At birth, 15% of body weight is organ mass, 25% is muscle mass, 14% is fat, and 15% is bone and connective tissue. Throughout infancy these organ systems continue to grow and mature at a rapid rate. Cell number, measured by increments of DNA, continues to increase rapidly in the brain, heart, kidney, liver, and spleen. The brain doubles in size by 1 year of age. Energy or nutrient deficiencies during this period of rapid cell replication may limit the number of cells formed and possibly cause permanent deficits in the developing brain and nervous system.

Organ Maturation

The number and magnitude of obstacles newborns face in maintaining nutrient balance are inversely related to gestational age. The gastrointestinal tract of the preterm and sometimes the term infant may not be ready to perform the vital functions of nutrient intake, processing, assimilation, metabolism, and distribution to other organs. The term infant has mature coordination of sucking and swallowing but poor coordination of esophageal motility, decreased lower esophageal sphincter pressure, (which enhances the risk of gastroesophageal reflux), limited gastric volume and delayed gastric emptying, and variable maturity of several enzymatic and hormonal systems.

The kidneys fine-tune water and electrolyte excretion in relation to intake to maintain a body-fluid composition that supports optimal functioning. The term infant has the full number of nephrons but a low glomerular filtration rate in the first 48 hours, a higher fractional excretion of sodium than in adults, relative difficulty excreting a high-acid load, and normal diluting but limited concentrating capabilities.

BREAST-FEEDING

Exclusive breast-feeding is adequate for the first 4 to 6 months of age in almost all infants. One of the U.S. Public Health Service's *Healthy People 2000* goals is "to increase to at least 75% the proportion of mothers who breast-feed their babies in the early postpartum period and to at least 50% the proportion who continue breast feeding until their babies are 5 to 6 months old."[3] Differences in energy requirements between breast-fed and formula-fed infants are a result of lower energy excretion in breast-fed infants and higher energy cost of tissue synthesis (greater fat deposition) in formula-fed infants. Some of the advantages and disadvantages of breast milk are presented in Table 4-2.

Nutritional Advantages of Breast Milk

Human milk is tailored precisely for the growth and development needs of the human infant. The protein content of breast milk is lower than that of other species (1% versus 3% in cow milk) whose young double their birth weight and wean quickly in days or weeks. The profile of amino

TABLE 4-2 Advantages and disadvantages of breast milk

Advantages (antibacterial and antiviral properties)	Comments
Humoral factors	
IgA	Confers passive mucosal protection of gastrointestinal tract against penetration of intestinal organisms and antigens
Bifidus factor	Supports growth of *Lactobacillus bifidus,* a microorganism that converts lactose to acetic and lactic acids; low resulting pH — inhibits growth of *E. coli* and protects against *Staphylococcus aureus, Shigella,* and protozoal infections
Lysozymes	Bacteriolytic enzymes that act against *Enterobacteriaceae* and gram-positive bacteria
Lactoferrin	Iron-binding whey protein; bacteriostatic effect on *S. aureus* and *E. coli* by limiting iron available for their growth
Interferon	Antiviral protein
Cellular factors	
Macrophages	Phagocytize bacteria and viruses in the gut; synthesize complement lysozyme, and lactoferrin
Lymphocytes	T-cells: may transfer delayed hypersensitivity from mother to infant; B-cells: synthesize Ig

Advantages (nutritional properties)	Comments
Protein quality	
60:40 whey/casein ratio	Forms small, soft, easily digestible curd in stomach; essential amino acids (cysteine) provided in higher concentrations by whey.

TABLE 4-2 Advantages and disadvantages of breast milk—cont'd

Advantages (nutritional properties)	Comments
Protein quality—cont'd	
Nucleotides	Nonprotein nitrogen postulated to play a role in anabolism and growth
Hypoallergenic	Reduces potential for allergenic reactions
Lipid quality	
High oleic acid content	Improves digestibility and absorbability of lipid by increasing lipolytic enzymes' ability to act stereospecifically
Lipolytic activity	Improves fat absorption
Cholesterol	Possibly facilitates formation of nerve tissue and synthesis of bile salts; necessary for optimal development of cholesterol regulatory mechanism
Mineral/electrolyte content	
Ca^{++}/P ratio = 2:1	Improves absorption of calcium in gut
Low renal solute load (one third of cow milk)	More suited to immature capacity for renal solute excretion
Iron	High bioavailability (40%-50% absorption) compared to commercial formulas (<10% absorption)
Other	
Infant-maternal bonding	Potential long-term advantage

Continued

TABLE 4-2 Advantages and disadvantages of breast milk—cont'd

Advantages (nutritional properties)	Comments
Other—cont'd	
Possible decreased risk for obesity	High lipid and protein content at the end of breast milk feedings may signal satiety and inhibit overconsumption; may postpone introduction of solids

Disadvantages	Comments
Possible nutrient inadequacies	May develop Vitamin D and iron deficiencies with prolonged breast feeding if supplements or a variety of solid foods are not initiated
Inborn errors of metabolism	Inappropriate nutrient composition
Maternal drugs (antithyroid, antimetabolite, anticoagulant)	May be hazardous to the nursing infant
Environmental contaminants (herbicides, pesticides, insecticides, radioisotopes)	Have unknown effects on exposed children; no practical way to monitor contamination of human milk

acids in human milk is ideal not only for absorption but for utilization, especially by the brain. The composition of human milk relative to infant needs for essential amino acids is shown in Table 4-3. The main protein in cow milk, casein, forms a somewhat indigestible curd and has high levels of phenylalanine, tyrosine, and methionine for which the infant has little digestive enzyme resources. Cow milk contains little lactalbumin and cysteine, which the infant can digest readily. Human milk contains taurine, an im-

TABLE 4-3 Essential amino acid composition of breast milk and a casein-based formula relative to infant requirements

| Essential amino acid | Intake (150 ml/kg/day) | | Requirement (mg/kg/day) |
	Breast milk	Casein-based formula	
Histidine	37	45	28
Isoleucine	90	112	70
Leucine	155	210	161
Lysine	105	155	103
Methionine and cystine	68	82	58
Phenylalanine and tyrosine	135	190	125
Threonine	75	100	87
Tryptophan	30	30	17
Valine	100	120	93
Taurine	7.5	7	—

portant nutrient for brain and nerve growth, whereas cow milk contains none, so taurine must be added to most infant formulas.

The fat profile of human milk is predominantly composed of polyunsaturated fats and a stable amount of cholesterol, regardless of the mother's cholesterol intake (Table 4-4). Cholesterol is an important constituent of brain and nerve tissue as well as many enzymes. Most formulas contain no cholesterol and have the animal fats of cow milk replaced with a variety of fats of varying quality. Animal studies suggest a strong relationship between docosahexaenonic acid (DHA) and brain growth; a current concern is that the DHA and omega-3 oils present in human milk and fish oils are absent in cow-milk and infant formulas. Adding DHA to the diet by using fish oils guarantees neither absorption nor utilization.

Human milk is rich in vitamins A, C, and E (Table 4-5). The vitamin B content depends on maternal intake and

TABLE 4-4   Fat composition of breast milk relative to a whey-based formula

	Breast milk	Whey-based formula
Total (g/dl)	3.5-4.5	3.8
Triglycerides (%)	98-99	99
Cholesterol (mg/dl)	10-15	—
Phospholipids (mg/dl)	15-20	30
Fatty acids (%)		
Oleic (18:1)	35	16
Palmitic (16:0)	22	10
Linoleic (18:2, n-6)	15	32
Myristic (14:0)	6	9
Lauric (12:0)	4	22
Linolenic (18:3, omega-3)	1	1
Medium-chain triglycerides	10	8

meets calculated standards. Because the primary source of vitamin B_6 and the only source of vitamin B_{12} is animal products, vegetarian mothers (especially strict vegans) may produce milk that is deficient in these vitamins unless they supplement their diets. The vitamin D content of human milk is lower than that of cow milk, and supplementation is advisable when sun exposure is restricted. All newborns should receive a 0.5- to 1-mg injection or a 2-mg oral dose of vitamin K immediately after birth, regardless of whether breast- or bottle-feeding will be used.

Variations in Composition

The composition of milk varies during each feeding and as the child matures. When a feeding is initiated, the mother's milk "lets down," and the first milk or foremilk is released from the ducts as the lacteal cells respond to the surge of prolactin. The first milk is lower in fat and slightly higher in cells, protein, and lactose. The hindmilk is high in fat because the fat globules take more time to form and

TABLE 4-5 Vitamin and trace mineral content of breast milk

Vitamin or trace mineral	Amount/L of breast milk	Infant RDA
A	500 µg	375 µg
Thiamin (B_1)	0.2 mg	0.3-0.4 mg
Riboflavin (B_2)	0.35 mg	0.4-0.5 mg
Niacin (B_3)	1.5 mg	5-6 mg
Pyridoxine (B_6)	0.2 mg	0.3-0.6 mg
Folate	50 µg	25-35 µg
B_{12}	0.5 µg	0.3-0.5 µg
C	40 mg	30-35 mg
D	0.55 µg	7.5-10 µg
E	3 mg	3-4 mg
Chromium	50 µg	10-60 µg
Copper	250 µg	40-70 µg
Fluoride	0.016 mg	0.1-1 mg
Iodine	110 µg	40-50 µg
Manganese	6 µg	30-100 µg
Molybdenum	1-2 µg	15-40 µg
Selenium	20 µg	10-15 µg
Zinc	1.2 mg	5 mg

pass across the cell membrane. Human milk goes through three phases: colostrum, transitional milk, and mature milk. Produced at delivery and the first few days postpartum, colostrum is high in protein, especially immunoglobulins such as secretory IgA, that provide the infant with initial protection against infection. Colostrum is also high in carotene, giving it a yellow color. Colostrum provides enzymes that stimulate gut maturation, facilitate digestion (especially of fats by lipase), and stimulate the gut to pass meconium. There is a gradual change from colostrum to transitional milk and then mature milk over the first 7 to 10 days postpartum. The profile of mature milk persists until about 6 months postpartum when there is a slight decrease in protein content. The immune properties are measurable throughout lactation. During weaning the milk increases in protein, sodium, and chloride as the supply diminishes. Mothers who are not fully lactating or are experiencing lactation failure have milk that is higher in sodium and chloride than mature milk.

Other Components of Human Milk

Living cells are present in concentrations of $4000/mm^3$ in colostrum and $1500/mm^3$ in mature milk. They include macrophages that phagocytize bacteria and viruses in the gut and lymphocytes from the mother's Peyer patches that also provide immunologic protection in the infant's intestines. The normal flora of the newborn gut include lactobacilli, whose growth is stimulated by the bifidus factor and slightly acidic pH of human milk. The growth of *Escherichia coli* is suppressed by lactoferrin in human milk, which binds the iron that *E. coli* need for survival, whereas growth of *E. coli* is enhanced by iron provided in the diet. Secretory IgA in human milk impedes translocation of organisms across the intestinal wall and mucous membranes from the mouth onward and has been shown in recent studies to reduce respiratory disease, diarrhea, and sepsis. Other humoral factors found in human milk (whose precise roles have not all been identified) include nucleotides, resistance factor, lysozyme, interferon, complement, and B_{12} binding protein. All these properties are unique to human milk, and attempts to fortify infant formulas with some of them (e.g., nucleotides) have not been shown to prevent disease.

Fully breast-fed infants experience a lower incidence of and morbidity from bacterial, especially respiratory, illnesses. Both retrospective and prospective epidemiologic studies also suggest that infants who are fully breast-fed for at least 4 to 6 months may be protected against childhood-onset diabetes, cancers (such as lymphoma), celiac disease, and Crohn's disease. The incidence of significant allergic disease (eczema, asthma, and allergic rhinitis) is significantly reduced in the first 2 years of life by breast-feeding, at least in part because of decreased intestinal permeability.

Contraindications to Breast-Feeding

Maternal infections in general do not contraindicate breast-feeding, and in most cases they even provide additional protection for the infant via the milk. At one time hepatitis B represented a contraindication to breast-feeding. However, now that all infants born to mothers with hepatitis B are given hepatitis B immune globulin in the first 12 hours of life and then a vaccine before hospital discharge, breast-feeding is safe even if the virus passes into the milk.

The disease that is currently causing significant concern is acquired immunodeficiency syndrome (AIDS). Not all infants born to HIV-positive mothers are infected with the virus at birth, but those who are infected cannot be identified immediately because they have passive maternal antibodies. In the United States where the survival of healthy bottle-fed babies is assured, mothers with HIV disease should not breast-feed. In contrast, breast-feeding is encouraged in developing countries where there is less than an 18% risk of an infant acquiring AIDS by breast-feeding from an HIV-positive mother but a greater than 50% chance of an infant dying in the first year of life if not breast-fed. Present data suggest that the virus may pass into the milk, but the milk suppresses the growth of the virus, at least *in vitro*.

Maternal Medications

Although medications pass into milk in varying amounts depending on the pharmacologic properties of the compound, most medications are safe for mothers to take if they are breast-feeding. Medications that are the most effective but deliver the lowest amounts to the infant should be selected. Over-the-counter drugs such as aspirin, acetaminophen, and ibuprofen are usually acceptable in moderate doses for temporary use. Although most antibiotics pass into milk to some degree, those that can be given directly to infants are safe for lactating mothers to take. A short list of drugs contraindicated during lactation is given in Table 4-6. In most cases acceptable substitutes are available.

Although drugs of abuse represent a risk to nursing infants, in the case of marijuana the risk-to-benefit ratio favors breast-feeding over bottle-feeding. The mother who is bottle-feeding and smokes marijuana in the presence of her infant creates risk in addition to losing the benefits of breast-feeding. Cigarette smoking has been associated

TABLE 4-6 Drugs contraindicated during breast-feeding

Drug	Rationale
Amethopterin, cyclophosphamide, cyclosporine, methotrexate	May suppress the immune system; unknown whether they affect growth or cause cancer in infants
Bromocriptine	Suppresses lactation
Cimetidine	Concentrated in breast milk; may suppress gastric acidity in infant, inhibit drug metabolism, and stimulate central nervous system
Clemastine	May cause drowsiness, irritability, refusal to feed, high-pitched cry, neck stiffness
Ergotamine	Causes vomiting, diarrhea, convulsions in doses used in migraine medications
Gold salts	Cause rash and inflammation of kidneys and liver
Methimazole	Potentially interferes with thyroid function
Phenindione	Causes hemorrhage
Thiouracil	Decreases thyroid function (does not apply to propylthiouracil)

with decreased breast-feeding duration, but breast-fed infants of smoking mothers have fewer respiratory infections than bottle-fed infants whose mothers smoke. Mothers should be cautioned never to smoke in the presence of the infant and not to smoke within 30 minutes before a feeding to avoid suppressing the let-down reflex and decrease the possibility of nicotine appearing in the milk.

A mother who has received radioactive pharmaceuticals as a single dose for clinical diagnosis should temporarily stop breast-feeding. The breasts should be pumped to maintain lactation, but the milk should be discarded. When radioactive drugs are used in multiple doses for treatment, breast-feeding must be completely discontinued, because no amount of radioactive material is safe for an infant.

Common Misunderstandings

Breast-feeding success is enhanced by early initiation. Ideally, the baby should be offered the breast immediately after birth. No test water is necessary when the Apgar scores are good and secretions modest. Subsequent feedings should be "on demand" but never more than 4 to 5 hours apart in the first week. This is important not only for nourishing and hydrating the infant but also for stimulating the breast to produce milk. Breast-feeding is an infant-driven process. Ending feedings with water, glucose water, and especially formula is a recipe for lactation failure. Carefully controlled studies have demonstrated clearly that infants who are given water, glucose water, or formula instead of human milk exclusively in the first week lose weight, regain it more slowly, and have higher bilirubin levels and fewer stools.

The average infant nurses every 2 hours for 10 to 12 feedings a day during the first few weeks. The stomach's emptying time with human milk is no more than 90 minutes, whereas with formula it is more than 3 hours and up to 6 hours with homogenized milk. Weight gain should be consistent, at least 1 oz per day after 10 to 14 days when the milk supply is well established. Initial weight loss should not exceed 10% of birth weight and usually averages about 8% when the mother is primiparous. An additional means of monitoring adequate breast milk intake is to count the number of the infant's urinary voidings, which should total at least six per day and include some soaking. Stools are an important indication of adequate food in the gut. In the first few weeks, infants produce stool every day, often with every feeding. Signs such as failure to thrive or infrequent stools and voidings should be evaluated.

Sore nipples are associated more with the position of the infant during breast-feeding than the length of feedings. When mothers complain of sore nipples, observe the infant when it is breast-feeding, taking particular note of positioning; the baby's abdomen should face the mother's abdomen, and the infant should directly face the breast.

INFANT FORMULAS

When breast-feeding is not feasible, commercially prepared infant formulas are an acceptable alternative. They are stable mixtures of emulsified fats, proteins, carbohydrates, minerals, and vitamins and come in ready-to-feed, concentrated-liquid, or powdered preparations. Standard infant formulas have an energy density of 20 kcal/oz and an osmolarity of 300 mOsm/L. The American Academy of Pediatrics suggests a caloric distribution of 30% to 55% fat (2.7% of the calories as linoleic acid), 7% to 16% protein, and the remaining 35% to 65% of energy from carbohydrate. The Infant Formula Act of 1980 regulates the composition of infant formulas sold in the United States. Table 4-7 lists a number of these formulas.

SOLID FOOD

A recommended schedule for introducing solid food is shown in the box on the top of p. 121.

The introduction of solid food should be based on the individual infant's growth, activity, and neuromuscular development. Infants do not have the oral motor skills to con-

Text continues on page 122.

TABLE 4-7 Formulas for infant feeding

Formula (manufacturer)	Indication	Osmolarity (mOsm/L)	Renal solute load (mOsm/L)
Mature human milk	Gold standard	300	80
Similac (Ross)	Routine feeding	290	108
Enfamil (Mead Johnson)	Routine feeding	300	100
SMA (Wyeth)	Routine feeding	300	128
Gerber	Routine feeding	290	132
Whole cow milk*	>12 months	288	240
LactoFree (Mead Johnson)	Lactose intolerance	200	100
Nursoy (Wyeth)	Vegetarian	296	172
Isomil (Ross)	Vegetarian	260	125
ProSobee (Mead Johnson)	Vegetarian	200	130
I-Soyalac or Alsoy (Carnation)	Vegetarian	270	130
Human Milk Fortifier [8.1kcal/g] (Mead Johnson)†	Supplement low birth infants	—	—
Similac Special Care 24 (Ross)	Low-birth weight infant	300	156
Enfamil Premature 24 (Mead Johnson)	Low-birth weight infant	300	130
Preemie SMA 24 (Wyeth)	Low-birth weight infant	268	175
Similac PM 60/40 (Ross)	Low-birth weight infant	280	97
Pregestimil (Mead Johnson)	Malabsorption, hypoallergenic	350	120
Nutramigen (Mead Johnson)	Hypoallergenic	480	130

Continued

TABLE 4-7 Formulas for infant feeding—cont'd

Formula (manufacturer)	Indication	Osmolarity (mOsm/L)	Renal solute load (mOsm/L)
Alimentum (Ross)	Malabsorption, hypoallergenic	370	123
Good Start (Carnation)	Hypoallergenic	263	100
Portagen (Mead Johnson)	Pancreatic and hepatic insufficiency	220	150
RCF (Ross)[†]	Carbohydrate intolerance (CHO added as tolerated)	74	—
3232A (Mead Johnson)[†]	Carbohydrate intolerance (CHO added as tolerated)	250	170
ProViMin (Ross)[†]	Malabsorption (Fat and CHO added as tolerated)	—	—

TABLE 4-7 Formulas for infant feeding—cont'd

Formula (manufacturer)	Protein (% weight/volume)	Protein profile (%)			Fat (% weight/volume)
		Whey	Casein	Soy	
Mature human milk	1.1	60	40	—	3.6
Similac (Ross)	1.5	18	82	—	3.6
Enfamil (Mead Johnson)	1.5	60	40	—	3.8
SMA (Wyeth)	1.5	60	40	—	3.6
Gerber	1.5	18	82	—	3.7
Whole cow milk°	3.6	18	82	—	3.7
LactoFree (Mead Johnson)	1.5	18	82	—	3.7
Nursoy (Wyeth)	2.1	—	—	100	3.6
Isomil (Ross)	1.8	—	—	100	3.7
ProSobee (Mead Johnson)	2	—	—	100	3.6
I-Soyalac or Alsoy (Carnation)	2.1	—	—	100	3.8
Human Milk Fortifier [8.1kcal/g] (Mead Johnson)†	0.7	60	40	—	<0.1
Similac Special Care 24 (Ross)	2.2	60	40	—	4.4
Enfamil Premature 24 (Mead Johnson)	2.4	60	40	—	4.1
Preemie SMA 24 (Wyeth)	2	60	40	—	4.4
Similac PM 60/40 (Ross)	2.4	60	40	—	5.4
Pregestimil (Mead Johnson)	1.9	—	Hydrolyzed 100	—	2.7
Nutramigen (Mead Johnson)	1.9	—	Hydrolyzed 100	—	2.6

Continued

TABLE 4-7 Formulas for infant feeding—cont'd

Formula (manufacturer)	Protein (% weight/volume)	Protein profile (%)			Fat (% weight/volume)
		Whey	Casein	Soy	
Alimentum (Ross)[†]	1.86	—	Hydrolyzed 100	—	3.75
Good Start (Carnation)	1.6	100	—	—	3.5
Portagen (Mead Johnson)	2.3	0	100	—	3.2
RCF (Ross)[†]	1.8	—	—	100	3.7
3232A (Mead Johnson)[†]	1.9	—	Hydrolyzed 100	—	2.7
ProViMin (Ross)[†]	2	100	—	—	0.04

TABLE 4-7 Formulas for infant feeding—cont'd

Formula (manufacturer)	Fat profile (%)					Predominant oil
	Polyun-saturated	Mono-saturated	Saturated	LCT[‡]	MCT[‡]	
Mature human milk	14.2	41.6	44.2	—	—	—
Similac (Ross)	37.3	17.6	45.1	—	—	Soy, coconut
Enfamil (Mead Johnson)	29	16	55	—	—	Coconut, soy
SMA (Wyeth)	14.5	41.3	44.2	—	—	Oleo, safflower, coconut, soy
Gerber	36	17.9	46.1	—	—	Soy, coconut
Whole cow milk[o]	3.8	30.4	65.8	—	—	—
LactoFree (Mead Johnson)	19	38	42.9	—	—	Palm olein, safflower, soy, coconut
Nursoy (Wyeth)	14.5	41.3	44.2	—	—	Oleo, coconut, safflower, soy
Isomil (Ross)	37.3	17.6	45.1	—	—	Soy, coconut
ProSobee (Mead Johnson)	29	16	55	—	—	Coconut, soy
I-Soyalac or Alsoy (Carnation)	60.5	23.7	15.8	—	—	Soy
Human Milk Fortifier [8.1kcal/g] (Mead Johnson)[†]	—	—	—	—	—	—
Similac Special Care 24 (Ross)	—	—	—	50	50	—
Enfamil Premature 24 (Mead Johnson)	—	—	—	60	40	—
Preemie SMA 24 (Wyeth)	—	—	—	87.5	12.5	—
Similac PM 60/40 (Ross)	—	—	—	94	6	—
Pregestimil (Mead Johnson)	—	—	—	60	40	—
Nutramigen (Mead Johnson)	—	—	—	100	—	—

Continued

TABLE 4-7 Formulas for infant feeding—cont'd

Formula (manufacturer)	Fat profile (%)					Predominant oil
	Polyun-saturated	Mono-saturated	Saturated	LCT[‡]	MCT[‡]	
Alimentum (Ross)	—	—	—	50	50	—
Good Start (Carnation)	31.9	25.6	42.5	—	—	Palm olein, safflower, coconut
Portagen (Mead Johnson)	—	—	—	20	80	—
RCF (Ross)[†]	—	—	—	100	—	—
3232A (Mead Johnson)[†]	—	—	—	60	40	—
ProViMin (Ross)[†]	—	—	—	—	—	—

TABLE 4-7 Formulas for infant feeding—cont'd

Formula (manufacturer)	Carbohydrate (% weight/volume)	Type carbohydrate	Sodium (mg/L)$
Mature human milk	7.2	Lactose	150
Similac (Ross)	7.2	Lactose	220
Enfamil (Mead Johnson)	6.9	Lactose	180
SMA (Wyeth)	7.2	Lactose	150
Gerber	7.2	Lactose	225
Whole cow milk°	4.8	Lactose	520
LactoFree (Mead Johnson)	6.9	Corn-syrup solids	200
Nursoy (Wyeth)	6.9	Sucrose	200
Isomil (Ross)	6.8	Corn-syrup solids, sucrose	320
ProSobee (Mead Johnson)	6.8	Corn-syrup solids	290
I-Soyalac or Alsoy (Carnation)	6.7	Sucrose, tapioca, dextrin	285
Human Milk Fortifier [8.1kcal/g] (Mead Johnson)[†]	2.7	Corn-syrup solids, lactose	70
Similac Special Care 24 (Ross)	8.6	Lactose-hydrolyzed starch	350
Enfamil Premature 24 (Mead Johnson)	8.9	Lactose-hydrolyzed starch	320
Preemie SMA 24 (Wyeth)	8.6	Lactose-hydrolyzed starch	320
Similac PM 60/40 (Ross)	11.5	Lactose	240
Pregestimil (Mead Johnson)	9	Partially hydrolyzed starch	315
Nutramigen (Mead Johnson)	9	Partially hydrolyzed starch	315

Continued

TABLE 4-7 Formulas for infant feeding—cont'd

Formula (manufacturer)	Carbohydrate (% Weight/Volume)	Type carbohydrate	Sodium (mg/L)§
Alimentum (Ross)	6.89	Sucrose, tapioca	300
Good Start (Carnation)	7.4	Lactose, maltodextrin	162
Portagen (Mead Johnson)	7.7	Hydrolyzed starch, sucrose, lactose	370
RCF (Ross)†	0	—	320
3232A (Mead Johnson)†	0	—	290
ProViMin (Ross)†	0.06	—	328

TABLE 4-7 Formulas for infant feeding—cont'd

Formula (manufacturer)	Potassium (mg/L)[§]	Calcium (mg/L)	Phosphorus (mg/L)	Iron (mg/l)
Mature human milk	550	340	140	0.5
Similac (Ross)	810	510	390	12
Enfamil (Mead Johnson)	720	460	320	13
SMA (Wyeth)	560	420	280	12
Gerber	730	510	390	12
Whole cow milk[*]	1480	1220	960	0.6
LactoFree (Mead Johnson)	730	540	365	12
Nursoy (Wyeth)	700	600	420	12
Isomil (Ross)	950	710	510	12
ProSobee (Mead Johnson)	780	630	500	13
I-Soyalac or Alsoy (Carnation)	790	690	475	13
Human Milk Fortifier [8.1kcal/g] (Mead Johnson)[†]	156	900	450	0
Similac Special Care 24 (Ross)	1000	1440	720	3
Enfamil Premature 24 (Mead Johnson)	900	950	470	1.3
Preemie SMA 24 (Wyeth)	750	750	400	3
Similac PM 60/40 (Ross)	850	600	300	4
Pregestimil (Mead Johnson)	730	630	415	12.5
Nutramigen (Mead Johnson)	730	630	415	12.5

Continued

TABLE 4-7 Formulas for infant feeding—cont'd

Formula (manufacturer)	Potassium (mg/L)§	Calcium (mg/L)	Phosphorus (mg/L)	Iron (mg/l)
Alimentum (Ross)	800	710	510	12
Good Start (Carnation)	662	433	243	10
Portagen (Mead Johnson)	840	630	470	12.5
RCF (Ross)†	950	710	510	12
3232A (Mead Johnson)†	730	630	415	12.5
ProViMin (Ross)†	904	658	464	5.8

From Mead Johnson, Evansville, IN; Ross Laboratories, Columbus, OH; Wyeth Laboratories, Philadelphia, PA, Gerber Products Company, Fremont, MI; Carnation, Glendale, CA.

*For comparison only. Whole cow milk should not be fed to infants until they are 12 months of age.
†These are not complete formulas.
‡LCT, Long-chain triglycerides; MCT, Medium-chain triglycerides.
§To determine mEq/L sodium, divide by 23; To determine mEq/L potassium, divide by 39.1.

AGE SCHEDULE FOR INTRODUCING SOLID FOOD

Ages 1 to 4 months

Breast milk or formula only

Ages 4 to 6 months

Iron-fortified cereal

Ages 6 to 7 months

Fruit (strained or mashed); cup introduced

Ages 7 to 8 months

Vegetables (strained or mashed)

Ages 8 to 9 months

Finger food (e.g., crackers, bananas) and chopped (junior) baby food

Age 9 months

Meat and citrus juice

Age 10 to 11 months

Bite-size cooked food

Age 12 months

All table food

sume solid food or eat from a spoon until 4 to 6 months of age. The potential disadvantages of introducing solid food before this time are shown in the box on top of p. 122.

When adding solid food to an infant's diet, one new, single-ingredient food should be introduced every 3 to 5 days. This allows the parent to watch for allergic reactions and gives the infant time to become accustomed to new tastes. Other suggested guidelines for introducing solids are shown in the box on the bottom of p. 122. The sequence of introducing food is not critical, although iron-fortified, dry baby cereal is usually added first. Rice cereal is commonly the first food added because rice is the least aller-

POTENTIAL DISADVANTAGES OF INTRODUCING SOLID FOOD BEFORE 4 TO 6 MONTHS OF AGE

Poor oral-motor coordination

Insufficient energy and nutrient replacement for breast milk or infant formula

Increased risk of food allergies

Increased renal solute load and hyperosmolarity

Disturbance of appetite regulation possibly encouraging overfeeding

Increased likelihood of infant desiring sugar and salt later in life

GUIDELINES FOR INTRODUCING SOLID FOOD

Begin with single-ingredient foods; add one at a time.

Introduce a small amount of each new food beginning with 1 to 2 tsp, and gradually increase the amount to 3 to 4 tsp per feeding.

Wait 3 to 5 days before adding another new food; discontinue the last food if an allergy is detected.

Ultimately, offer a wide variety of food. For older infants include meat, milk, fruit, vegetables, bread, and cereal for nutritional adequacy and diversity.

Avoid mixing solids with fluids so that the infant can learn textures and flavors and develop facial muscles. (EXCEPTION: For infants with reflux, add rice cereal to thicken feedings.)

Never put a baby to bed with a bottle or allow a baby to suck a bottle continuously during the day. This practice increases the risk of dental caries and may affect tooth eruption.

Provide solids with textures that are compatible with the infant's ability to chew and swallow.

FINGER FOOD FOR INFANTS

Preferred

Bread: bread, toast, unsalted crackers

Fruit: items that are fresh or canned (unsweetened), soft, and without seeds or peels (bananas, apples, peaches, apricots)

Meat, poultry, fish: items that are tender and in small cooked pieces or strips without bones (meatballs, meat sticks, hamburger, meat loaf, chicken nuggets, turkey, fish sticks)

Vegetables: items that are tender and in cooked whole pieces or chunks (carrots, green beans, squash, potato)

Avoid

Popcorn, nuts, seeds, unmashed peas, raisins, potato chips, corn kernels (potential for choking and aspiration)

genic. Eggs and wheat should be avoided during the first 6 to 9 months of age to minimize the possibility of an allergic reaction. Combination food such as strained cereal with fruit, vegetables with meat, high-meat dinners, and other infant or toddler food may be introduced after single-ingredient food is well tolerated. Unsweetened fruit juice should be introduced when the infant can drink from a cup. Juice should be given in a cup and not a bottle, as the latter may predispose the infant to nursing-bottle caries. The protein content of breast milk decreases gradually as lactation duration increases. High-protein baby food intake should be encouraged. Sugar and salt should not be added during the preparation of homemade baby food, and frozen or canned food containing sugar and salt should be avoided.

Between 6 and 12 months of age, infants show increasing interest in self-feeding and develop the ability to grasp and pick up food. Finger food should be offered once the ability to chew is acquired. These should be carefully selected to allow for easy manipulation in the mouth and minimize the potential for choking and aspiration (box above).

The products listed in Table 4-8 were developed to help physicians treat infants and children with med-

TABLE 4-8 Commercial modular feeding components

Product	Manufacturer	Composition	Energy content
Moducal	Mead Johnson	Maltodextrin	3.8 kcal/g
Polycose liquid	Ross Laboratories	Glucose polymer	2 kcal/ml
Polycose powder	Ross Laboratories	Glucose polymer	3.8 kcal/g
Corn oil	—	—	9 kcal/ml
Microlipid	Sherwood	Emulsified long-chain triglycerides	4.5 kcal/ml
Medium-chain triglyceride oil	Mead Johnson	Fractionated coconut oil	7.7 kcal/ml
Casec	Mead Johnson	Calcium caseinate, egg-white solids	3.7 kcal/g

ical problems. Most of these products are not complete diets, so use care to avoid producing nutrient deficiencies.

NUTRITIONAL REQUIREMENTS OF INFANTS

The Recommended Dietary Allowances (RDAs) are the intake levels of essential nutrients that are adequate to meet the known nutritional needs of practically all healthy persons. These recommendations are based on the average daily amount of nutrients that population groups should consume over time and are not requirements for specific individuals. The RDAs for infants up to 6 months of age are based primarily on the amount of nutrients known to be provided by breast milk. Those for infants from 6 months to 1 year of age are based on the consump-

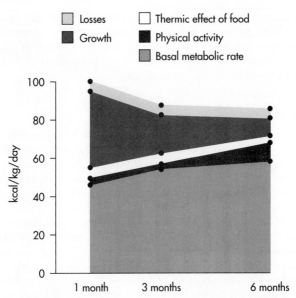

FIGURE 4-1 Changes in energy requirements in the first 6 months.

tion of formula and increasing amounts of solid food (see Tables 2-1 and 2-3).

Energy

The energy balance of infants may be described simply as

Gross energy intake = Energy excreted + Energy expended + Energy stored.

The components of energy expenditure are basal metabolic rate (energy needed to maintain body temperature; support the minimal work of the brain, heart, and respiratory muscles; and supply the minimal energy requirements of tissues at rest), thermic effect of feeding (energy used for digestion, transport, and conversion of absorbed nutrients into their respective storage forms), and physical activity. The changes in the partitions of energy requirements during the first 6 months of life are shown in Figure 4-1. Energy requirements per kilogram of body weight gradually decline throughout infancy as a result of decreases in basal metabolic rate per kilogram and growth rate. Fomon estimates that the percent of energy intake used for growth decreases from about 27% at birth to about 5% by 1 year of age.[4]

Water

Water is necessary for the infant to replace losses from the skin and lungs (evaporative loss), feces, and urine; a small amount is also needed for growth. Under most conditions water intake exceeds the requirements for evaporative losses, renal excretion of solutes, and growth, and any excess is excreted in the urine.

Human milk, cow milk, and infant formulas of conventional energy density (67 kcal/100 ml) provide approximately 89 ml of preformed water in each 100 ml of milk or formula consumed. In addition, food yields water when oxidized; the combustion of 1 g of protein, fat, and carbohydrate yields 0.41 ml, 1.07 ml, and 0.55 ml of water respectively. In milks and formulas, preformed water and oxidation water amount to approximately 95% of the volume consumed.

Carbohydrates

Carbohydrates should comprise 35% to 65% of the total energy intake of the term infant and are usually in the form of disaccharides or glucose polymers. Glucose is the principal nutrient the neonatal brain utilizes, and inadequate carbohydrate intake can lead to hypoglycemia, ketosis, and excessive protein catabolism. Most milk-based formulas contain lactose as the principal carbohydrate in amounts similar to that of human milk (6 to 7 g/100 ml). As shown in Table 4-7, several hypoallergenic formulas contain sucrose, maltose, fructose, dextrins, and glucose polymers as their carbohydrate sources. Because they are lactose free, they are also useful in managing disorders such as galactosemia and primary lactase deficiency and recovering from secondary lactose intolerance.

Fat

Dietary fat serves as a concentrated source of energy, carries fat-soluble vitamins, and provides essential fatty acids (EFAs). EFAs are precursors for the synthesis of prostaglandins and serve other essential functions. The American Academy of Pediatrics recommends that 30% to 55% of total energy intake be from fat and 2.7% from linoleic acid. Table 4-4 compares the fat composition of breast milk with that of a whey-based formula.

Breast milk is unique in containing maternal lipases that aid in fat digestion. Fat digestion begins in the stomach with the additional action of lingual lipase, an enzyme secreted from lingual serous glands, and gastric lipase secreted from glands in the gastric mucosa. Further digestion takes place in the small intestine through the action of pancreatic and intestinal lipases.

The fat content of infant formulas (see Table 4-7) is derived from a variety of long-chain vegetable triglycerides such as soy, corn, and safflower oil and from medium-chain triglycerides (MCTs). Linoleic acid is found only in the long-chain vegetable oils in various concentrations. Breast milk contains 8% to 10% of total calories as linoleic acid, and most infant formulas have at least 10%. Some special formulas contain MCTs (fatty acids from 6 to 12 carbons in length) compared with long-chain triglycerides (fatty acids more than 16 carbons long). MCTs are partially soluble in water and not dependent on bile acids for solubilization, so they can be absorbed by patients with malabsorption and hepatobiliary disease. Because of their solubility, MCTs can appose the mucosal surface and be hydrolyzed by mucosal lipases. This obviates the need for pancreatic lipase, which is deficient in patients with pancreatic insufficiency. A large percentage of absorbed MCTs are transported directly into the portal circulation, bypassing the lymphatic channels necessary to transport long-chain triglycerides. For this reason, MCT oil is useful in managing diseases such as intestinal lymphangiectasia. The disadvantages of MCTs are that they are not very palatable, have a cathartic effect when given in large amounts, are expensive, and do not contain EFAs.

Protein

Protein provides nitrogen and amino acids for the synthesis of body tissues, enzymes, hormones, and antibodies that regulate and perform physiologic and metabolic functions. Excess dietary proteins are metabolized for energy, increasing the renal solute load and water requirements. The American Academy of Pediatrics recommends that 7% to 16% of total energy be from protein or 1.6 to 2.2 g/kg/day. Healthy term infants may grow well with a protein intake (from breast milk) slightly below 1.6 g/kg per day.

The protein in commercial formulas was originally from cow milk, which has a whey/casein ratio of 20:80. Several recently developed infant formulas contain whey/casein ratios of 60:40, which is closer to the 65:35 or 70:30 ratio and amino acid composition of human milk. The curd formed from whey in an acidic stomach is small, soft, easily digestible, and emptied quickly. Table 4-3 compares the essential amino acid compositions of breast milk and a casein-based formula with requirements.

Other protein sources used in infant formulas (see Table 4-7) include soy-protein isolates and protein hydrolysates. Infant formulas containing soy protein are well received by vegetarian families who wish to avoid cow milk and animal products. Soy proteins contain trypsin inhibitors that may interfere with absorption. These inhibitors are largely inactivated by heat treatment of the protein isolate. Soy also produces tightly bound protein-phytate mineral complexes that may reduce the bioavailability of some minerals. For these reasons, soy formulas are not recommended for routine infant feedings.

Between 20% and 80% of infants who are allergic to casein are also allergic to soy, so hydrolyzed casein is the protein of choice for these infants. The enzymatic hydrolysis process results in a mixture of amino acids and peptides of various chain lengths and destroys its allergenicity, making it ideal for treating protein hypersensitivity.

Vitamins

Many of the vitamins play important roles as cofactors and catalysts for cell function and replication. Table 4-5 shows the vitamin and trace mineral content of breast milk. The content of most commercial infant formulas is also adequate to meet the requirements of most healthy infants when they consume approximately 750 ml (26 oz) of formula each day. Vitamin supplementation may be necessary for infants whose intake is less than this, when steatorrhea is present (hepatobiliary disease, pancreatic insufficiency, or small intestinal disease causing malabsorption), or when prescribed medications affect vitamin absorption or utilization. Table 4-9 provides guidelines for using vitamin and mineral supplements in healthy infants and children.

Minerals

The RDAs for minerals in term infants are presented in Table 2-1. The mineral content of commercial formulas (see Table 4-7) warrants special consideration. The American Academy of Pediatrics recommends a dietary calcium/phosphorus ratio between 1:1 and 1:2 for optimal calcium absorption. The ratio declines during infancy with the introduction of solid food. There are also minimum and maximum levels for sodium, potassium, and chloride in formulas, which will meet growth needs and leave little residue to be excreted in the urine. The sodium/potassium ratio should not exceed 1, and the (sodium + potassium)/chloride ratio should be at least 1.5.

Iron deficiency is the most common cause of anemia in infants and children. In the healthy term infant there is no need for exogenous iron between birth and 4 months of age. The usually abundant neonatal iron stores gradually decline during this period to provide for the synthesis of hemoglobin, myoglobin, and enzymes, but iron deficiency is rare in the first several months unless there has been substantial loss of iron through perinatal or subsequent blood loss.

There are two broad categories of iron in food—heme iron and nonheme iron (see Chapter 24). Because infant diets contain little meat, the vast preponderance of iron is in the nonheme form. The extent of nonheme iron absorption depends on how soluble it becomes in the duode-

TABLE 4-9 Guidelines for use of vitamins and mineral supplements in healthy infants and children[a,b]

Group	Multivitamins	Individual vitamins			Minerals	
		Vitamin D	Vitamin E	Folate	Iron	Fluoride
Preterm infants						
Breast-fed[c]	+	+	±	±	+	—
Formula-fed	+	+	±	±	+	—
Term infants (0-6 mo)						
Breast fed	—	+	—	—	—	—
Formula-fed	—	—	—	—	—	—
Infants > 6 mo[d]	—	+	—	—	±[e]	±[e]
Children > 1 year	—	—	—	—	—	±
Pregnant women	±	—	—	±	+	—
Lactating women	±	—	—	—	±	—

[a]Vitamin K is not shown but should be given to all newborn infants.
[b]Extra calcium for pregnant and lactating women is not shown.
[c]The sodium content of human milk is marginal for preterm infants.
[d]If high risk (poor intake, steatorrhea, or medication use that affects vitamin absorption or utilization), multivitamins and multiminerals (including iron) are preferred.
[e]See discussion in text.

num, determined by the composition of food consumed in a given meal. The most important enhancers of nonheme iron absorption are ascorbic acid and meat, fish, and poultry. Major inhibitors are bran (whole-grain cereal), oxalates (spinach), polyphenols (tannates in tea), and phosphates (cow milk, egg yolks). Absorption of the small amount of iron in breast milk is uniquely high at 50% on average, in contrast to 10% from unfortified cow-milk formula and 4% from iron-fortified cow-milk formula and dry infant cereal (Figure 4-2). The box below suggests ways to optimize iron status in infants.

OPTIMIZING IRON STATUS IN INFANTS

Unfortified food

Maintain breast-feeding for at least 4 months.

Do not give fresh cow milk until after about 9 months.

Use vitamin C-rich food and fruit juice and/or meat with meals of solid food after about 6 months.

Iron- and vitamin C-fortified food

If cow-milk formula is used, choose one fortified with iron and vitamin C.

Use infant cereal or milk-cereal products fortified with iron ± vitamin C.

Use vitamin C-fortified fruit juice with meals of solid food.

Iron supplementation (ferrous sulfate or similarly bioavailable compounds)

Supplement low-birth weight infants with the following amounts of iron from formula and/or drops, beginning no later than 2 months of age and continuing through the sixth month:

Birth weight; supplemental iron dose

1500-2500 g; 2 mg/kg/day

1000-1500 g; 3 mg/kg/day

<1000 g; 4 mg/kg/day

For established iron deficiency: 3 mg/kg/day

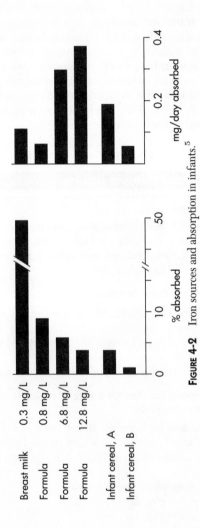

Figure 4-2 Iron sources and absorption in infants.[5]

Trace Minerals

The trace mineral content of breast milk and the infant RDAs are shown in Table 4-5. Normal volumes of commercial formulas also provide adequate amounts for full-term infants. The fluoride concentration of breast milk ranges between 3 and 10 µg/L. Fluoride is poorly transported from plasma to milk, and concentrations in milk remain low even if the mother consumes fluoridated water. There is no convincing evidence that orally ingested fluoride is important in preventing dental caries (i.e., by altering the composition of the dental enamel). However, there is clear evidence that oral consumption may contribute to fluorosis of the permanent dentition. Therefore *no* fluoride supplements are recommended for infants until after teeth have erupted, when it is recommended that fluoridated water be offered (when feasible) several times daily to infants fed by breast milk, cow milk, or formulas prepared with water that contain no more than 0.3 mg/L.

References

1. Fomon SJ et al: Body composition of reference children from birth to age 10 years, *Am J Clin Nutr* 35:1169, 1982.
2. Hamil PV et al: Physical grwoth: National Center for Health Statistics percentiles, *Am J Clin Nutr* 32:607, 1979.
3. US DHHS: *Healthy People 2000: national health promotion and disease prevention objectives,* Washington, DC, 1990, US Government Printing Office.
4. Fomon SJ, ed: *Nutrition of normal infants,* St Louis, 1993, Mosby.
5. Tsang RC, Nichols BL, eds: *Nutrition during infancy,* St Louis, 1988, Mosby.

Suggested Readings

American Academy of Pediatrics, Committee on Drugs: Transfer of drugs and other chemicals into human milk, *Pediatrics* 84:924,1989.

Grand RA, Sutphen JL, Dietz WH Jr, eds: *Pediatric nutrition: theory and practice,* Stoneham, Mass, 1978, Butterworths.

Huggins K: *The nursing mother's companion,* rev ed, Boston, 1990, The Harvard Common Press.

Lawrence RA, ed: *Breastfeeding: A guide for the medical profession,* ed 3, St Louis, 1989, Mosby.

National Research Council, Food and Nutrition Board: *Recommended dietary allowances,* ed 10, Washington, DC, 1989, National Academy Press.

5

Childhood and Adolescence

The periods of childhood (ages 1 to 10) and adolescence (ages 11 to 18) are characterized by changes in growth rates, body composition, and nutrient requirements. Between infancy and adolescence, body fat decreases and fat-free body mass (FFBM) increases. Growth proceeds at a slower rate as energy and protein requirements decrease.

NORMAL GROWTH RATES

Growth is predictable in a normal child. The rate of growth varies with age and can be quantitated using standard-height velocity charts for males and females. Children's stature should be measured in the supine position until they are 24 to 36 months of age. Two people are needed to make an accurate measurement, with one holding the child in the proper position while the other measures. Children from 2 to 18 years are measured standing.

Figures 5-1 through 5-8 show national growth curve percentiles according to gender and age. A normal child's weight triples by 12 months of age and quadruples by 2 years of age. Thereafter the weight gain slows to a relatively steady yearly increase of 2 to 3 kg (4 to 6 lb) until the onset of the adolescent growth spurt. After the first year of life the linear growth velocity decreases more gradually than weight gain (Figure 5-9, *A*, p. 144). Between 3 and 10 years of age the height gain by girls and boys is consis-

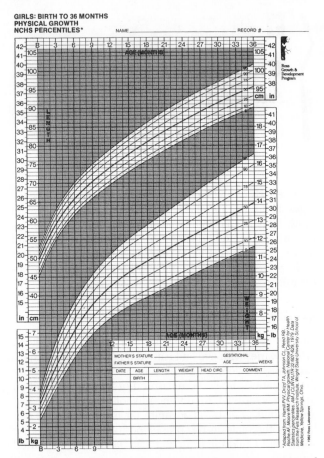

GIRLS: BIRTH TO 36 MONTHS
PHYSICAL GROWTH
NCHS PERCENTILES*

FIGURE 5-1 Girls: birth to 36 months; weight-for-age percentiles.[1]
(Data from Fels Research Institute, Wright State University School
of Medicine, Yellow Springs, Ohio.)

tently between 5 and 8 cm per year. A normal 2-year-old
has reached 50% of adult height, and a normal 10-year-old
has reached about 80%. The head circumference of a
newborn in the United States is about 34 cm. The brain
normally doubles in size during the first year of life, and by

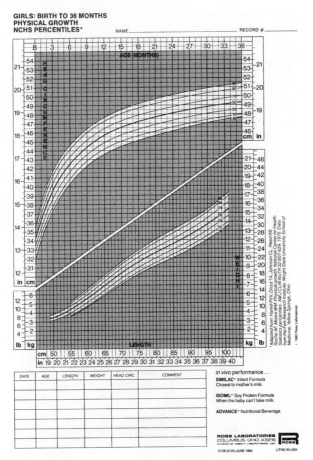

GIRLS: BIRTH TO 36 MONTHS
PHYSICAL GROWTH
NCHS PERCENTILES*

FIGURE 5-2 Girls: birth to 36 months; weight-for-height percentiles.[1] (Data from Fels Research Institute, Wright State University School of Medicine, Yellow Springs, Ohio.)

3 years of age the head circumference has increased to approximately 50 cm. Thereafter head circumference does not change markedly.

Figure 5-9, *B* (p. 145) shows the growth velocity curve, which is calculated by dividing the difference be-

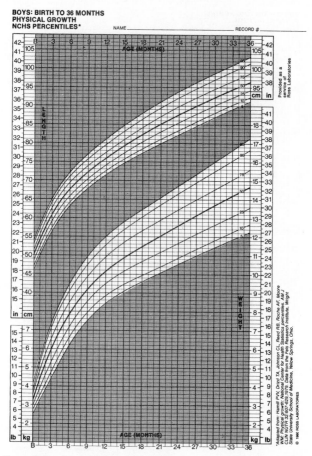

FIGURE 5-3 Boys: birth to 36 months; weight-for-age percentiles.[1] (Data from the Fels Research Institute, Wright State University School of Medicine, Yellow Springs, Ohio.)

tween two height measurements as near to 1 year apart as possible by the exact time elapsed between them. It is plotted at the midpoint of the time interval. There are three epochs of growth: early (rather fast growth before the age of 2 years), a relatively unchanging pattern of

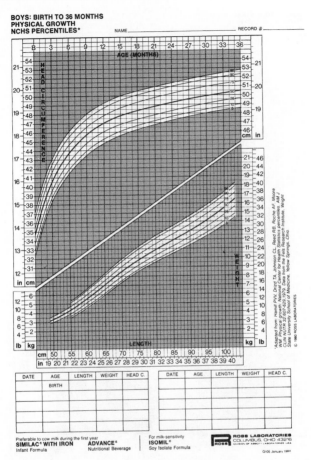

FIGURE 5-4 Boys: birth to 36 months; weight-for-height percentiles.[1] (Data from the Fels Research Institute, Wright State University School of Medicine, Yellow Springs, Ohio.)

growth during preschool and primary school years, and an adolescent growth spurt. There is little difference in growth between boys and girls before 10 years of age, but then the typical girl starts her adolescent growth spurt and for a few years is taller than a boy of the same age. Ap-

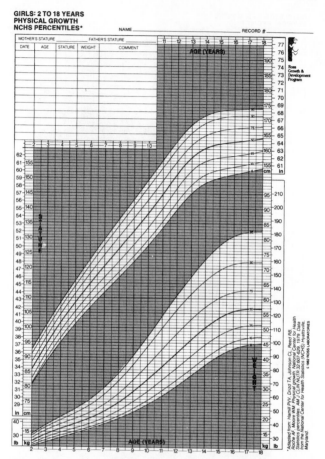

FIGURE 5-5 Girls: 2 to 18 years; weight-for-age percentiles.[1] (Data from National Center for Health Statistics, Hyattsville, Md.)

proximately 2 years later the boy starts his growth spurt and by the age of 14 is taller than the girl. The mean difference in ma-ture height between men and women in the United States is 12.5 cm.

Figure 5-10 (p. 146) shows the interrelationship between maturity stages and the adolescent growth spurt to-

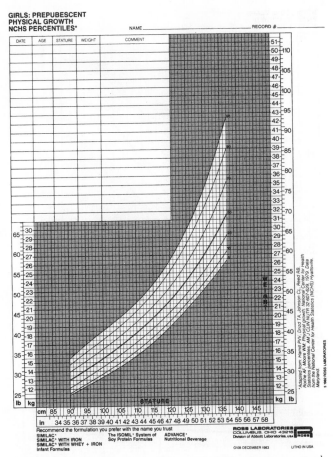

FIGURE 5-6 Girls: prepubescent; weight-for-height percentiles.[1] (Data from National Center for Health Statistics, Hyattsville, Md.)

gether with testicular volume in boys and the mean age of menarche in girls. The development of breasts and male genitalia and the growth of pubic hair in both genders are graded in stages 1 (prepubescent) through 5 (mature) and utilize convenient and reasonably objective anatomic cri-

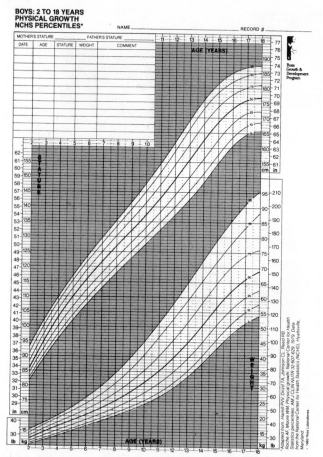

FIGURE 5-7 Boys: 2 to 18 years; weight-for-age percentiles.[1] (Data from National Center for Health Statistics, Hyattsville, Md.)

teria. In general, girls experience adolescence earlier than boys; this is most striking in terms of the growth spurt. In girls, puberty has begun when breast stage 2 is reached, although in a small percentage the adolescent growth spurt has already started. The peak of the growth spurt is usually

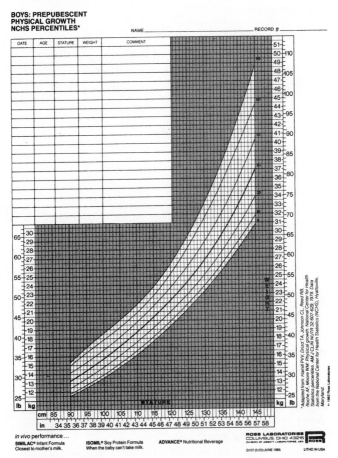

**BOYS: PREPUBESCENT
PHYSICAL GROWTH
NCHS PERCENTILES***

FIGURE 5-8 Boys: prepubescent; weight-for-height percentiles.[1]
(Data from National Center for Health Statistics, Hyattsville, Md.)

reached by breast stage 3, and by the time a girl is menstruating her growth spurt is virtually always waning. In boys, testicular enlargement to a 4-ml capacity from a prepubertal 2- to 3-ml capacity is usually the first evidence of puberty, although this small change is not evident during a

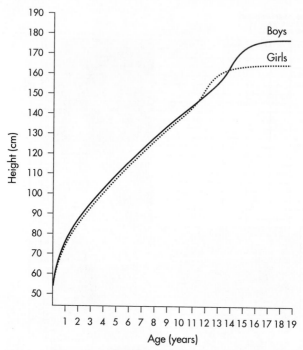

FIGURE 5-9 The height-distance curve (**A**) and the velocity curve (**B**) of a typical boy *(solid line)* and girl *(broken line)*.[2]

cursory examination. The adolescent growth spurt is a late event, seldom starting before genitalia stage 3 and peaking between genitalia stages 4 and 5.

Table 5-1 (p. 147) shows the typical body compositions of children aged 1 to 10 years. The proportion of body weight represented by fat decreases from 23% to 13% in boys between the ages of 1 and 7 with a concurrent increase in FFBM. Preadolescent girls have a higher percentage body fat than boys; it decreases (from 24% to 16%) by age 6. After that time, girls once again begin to have a higher proportion of their weight as fat, a trend that continues into adulthood. The percentage of FFBM changes in a reciprocal manner.

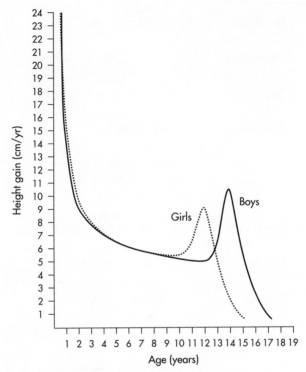

FIGURE 5-9 For legend see opposite page.

NUTRIENT REQUIREMENTS

An adequate intake of energy, protein, and all other essential nutrients is required for the rapid growth and development of a young child. As shown in Table 5-2 (p. 148), children require less protein and energy per kilogram of body weight as growth decelerates. The recommendation for protein is intended to be adequate for 95% of the population, whereas the recommendation for energy is expressed as the population mean. Actual energy requirements vary with the individual growth and physical

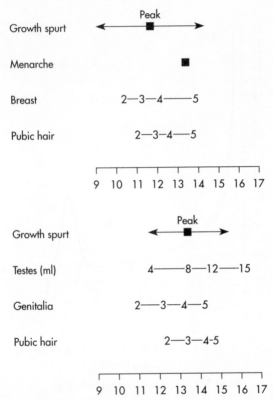

FIGURE 5-10 The interrelationships between events at puberty (girls, upper panel; boys, lower panel). The mean attainment ages of the breast, genitalia, and pubic hair stages are indicated by the numbers 2 to 5. For testes the numbers indicate the volume in milliliters of a single testis at the mean attainment age. The peaks for growth spurt and menarche are at the mean age and are indicated by solid blocks. The horizontal arrows represent the typical span of the growth spurt for an average child.[3]

activity of the child. Insufficient dietary carbohydrate and fat will cause dietary protein and lean body mass to be utilized to provide energy needs. Minerals such as calcium, iron, and zinc are also essential for normal growth and development. For the following discussion, it will be help-

TABLE 5-1 Body composition of reference children (1 - 10 years)[4]

Age (years)	Length (cm)	Weight (kg)	Fat (kg)	Fat (%)	FFBM (kg)	FFBM (%)
Boys						
Toddlers						
1	76.1	10.2	2.3	23	7.9	77
2	87.2	12.6	2.5	20	10.2	80
3	95.3	14.7	2.6	18	12.1	82
Preschoolers						
4	102.9	16.7	2.7	16	14	84
5	109.9	18.7	2.7	15	16	85
6	116.1	20.7	2.8	14	17.9	86
Preadoles- cents						
7	121.7	22.9	3	13	20	87
8	127	25.4	3.3	13	22	87
9	132.3	28.2	3.7	13	24.4	87
10	137.7	31.4	4.3	14	27.1	86
Girls						
Toddlers						
1	74.3	9.2	2.2	24	7	76
2	85.5	11.9	2.4	20	9.5	80
3	94.1	14.1	2.6	19	11.5	81
Preschoolers						
4	101.6	16	2.8	17	13.2	83
5	108.4	17.7	3	17	14.7	83
6	114.6	19.5	3.2	16	16.3	84
Preadoles- cents						
7	120.6	21.8	3.7	17	18.2	83
8	126.4	24.8	4.3	17	20.5	83
9	132.2	28.5	5.2	18	23.3	82
10	138.3	32.6	6.3	19	26.3	81

TABLE 5-2 Recommended energy and protein intakes for children[5]

	Toddlers (1-3 years)	Preschoolers (4-6 years)	Preadolescents (7-10 years)
Energy intake			
kcal/day	1300	1800	2000
kcal/kg	102	90	70
Protein intake			
g/day	16	24	28
g/kg	1.2	1.1	1

ful to refer to the age-specific RDAs listed in Tables 2-1, 2-2, and 2-3.

Toddlers (1 to 3 years)

Developmental stages, behavioral characteristics, and food-selection choices must be considered when providing food for toddlers. Between ages 1 and 3 the annual weight gain decreases from 6.5 kg to 2.5 kg, and height gain declines from 25 cm to 7 cm. The growth in head circumference also slows down to 0.5 to 1.2 cm per year by age 3. There is a concurrent decrease in energy and protein needs to approximately 100 kcal/kg and 1.2 g protein/kg.

Feeding behavior changes throughout the toddler years (Table 5-3). Oral and neuromuscular development improves eating ability. Increased refinement of hand and finger movement occurs, and the appearance of most of the primary teeth leads toddlers to self-feeding. As children gain proficiency in coordinating arm, wrist, and hand movements, they demand increased responsibility for feeding themselves and may reject offers of assistance. Finger foods and use of spoons and cups should be encouraged to help continue development of manual dexterity and coordination.

Although three meals and two snacks each day should be offered to toddlers, their food intake will vary. Avoid foods likely to be aspirated, such as hot dogs, nuts, grapes,

TABLE 5-3 Development of feeding behavior[6]	
Age	Typical feeding behavior
12 months	Chews solid food
	Begins to use spoon but turns it before reaching mouth
	May hold cup; likely to tilt cup causing spilling
18 months	Uses spoon well with frequent spilling
	Turns spoon in mouth
	Holds glass with both hands
24 months	Feeds self without inverting spoon
	Uses spoon well with moderate spilling
	Holds glass with one hand
	Plays with food
	Distinguishes between food and inedible materials
36 months	Self-feeding complete with occasional spilling
	Can manage knife and fork with some help on hard foods
	Obtains drink of water from faucet
	Pours from pitcher

round candies, popcorn, and raw carrots. Set limits so that demands for food and drink do not become attention-getting devices that might lead to inappropriate intake.

The eating patterns of most toddlers are characterized by decreased food intake relative to body size. This change in food consumption after infancy often worries parents but is normal and related to the dramatic reduction in growth rate. Needless conflicts often occur because of discrepancies between a child's food intake and parents' expectations of what and how much should be eaten. The box lists suggestions to facilitate the feeding of toddlers. They should be offered a variety of foods from the basic

HINTS FOR FEEDING TODDLERS

Try to relax; feeding/eating and mealtimes should be pleasant for everyone.

Avoid battles about eating. Encourage your child but avoid forced feeding or punitive approaches.

Withholding food is not appropriate.

Although you are responsible for deciding when, where, and what food your child is offered (with consideration for your child's preferences), your child decides *how much* to eat.

Use positive reinforcement (e.g., praise for eating well).

Grant children's requests to feed themselves. Accept that there will be messes and be prepared (e.g., with newspaper on the floor).

Try to eat together as a family. Good eating behavior can be modeled, and young children like to mimic older siblings and parents.

Allow about 1 hour without food or drink (except water) before a meal to stimulate the appetite.

Consumption of an excess of fluids reduces the intake of solid food; offer solids first and limit juice intake to 4 to 8 oz per day.

Establish a routine of meals and snacks at set times (with some flexibility); avoid providing snacks right after an unfinished meal.

Recognize your child's cues indicating hunger, satiety, and food preferences.

Limit possible distractions (e.g., television) during meals.

food groups at regular intervals. Food preferences may be erratic, with food being readily accepted one day and totally rejected the next. Milk consumption usually decreases as solid food intake increases. To foster sound eating habits the child's mealtime environment should be pleasant and enjoyable. The child should be allowed to eat with other family members when possible and should not be punished for spilling milk or being messy with food.

Quiet surroundings (e.g., having the television turned off) decrease distractions and enhance food intake.

Preschoolers (4 to 6 years)

Children in this age group pose fewer nutritional problems. Mealtime is more pleasant for all family members. Preschool children are able to eat without assistance, have more coordinated gross motor skills, and have changing and varied interests. The appetite tends to be sporadic and parallels weight gain. Food becomes a secondary interest. More time is spent away from home at day-care centers, with baby-sitters, or at friends' homes, and food consumption between meals increases. To promote sound nutritional habits and prevent nutritional deficiencies or excesses, parents should be informed of the basic principles of nutrition and meal planning and serve as role models for the preschool child. Foods from the six basic food groups should be emphasized. To prevent obesity and dental caries and promote sound nutritional habits, snacks or desserts high in concentrated sweets or low in nutritional value should be discouraged. Skim or low-fat milk may be substituted for whole milk, especially if the child is overweight.

Preadolescents (7 to 10 years)

This age group is characterized by a moderate growth rate of about 2 to 4 kg per year and 5 to 6 cm per year. Nutrient and energy intakes are important because preadolescents are laying down reserves in preparation for the adolescent growth spurt. However, excessive weight gain in anticipation of this growth spurt may result in childhood obesity. The eating habits of preadolescents are often influenced more by peer pressure than by parents' actions. Adaptation to school may likewise present nutritional problems. Breakfast may be eaten alone or skipped altogether, and snacks after school are often unsupervised. These adaptations may be less of a problem if sound eating habits are established early in life.

Nutrition education should be integrated into the school curriculum and encourage children to learn and incorporate into their daily lives the principles of basic nutrition. This training will allow children to accept more responsibility for their health and hopefully optimize their dietary habits in adulthood.

Adolescents (11 to 18 years)

Nutrient requirements increase markedly during adolescence because of the virtual doubling of body mass. The recommendations for energy intake are based on estimation of energy expenditure or surveys relating energy intake to average body weights. Adolescents often show considerable variation in energy expenditure, and recommendations represent average rather than individual requirements. Dietary proteins are essential for providing the amino acids needed for growth, but they will be oxidized for energy and unavailable for growth if energy needs are not met by carbohydrate and fat in the diet. The greatest demand for calcium occurs during the adolescent growth spurt, and increased intake should allow for variation in the timing of this event. The adolescent requirement for iron is related to increases in blood volume as well as hemoglobin and myoglobin synthesis; in girls, losses increase with the onset of menstruation. The timing of the increased need for iron will be subject to the enormous variation of pace at which puberty occurs. Iron losses before menarche are approximately 0.5 to 1 mg per day, and the recommendations assume that 10% of dietary iron is absorbed.

The food habits of the adolescent differ from those of any other age group and are characterized by an increase in skipping meals, snacking, inappropriately consuming fast foods, and fad dieting. This behavior can be explained by the teen's newly found independence, questioning of existing values, poor body image, and search for self-identity, peer acceptance, and desire for conformity of lifestyle. To counsel a teenager properly regarding diet, it is necessary to understand these factors. Take particular care that teens receive adequate levels of calcium, iron, and zinc, which are frequently marginal in the adolescent's diet. Dental caries, obesity, and anorexia nervosa are common in adolescents. A vegetarian teenager who eats eggs and/or dairy products (e.g., milk, cheese, yogurt) is likely to have adequate nutrient intake as long as a variety of foods including fruit and vegetables are eaten. Teenagers who are pure vegetarians (i.e., who avoid all animals products) may be at risk for developing certain nutrient deficiencies and should be counseled by a dietitian or other nutrition specialist.

References

1. Hamill PVV et al: Physical growth: National Center for Health Statistics percentiles, *Am J Clin Nutr* 32:607, 1979.
2. Tanner JM, Whitehouse RH, Takaishi M: Standards from birth to maturity for height, weight, height velocity, and weight velocity: British children, 1965, *Arch Dis Child* 41:454, 1966.
3. Falkner F, Tanner JM, eds: *Human growth,* vol 2, New York, 1978, Plenum Press.
4. Fomon SJ et al: Body composition of reference children from birth to age 10 years, *Am J Clin Nutr* 35:1169, 1982.
5. National Research Council, Food and Nutrition Board: *Recommended dietary allowances,* ed 10, Washington, DC, 1989, National Academy Press.
6. Grand RJ, Sutphen JL, Dietz WH, eds: *Pediatric nutrition: theory and practice,* Stoneham, Mass, 1987, Butterworths.

Suggested Readings

Fomon SJ, ed: *Nutrition of normal infants,* St Louis, 1993, Mosby.
Suskind RM, Lewinter-Suskind L, eds: *Textbook of pediatric nutrition,* ed 2, New York, 1993, Raven Press.

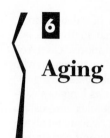

6

Aging

In 1989 there were 31 million persons in the United States who were 65 years of age or older, accounting for 12.5% of the population. Given the increased life expectancy in the United States, this number will increase dramatically in the next 40 years. By the year 2040, there will be 68 to 80 million individuals 65 and older comprising 22% to 25% of the population. The group expanding fastest is made up of individuals more than 85 years of age; this group tends to be more frail, often has comorbid illnesses, and is at the highest nutritional risk.

The prevalence of nutritionally-related disorders in older adults depends on the population studied. Approximately 30% to 40% of men and women over 75 years of age are at least 10% underweight. About 25% of males and 50% of females over 65 are obese, i.e., have a body mass index (BMI) of greater than 25. In dietary intake studies, 10% of men and 20% of women have intakes of protein below the recommended dietary allowance (RDA); one third consume less than the RDA of calories. Fifty percent of older adults who live at or near the poverty line have intakes of minerals and vitamins less than the RDA. Approximately 10% to 30% of all older adults have subnormal levels of minerals and vitamins.

Major nutritional deficits are rarely seen among community-dwelling, healthy older adults. In acutely ill hospitalized older adults the prevalence of malnutrition ranges between 32% and 50%. The highest prevalence of protein-energy malnutrition (PEM) is seen among nursing home residents where estimates range from 23% to 85%. Intakes of both calories and protein are frequently low. Body weight, midarm muscle circumference, and visceral protein levels are low in at least 50% of nursing home patients. Blood levels of both water-soluble and fat-soluble vitamins are also frequently low.

AGING CHANGES THAT INCREASE NUTRITIONAL RISK

Much of the variation in nutritional status results from the heterogeneity of the older adult population and physiologic changes associated with aging. Normal aging involves a steady erosion of certain organ system reserves and homeostatic controls. The loss of homeostatic reserves is most evident during periods of maximal exertion or physiologic stress.

Physiologic Factors

Both physiologic and pathophysiologic factors influence nutritional status in aging individuals. There is a decrease in lean body mass and a relative increase in body fat, so between the ages of 25 and 70 body fat doubles as a proportion of total body mass (Figure 6-1). Exercise programs may prevent or reverse some of the decrease in lean body mass. These changes in body composition have several important implications. As muscle mass decreases energy requirements decline. Protein reserves needed during periods of stress are diminished. Because body water is associated with lean body mass, there is a decrease in total body water and an increased susceptibility to dehydration. The distribution volume of fat-soluble drugs increases and their elimination is delayed.

Alterations in endocrine function that affect nutritional status include an increased incidence of insulin resistance and a change in water metabolism. Increased insulin resistance may be due in part to the proportional increase in body fat. This contributes to higher fasting

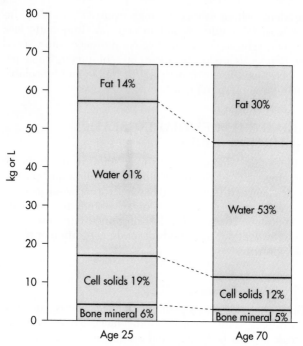

FIGURE 6-1 A comparison of major body compartments and their changes during the aging process.[1]

blood-glucose levels with increasing age and higher incidence of Type II diabetes mellitus. Alterations in water metabolism (dehydration and hypernatremia) occur because older adults do not have an appropriate thirst response. Older subjects also have a decrease in free water clearance in response to vasopressin.

One third of individuals over age 70 have a significantly diminished capacity to secrete stomach acid, which may lead to decreased absorption of vitamin B_{12}, calcium, iron, folic acid, and possibly zinc and may account for the increased tendency for depletion of these nutrients with age. The prevalence of lactose intolerance also rises with age and may contribute to a decreased intake of dairy products and thus of calcium and vitamin D.

Sensory changes that occur with aging include decreased ability to smell, alterations in taste, and often a decline in visual and auditory function. Because smell is an important part of food appreciation, declines in olfactory perception can affect appetite and food intake. Many medications also affect smell and may magnify this decline. Whether a decrease in taste sensation occurs with aging is controversial. Sensitivity to sweet and salty tastes decrease. This contributes to a relative increase in sweet-and/or salty-food intake by some to get the same "taste" they experienced when younger. Visual impairment, often due to cataracts, glaucoma or macular degeneration, may affect a person's ability to prepare food and remain independent. A deterioration in hearing may impact on the social aspects of eating.

Pathophysiologic Factors

Comorbid conditions commonly seen in and affecting the nutritional status of older adults include oral disease, renal impairment, and diseases that increase metabolic demands. Forty percent of older adults are edentulous. Only 17% to 20% of these individuals have dentures and many of them do not fit properly. Between 60% and 90% of older adults have severe periodontal disease, leading to gum recession, tooth loss, and oral pain, all of which may contribute to poor food intake.

Changes in renal function include a steady decline in glomerular filtration rate and a decreased ability to concentrate urine and conserve sodium. The fall in glomerular filtration rate leads to a reduction in both urinary acidification and renal clearance of many drugs. Hydroxylation of vitamin D to its active form is also diminished. The renin-angiotensin-aldosterone axis is less sensitive to volume depletion, placing older adults at greater risk for dehydration.

A number of disease conditions may increase metabolic demands. One half to two thirds of cancer patients present with cachexia, probably caused by both anorexia and increased metabolic rate. Other hypermetabolic conditions such as hyperthyroidism are common in older populations and often present atypically, making them more insidious.

Chronic Disease and Disability Factors

Older people have fewer episodes of acute illness than younger people. However, 85% of the elderly have one or more chronic afflictions, ranging from three to seven per person. Arthritis is the most common, followed by impairments in hearing and vision, heart disease, and hypertension. Almost 60% of persons over age 75 have some limitation of activity, compared to 8.5% of persons aged 17 to 44. Alzheimer's disease and senile dementia are almost epidemic; 20% of community-dwelling elderly persons and 50% of nursing-home residents are affected by a dementing illness. The net effect of these chronic conditions may be that affected individuals' ability to acquire, prepare, and enjoy food is limited; restrictive diets may also be imposed. When several conditions are present, a diet that has combined restrictions, such as being low in salt, low in fat, and restricted in carbohydrates, may render the diet unpalatable.

Medications

A number of medications can influence food consumption. Drugs may alter appetite, taste, or smell; directly interact with nutrients; or produce side effects such as nausea, vomiting, or diarrhea. Examples of these interactions are listed in Table 6-1.

Socioeconomic Factors

Social factors influencing nutritional status in older adults include the increased likelihood of isolation at mealtimes and financial limitations affecting food acquisition. One

TABLE 6-1 Nutritional complications of drug therapy in elderly persons

Drugs	Complications
Alcohol	Depletion of thiamin, folate, vitamin B_6, magnesium, phosphorus, protein
Analgesic agents (NSAIDs*)	Gastric irritation, nausea, dyspepsia
Antacids (Mg-containing)	Hypermagnesemia
Anticoagulants	Nausea, vomiting, diarrhea
Cholestyramine	Malabsorption of fat-soluble vitamins, vitamin K
Digoxin	Anorexia
Diuretics	Anorexia, decreased taste, altered excretion of calcium, potassium, magnesium
Hypotensive agents	Anorexia, nausea, diarrhea
Mineral oil, laxatives	Malabsorption of fat-soluble vitamins
Penicillamine	Decreased taste
Phenytoin	Increased vitamin D metabolism, folic acid deficiency
Serotonin-uptake inhibitors, (e.g., fluoxetine)	Anorexia, gastrointestinal distress
Theophylline	Anorexia, gastrointestinal distress

*NSAIDs, Nonsteroidal antiinflammatory drugs.

third of persons over 65 and half over 85 live alone, which typically decreases food enjoyment. Older people also have significantly lower incomes than those under 65. Although the elderly are about as likely as those who are not elderly to be poor, a greater proportion of the elderly live near the poverty line. Individuals with fixed incomes may use money previously spent on food for medications and other needed items.

DIETARY REQUIREMENTS OF OLDER ADULTS
Energy

Energy requirements decrease over the life span largely because of the decline in metabolically active lean body mass and decreased physical activity. The decrease in lean body mass reduces the basal metabolic rate by about 1% to 2% per decade from age 20 to 75. Recommended intakes based on the 1989 RDA are 2300 kcal for males and 1900 kcal for females age 51 and over. However, generalized estimates should be used cautiously, as they do not take into account individual activity levels or concurrent disease.

Protein

Protein needs do not change with age, but because energy requirements decline the percentage of calories from protein must increase. A range of 0.8 to 1 g/kg per day (14% to 16% of daily caloric intake) is recommended as a safe level for healthy older persons. However, half of chronically ill elderly persons are unable to maintain a nitrogen balance at this level.[2] Increasing the protein intake to beyond 1.5 g/kg per day may not increase protein synthesis and may cause dehydration.[3] Thus a reasonable protein allowance is probably between 1 and 1.5 g/kg per day. During periods of stress such as infection or trauma, protein intake should be increased to 1.2 to 1.5 g/kg per day to provide a cushion against progressive protein depletion.

Fiber

There is no RDA for fiber, and it is unclear how much fiber should be recommended in the diet of older persons. The National Cancer Institute recommends intakes of 25 to 35 g per day to reduce the risk for colon cancer. This amount is achievable with 5 servings of fruit or vegetables and a supplement of bran. Adequate fluid intake is essential, as a high-fiber diet without additional fluids can cause dehydration and constipation. Abdominal discomfort and flatulence are common during adaptation to increased fiber intake. Negative mineral balance (Ca, Mg, Fe, Zn) may also result if mineral intake is marginal.

Water

Changes in thirst mechanisms, the decreased ability to concentrate urine, and the reduction in total body water that occur with aging put older adults at high risk for dehydration. Fluid-intake prescriptions should be written for at-risk patients, particularly those who are institutionalized, with a goal of at least 1500 to 2000 ml per day (or 1 ml/kcal ingested or 30 ml/kg of body weight). Another approach is to provide enough fluids to keep urine osmolality below 800 mOsm/L.

Vitamins

In general, vitamin requirements are the same in older adults as in younger adults. Exceptions include vitamins D and B_{12}; for certain groups of elderly people higher intake may be indicated. Lack of sun exposure, impaired skin synthesis of previtamin D, and decreased hydroxylation in the kidney with advancing age contribute to marginal vitamin D status in many older adults. In all older adults increased consumption of dietary sources of vitamin D should be encouraged. In elderly people who are not exposed to sunlight, use of a low-dose vitamin supplement (10 µg or 400 IU per day) may be warranted.

The prevalence of B_{12} deficiency in older adults ranges between 10% and 20%. Some persons with mild deficiencies including neurologic signs have normal serum B_{12} levels, in which case an elevated serum methylmalonic acid level is diagnostic. In the past a majority of B_{12} deficiencies were thought to be results of an intrinsic factor deficiency. It is now known that many older adults poorly absorb only protein-bound B_{12}. This is a result of the maldigestion of the food-protein-B_{12} complex in the stomach in addition to B_{12} uptake by greater numbers of bacteria in the stomach, particularly when atrophic gastritis is present. These patients can generally be treated with oral

B_{12} rather than injections and may benefit from increasing the intake of B_{12} in food to overwhelm the binding capacity of the bacteria. Given the potentially significant effects of vitamin B_{12} deficiency on the nervous system, it is prudent to advocate a daily intake of 3 µg or more. (The RDA is 2 µg).

In addition to vitamin deficiencies, hypervitaminosis is seen in older adults as a result of the consumption of megadoses of vitamins. Malaise, liver dysfunction, headaches, hypercalcemia, and leukopenia may be seen with high doses of vitamin A. Diarrhea, false-negative fecal occult blood tests, and renal stones can occur with vitamin C megadoses. Peripheral neuropathy can result from excessive use of vitamin B_6.

Minerals and Trace Elements

Except for iron and calcium, aging probably does not significantly alter the requirements for minerals and trace elements. The RDA for iron declines from 15 mg to 10 mg in women who are no longer menstruating. When iron deficiency occurs in older adults, it is usually from gastrointestinal blood loss rather than poor diet.

Calcium nutrition is strongly influenced by age. The efficiency of calcium absorption from the gastrointestinal tract decreases significantly after age 60 in both sexes. Individuals between 70 and 90 years of age absorb about one third less calcium than do younger adults. Given the impact of calcium deficiency on cortical bone loss, it is recommended that women consume 1000 to 1500 mg per day and men 800 to 1000 mg per day. (Five calcium carbonate tablets provide 1000 mg of elemental calcium.)

Marginal zinc status is common in older adults. Institutionalized and hospitalized persons are at particularly high risk for zinc deficiency, especially those stressed by infection, trauma, or surgery. Deficiency may impair wound healing, immune function, taste, and smell. Zinc supplementation has only been shown to accelerate wound healing in zinc-deficient patients; however, excessive zinc supplementation may interfere with immune function and copper metabolism.

FACTORS AFFECTING DIETARY PRESCRIPTIONS IN OLDER ADULTS

Dental State

Many older adults have periodontal disease and poor dentition. Pay close attention to the patient's oral status so that appropriate diets will be prescribed. In persons with oral pain, a soft-mechanical, dental-soft, or pureed diet (although the latter is generally unpalatable) may be preferred over a regular diet.

Changes in Taste Sensitivity

As previously mentioned, sensitivity to salty and sweet tastes decreases with age, so older persons tend to overcompensate with a higher intake of salty and sweet foods. Diets restricting these may thus result in decreased food consumption. Much of the flavor in food results from its fat content. When fats are restricted, calorie consumption may fall to unacceptable levels. In home settings, patients have the option to ignore the restrictions, but in institutional settings forced compliance may simply reduce their intake.

Swallowing Disorders

Disorders of swallowing usually result from disease, the most common being cerebrovascular accidents. The loss of voluntary initiation of swallowing is a frequent finding in late-stage dementia. Because 60% of long-term care residents have dementia, difficulties with oral feeding are common in this setting. Bedside swallowing examinations should be routine in this population. Many individuals with oropharyngeal dysphagia will benefit from specific dysphagia diets designed in collaboration with a speech pathologist and a dietitian. Failure of the swallowing mechanism and inadequate protection of the airway can cause aspiration pneumonia and death.

Weight Maintenance

Although tables of desirable weights often imply that the weight distribution of 20- to 25-year-old persons is ideal for all subsequent ages, this concept has been discarded. Age-specific desirable weights should be used for older persons (Table 6-2). When plotted against body weight, mortality rates appear to be lowest with leanness in the twenties and moderately higher weights in middle age. The distribution of body fat also plays an important part in weight recommendations. When body fat is distributed primarily in the buttocks, hips, and thighs, obesity is relatively benign. In contrast, intraabdominal fat, or distribution in the abdominal areas is epidemiologically more risky. A simple measure of this distribution is the waist-hip circumference ratio (see Chapter 15).

The involuntary loss of more than 5% to 10% of an older person's usual weight during one year is an ominous clinical sign associated with increased risk for mortality. Weight loss should thus be met with concern and prompt a search for the cause. Causes of weight loss in the elderly are shown in Table 6-3.

Cultural and Societal Habits

Most persons old or young define food culturally rather than nutritionally. Food is a cultural symbol of love, status, hospitality, and friendship and is also strongly associated with emotional states. Foods can be a link to the past for elderly persons and provide security in unfamiliar surroundings. Under stress, people often regress to eating foods selected in childhood. Specific cultural factors influence food selections, including religion, ethnic origin, and social pressures. When menus are planned centrally, as in institutional settings, malnutrition may result. Breakfast is the meal most enjoyed and completely eaten by elderly people.

Compliance

Contrary to popular notions, compliance with drug and dietary therapy is higher in the elderly than in younger populations. Even so, about one third of prescription drugs are never filled by this group, and noncompliance with dietary restrictions may be even higher. Diets prescribed for elderly persons are usually not followed unless cultural,

TABLE 6-2 Body weight (lb) for persons age 55 to 74 (95th percentiles)

Height (in)	Small frame	Medium frame	Large frame
Males			
62	169	187	220
63	174	191	222
64	176	200	224
65	198	196	227
66	185	196	231
67	194	207	246
68	189	222	244
69	194	218	231
70	196	222	257
71	200	222	244
72	202	222	246
73	207	227	249
74	209	229	251
Females			
58	156	187	229
59	163	189	231
60	161	189	231
61	156	189	233
62	161	194	244
63	163	196	260
64	165	191	262
65	165	194	244
66	167	194	240
67	169	196	240
68	169	198	242
69	172	200	242
70	174	202	244

Modified from NHANES I and II data sets.[4] For extended information on anthropometry, see first Suggested Reading.

ethnic, and socioeconomic factors are accounted for. Compliance with dietary prescriptions can be improved by taking a dietary history, factoring in cultural bias, and evaluating the economic resources available. On the whole, foods that are restricted in salt, fat, or carbohydrates are more expensive than unrestricted foods.

TABLE 6-3 Causes of weight loss in the elderly

Cause	Estimated frequency
No etiology determined	24%
Poor intake	22%
Depression	18%
Cancer (predominately lung)	16%
Peptic ulcers	11%
Medications	9%

References

1. Fryer JH: Studies of body composition in men aged 60 and over. In Shock NW, ed: *Biological aspects of aging*, New York, 1962, Columbia University Press.

2. Gersovitz M et al: Human protein requirements: assessment of the adequacy of the current recommended dietary allowance for dietary protein in elderly men and women, *Am J Clin Nutr* 35:6, 1982.

3. Long CL et al: A physiologic basis for the provision of fuel mixtures in normal and stressed patients, *J Trauma* 30:1077, 1990.

4. Frisancho AR: New standards of weight and body composition by frame size and height for assessment of nutritional status of adults and the elderly, *Am J Clin Nutr* 40:808, 1984.

Suggested Readings

Frisancho AR: *Anthropometric standards for the evaluation of growth and nutritional status*, Ann Arbor, Mich, 1992, University of Michigan Press.

Morley JE, Glick Z, Rubenstein LZ, eds: *Geriatric nutrition: a comprehensive review*, New York, 1990, Raven Press.

Russell RM, Suter PM: Vitamin requirements of elderly people: an update, *Am J Clin Nutr* 58:4,1993.

Watson RR, ed: *Handbook of nutrition in the aged*, ed 2, Ann Arbor, 1994, CRC Press.

PART II

Nutritional Support in Patient Management

Hospital-Associated Malnutrition

PREVALENCE

Malnutrition can arise from primary causes such as inadequate or poor-quality food intake or secondary causes such as diseases that alter food intake, nutrient requirements, metabolism, or absorption. Primary malnutrition occurs mainly in developing countries and is unusual in the United States, so it will not be discussed here. Secondary malnutrition is the main form encountered in developed countries. Probably because of a narrow concept of nutrition, it was largely unrecognized until the late 1960s or early 1970s. Teaching in medical schools was limited to the basics of primary malnutrition, and it was not well appreciated that persons with adequate food supplies could become malnourished as a result of acute or chronic diseases that altered their nutrient intake or metabolism. This phenomenon can occur in any setting, but the acute-care hospital dramatically illustrates the integral relationship between nutrition and illness and the vital role nutritional support plays in influencing the outcome of the disease process.

In 1974, Butterworth called attention to the "skeleton in the hospital closet" and focused on iatrogenic (physician-induced) malnutrition in the United States.[1] Since that time, various studies have shown that protein-energy malnutrition (PEM) affects one third to one half of the patients on general medical and surgical wards in U.S. teaching hospitals. In a study of consecutive admissions to a general medical ward in 1976, 48% of patients had a high likelihood of malnutrition; nutritional parameters tended to deteriorate in patients hospitalized for 2 weeks or longer.[2] A follow-up study in the same institution in 1988 found a slightly lower likelihood of malnutrition on admission (38%) and a slight improvement in nutritional status in patients hospitalized for 2 or more weeks.[3] These and many other studies have shown that patients with evidence of malnutrition have significantly longer mean hospital stays and higher mortality and morbidity resulting from factors such as surgical complications.

The question of whether treatment of hospital-associated malnutrition can improve patient outcome is discussed in Chapter 9. However, the consistent finding that nutritional status influences a patient's prognosis underlines the importance of preventing as well as detecting and treating malnutrition. The terms *iatrogenic* and *hospital-induced* used in connection with malnutrition do not imply malicious intent or disregard for a patient's welfare. However, malnutrition can occur as a result of a physician's actions. To a considerable extent, iatrogenic malnutrition is caused by an emphasis on complex modern treatment over the fundamental principles of nutrition. Physicians too often lose sight of the facts that antibiotics cannot replace host defenses, that sutures and sterile gauze cannot heal wounds, and that the most advanced, sophisticated life-support systems cannot revitalize a malnourished patient. It is paradoxical that many cases of nutritional failure in hospitalized patients are the result of spectacular successes in other fields. Patients are kept alive longer only to exhaust their nutritional reserves and succumb to nutritional deprivation. Whatever the cause the end result is the same—many patients fail to receive the full benefits of current nutritional knowledge and technology.

PROTEIN-ENERGY MALNUTRITION

The two major types of PEM are marasmus and kwashiorkor. These conditions are compared in Table 7-1, and

	Marasmus	Kwashiorkor
TABLE 7-1 Comparison of marasmus and kwashiorkor		
Clinical setting	Decreased energy intake	Decreased protein intake during stress state
Time course to develop	Months or years	Weeks
Clinical features	Starved appearance	Well-nourished appearance
	Weight < 80% standard for height	Easy hair pluckability
	Triceps skinfold < 3 mm	Edema
	Midarm muscle circumference < 15 cm	
Laboratory findings	Creatinine-height index < 60% standard	Serum albumin < 2.8g/dl
		Total iron binding capacity < 200 µg/dl
		Lymphocytes < 1500/mm³
		Anergy
Clinical course	Reasonably preserved responsiveness to short-term stress	Infections
		Poor wound healing, decubitus ulcers, skin breakdown
Mortality	Low unless related to underlying disease	High

the criteria for diagnosing them are listed in Table 7-2. Marasmus and kwashiorkor can occur singly or in combination as marasmic kwashiorkor. Kwashiorkor can occur rapidly, whereas marasmus is the end result of a gradual wasting process that passes through several stages (an un-

TABLE 7-2 Minimum criteria for the diagnosis of marasmus and kwashiorkor

Kwashiorkor*	Marasmus
Serum albumin < 2.8 g/dl	Triceps skinfold < 3 mm
At least one of the following:	Midarm muscle
• Poor wound healing, decubitus ulcers, or skin breakdown	circumference < 15cm
• Easy hair pluckability†	
• Edema	

*The findings used to diagnose kwashiorkor must be unexplained by other causes.

†Test by *firmly* pulling a lock of hair from the top of the head (not the sides or back), grasping with the thumb and forefinger. An average of three or more hairs removed easily and painlessly is considered abnormal hair pluckability.

derweight stage followed by stages of mild, moderate, and severe cachexia; Figure 7-1).

Marasmus

Marasmus is the most severe or "end stage" in the cachexia process; virtually all available body fat stores have been exhausted because of starvation. Illnesses that produce marasmus in the United States are chronic and indolent, such as cancer and chronic pulmonary disease. Marasmus is easy to detect because of the patient's starved appearance. The diagnosis is based on severe fat and muscle wastage resulting from prolonged calorie deficiency. Diminished skinfold thickness reflects the loss of fat reserves; reduced arm-muscle circumference with temporal and interosseous muscle wastage reflects the resorption of protein throughout the body, including in vital organs such as the heart, liver, and kidneys.

The laboratory picture in marasmus is relatively unremarkable. The creatinine-height index (the 24-hour uri-

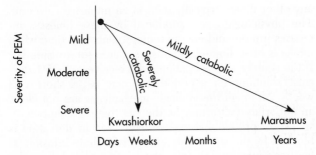

FIGURE 7-1 Time course of PEM. (*Marasmus,* End-stage energy deficiency; *Kwashiorkor,* Maladaptive state during catabolic stress with protein deficiency.)

nary creatinine excretion compared with normal values based on height) is low, reflecting the loss of muscle mass noted on clinical examination. Occasionally the serum albumin level is reduced, but it does not usually drop below 2.8 g/dl in uncomplicated cases. Immunocompetence, wound healing, and the ability to handle short-term stress are reasonably well preserved in most patients with marasmus despite their morbid appearances.

Rather than an acute illness, marasmus is a chronic, fairly well-adapted form of starvation; it should be treated cautiously in an attempt to gradually reverse the downward trend. Although nutritional support is necessary, overly aggressive repletion can result in severe and even life-threatening metabolic imbalances such as hypophosphatemia and cardiorespiratory failure (see Chapter 9). When possible, enteral nutritional support is preferred; treatment started slowly allows readaptation of metabolic and intestinal functions.

Kwashiorkor

In contrast to marasmus, kwashiorkor in the United States occurs mainly in connection with acute, life-threatening stresses or conditions such as trauma and sepsis or almost any other illness typically seen in an intensive care unit. The physiologic stress produced by these illnesses increases protein and energy requirements at a time when intake is often limited. A classic scenario for kwashiorkor is the acutely stressed patient who receives only 5% dextrose solutions for a period that may be as short as 2 weeks. Although the etiologic mechanisms are not clear, an important factor may be the fact that the adaptive response of protein sparing normally seen in starvation is blocked by the stress state and carbohydrate infusion. It has been suggested that this state differs enough from the kwashiorkor typically seen in children in developing countries that it should be given a different label such as "hypoalbuminemic stress state."

In its early stages the physical findings of kwashiorkor are few and subtle. Fat reserves and muscle mass may be normal or even above normal, giving the deceptive appearance of adequate nutrition. Signs that support the diagnosis of kwashiorkor include easy hair pluckability, edema, skin breakdown, and poor wound healing. The *major* sign in the diagnosis is severe reduction of levels of serum proteins, such as albumin (less than 2.8 µg/dl) and transferrin (less than 150 mg/dl) or iron-binding capacity (less than 200 µg/dl). Cellular immune function is depressed, reflected by lymphopenia (less than 1500 lymphocytes/mm^3 in adults and older children) and lack of response to "recall" skin test antigens (anergy).

The prognosis of adult patients with full-blown kwashiorkor is guarded even with aggressive nutritional support. Surgical wounds often dehisce (fail to heal), pressure sores develop, gastroparesis and diarrhea can occur with enteral feeding, the risk of gastrointestinal bleeding from stress ulcers is increased, host defenses are compromised, and death from overwhelming infection may occur despite antibiotic therapy. Unlike treatment in patients with marasmus, aggressive parenteral feeding is often necessary to more rapidly restore better metabolic balance. Although kwashiorkor in children is often less foreboding (perhaps because of the lower degree of stress required to precipitate the disorder), it is still a serious condition.

Kwashiorkor is much more easily prevented than treated. Prevention requires early recognition of the severely stressed (hypermetabolic) state and daily provision for energy and protein needs.

Marasmic Kwashiorkor

Marasmic kwashiorkor, the combined form of PEM, develops when the cachectic or marasmic patient is subjected to an acute stress such as surgery, trauma, or sepsis, superimposing kwashiorkor onto chronic starvation. An extremely serious, life-threatening situation can occur because of the high risk of infection and other complications. If kwashiorkor predominates, the need for vigorous nutritional therapy is urgent. It is important to determine the major component of PEM so that the appropriate nutritional plan can be developed; the starved, unstressed, hypometabolic patient is at risk for the complications of overfeeding, and the stressed, hypermetabolic patient is more likely to suffer the consequences of underfeeding.

Body Defenses in Persons with Protein-Energy Malnutrition

The body has three main types of defenses against infection: mechanical, cellular, and humoral. Mechanical defenses include epithelial surfaces, mucous barriers, and digestive enzymes. Cellular defenses are mediated by lymphocytes, plasma cells, and polymorphonuclear leukocytes, which ingest and destroy bacteria and foreign bodies. Humoral defenses include immunoglobulins and other plasma proteins involved in destruction of microorganisms. Some antibodies appear in secretions such as tears, colostrum, and intestinal mucus.

There is ample evidence that all of these defense systems are impaired in PEM. Like all other cells, epithelial cells require adequate nutrients for growth, turnover, and function. Kwashiorkor is commonly associated with low lymphocyte counts and nonreactivity to skin recall antigens (impaired cellular immunity) and low circulating protein levels that usually include immunoglobulins (humoral immunity). With nutritional repletion, immunocompetence can often be restored. However, tests of immune function cannot always be directly related to nutritional status, and the use of skin tests to demonstrate anergy adds little to the diagnosis or treatment of kwashiorkor. These issues are discussed further in Chapter 27.

PHYSIOLOGIC CHARACTERISTICS OF HYPOMETABOLIC AND HYPERMETABOLIC STATES

The metabolic characteristics and nutritional needs of hypermetabolic patients who are stressed from injury or infection are considerably different from those of hypometabolic patients who are unstressed but chronically starved. In both cases, nutritional support is of utmost importance, but misjudgments in selecting the appropriate approach may have disastrous consequences.

The hypometabolic patient is typified by the relatively unstressed but mildly catabolic and chronically starved individual who with time will develop marasmus (see Figure 7-1). The hypermetabolic patient stressed from injury or infection is catabolic (experiencing a rapid breakdown of body mass) and at high risk for developing kwashiorkor if nutritional needs are not met and/or the illness does not resolve quickly. As shown in Table 7-3 the two states are distinguished by differing alterations in metabolic, protein breakdown (proteolysis), and gluconeogenesis rates. These differences appear to be mediated largely by alterations in cytokines and counterregulatory hormones—tumor necrosis factor, interleukin-1, catecholamines (epinephrine and norepinephrine), glucagon, and cortisol—that are relatively reduced in hypometabolic patients and increased in hypermetabolic patients. Although insulin levels are also elevated in stressed patients, insulin resistance in the target tissues prevents the expression of insulin's anabolic properties.

TABLE 7-3 Physiologic characteristics of hypometabolic and hypermetabolic states

Physiologic characteristics	Hypometabolic, nonstressed patient (cachectic, marasmic)	Hypermetabolic, stressed patient (kwashiorkor risk*)
Cytokines, catecholamines, glucagon, cortisol, insulin	↓	↑
Metabolic rate	↓	↑
Proteolysis, gluconeogenesis	↓	↑
Urea excretion	↓	↑
Fat catabolism, fatty-acid utilization	↑	↑
Adaptation to starvation	Normal	Abnormal

* These changes characterize the stressed, kwashiorkor-risk patient commonly seen in intensive care units and differ in some respects from primary kwashiorkor seen in other settings (see Suggested Readings).

Metabolic Rate

In starvation and semistarvation the resting metabolic rate falls between 10% and 30% as an adaptive response to energy restriction, slowing the rate of weight loss. By contrast, the resting metabolic rate rises in the presence of physiologic stress in proportion to the degree of the insult. For example, the rise may be about 10% after elective surgery, 20% to 30% after bone fractures, 30% to 60% for severe infections such as peritonitis or gram-negative septicemia, and as much as 110% after major burns. Because the rise in metabolic rate is a generalized response and not isolated to any one organ system or injury site, the accompanying increase in oxygen consumption affects the entire body, including the splanchnic bed, skeletal muscle, and kidneys.

Weight loss results in both states—slowly in hypometabolic patients and quickly in hypermetabolic patients—if the metabolic rate (energy requirement) is not matched by energy intake. Losses of up to 10% of body weight are unlikely to have an adverse effect; however, losses greater than this in acutely ill hypermetabolic patients may be associated with a rapid deterioration in body function.

Protein Catabolism

The rate of endogenous protein breakdown (catabolism) to supply energy needs normally falls during uncomplicated energy deprivation. After about 10 days of total starvation an unstressed individual will have protein losses amounting to only 12 to 18 g per day (equivalent to approximately 2 oz of muscle tissue or 2 to 3 g of nitrogen). By contrast, protein breakdown in patients with an injury or sepsis accelerates in proportion to the degree of stress to 30 to 60 g per day after elective surgery, 60 to 90 g per day with infection, 100 to 130 g per day with severe sepsis or skeletal trauma, and at times over 175 g per day with major burns or head injuries. These losses are reflected by proportional increases in the excretion of urea, the major by-product of protein breakdown (see Table 8-5).

Protein catabolism occurs throughout the body and not solely at the site of injury. Because protein represents approximately 25% of the weight of muscle tissue, if protein losses are not offset by intake, the amount of muscle wasted each day can be estimated as 4 times the amount of protein catabolized. Consider this example of the potential magnitude of muscle wastage: a patient with multiple long-bone fractures without any protein intake had a 24-hour urinary urea nitrogen (UUN) excretion of 17 g. As described in Chapter 8, estimated protein losses are calculated as follows:

$$
\begin{aligned}
\text{Protein catabolic rate (g/day)} &= (\text{24-hour UUN} + 4) \times 6.25 \\
&= (17 + 4) \times 6.25 \\
&= 131 \text{ g/day}
\end{aligned}
$$

The breakdown of 131 g protein per day is equivalent to about 4 times that amount of muscle mass, i.e., with this degree of stress and protein catabolism, 524 g or over 1 lb of muscle tissue will be wasted each day if not offset by protein intake.

Gluconeogenesis

The major aim of protein catabolism during a state of starvation is to provide the "glucogenic" amino acids (especially alanine and glutamine) that serve as substrates for endogenous glucose production (gluconeogenesis) in the liver. In the hypometabolic/starved state, protein breakdown for gluconeogenesis is minimized, especially as ketones become the substrate preferred by certain tissues. In the hypermetabolic/stress state, gluconeogenesis increases dramatically and in proportion to the degree of the insult to increase the supply of glucose (the major fuel of reparation). Glucose is the only fuel that can be utilized by hypoxic tissues (during anaerobic glycolysis), by phagocytosing (bacteria-killing) white cells, and by young fibroblasts.

Infusions of glucose partially offset a negative energy balance but do not significantly suppress the high rates of gluconeogenesis in the hypermetabolic patient. Hence, adequate supplies of protein are needed to replace the amino acids utilized for this metabolic response.

In summary, the two physiologic states represent very different responses to starvation. The hypometabolic patient, who conserves body mass by reducing the metabolic rate and using fat as the primary fuel (rather than glucose and its precursor amino acids), is well adapted to starvation. The hypermetabolic patient also uses fat as a major fuel but rapidly breaks down body protein to produce glucose, the fuel of reparation, thereby causing loss of muscle and organ tissue and endangering vital body functions.

MICRONUTRIENT MALNUTRITION

PEM is not the only type of malnutrition found in hospitalized patients. The same illnesses and reductions in nutrient intake that lead to PEM can produce deficiencies of vitamins and minerals. Deficiencies of nutrients that are only stored in small amounts (such as the water-soluble vitamins) or are lost through external secretions (such as zinc in diarrhea fluid or burn exudate) are probably quite common. If levels of these nutrients were measured more routinely, deficiencies would probably be diagnosed more frequently.

In the authors' experience, deficiencies of vitamin C, folic acid, and zinc are common in hospitalized patients. For instance, signs of scurvy such as corkscrew hairs on the lower extremities are found with surprising frequency in chronically ill and/or alcoholic patients hospitalized for acute illnesses. The diagnosis can be confirmed with plasma vitamin C levels. Folic acid intakes and blood levels are often less than optimal even among healthy persons; when factors such as illness, alcoholism, poverty, or poor dentition are present, deficiencies are common. Low blood-zinc levels are also prevalent in patients with malabsorption syndromes such as inflammatory bowel disease. Patients with zinc deficiencies often exhibit poor wound healing, decubitus ulcer formation, and impaired immunity. Thiamin deficiency is a common complication of alcoholism, but it may be seen less commonly than the previously mentioned deficiencies because of the frequent use of therapeutic doses of thiamin after patients are admitted for alcohol abuse.

Patients with low plasma vitamin C levels usually respond to the doses found in multivitamin preparations, but patients with deficiences should be supplemented with 250 to 500 mg per day. Folic acid is absent from some oral multivitamin preparations; patients with deficiencies should be supplemented with about 1 mg per day. Patients with zinc deficiencies resulting from large external losses sometimes require oral daily supplementation with 220 mg of zinc sulfate 1 to 3 times daily. For these reasons, laboratory assessments of the micronutrient status of patients who are at high risk are desirable.

Hypophosphatemia (low serum phosphorus level) develops in hospitalized patients with remarkable frequency and generally results from rapid intracellular shifts of phosphate in cachectic or alcoholic patients receiving intravenous glucose or from taking antacids. The adverse clinical sequelae are numerous, and some such as acute cardiopulmonary failure can be life-threatening (see Table 9-1).

For more information on the functions of these micronutrients, and common causes and physical findings of deficiencies, see Tables 2-4, 8-2, and 8-3. Table 2-5 lists recommended daily dose ranges of the vitamins for prevention and treatment of various diseases.

References

1. Butterworth CE: The skeleton in the hospital closet, *Nutr Today* 9:4, 1974.
2. Weinsier RL et al: Hospital malnutrition: a prospective evaluation of general medical patients during the course of hospitalization, *Am J Clin Nutr* 32:418,1979.
3. Coats KG et al: Hospital-associated malnutrition: a reevaluation 12 years later, *J Am Dietetic Assoc* 93:27,1993.

Suggested Readings

Cahill GF: Starvation in man, *N Engl J Med* 282:668,1970.

Torosian MH, ed: *Nutrition for the hospitalized patient,* New York, 1995, Marcel Dekker.

Torún B, Chew F: Protein-energy malnutrition. In Shils ME, Olson JA, Shike M, eds: *Modern nutrition in health and disease,* ed 8, Philadelphia, 1994, Lea & Febiger.

Nutritional Assessment

Because the interaction between illness and nutritional status is complex, many physical and laboratory findings are a reflection of underlying disease as well as nutritional status. Therefore the nutritional evaluation of a patient requires an integration of the history, physical examination, anthropometrics, and laboratory studies. Although this approach helps detect nutritional problems, it also helps to avoid concluding that isolated findings indicate nutritional problems when they actually may not. (For example, hypoalbuminemia caused by an underlying illness does not necessarily indicate malnutrition.)

Each medical and surgical subspecialty focuses on its medical history and clinical and laboratory assessments in a way that is directly relevant to the particular subspecialty. Similarly, clinical nutrition has specialized history reviews, physical examinations, and laboratory approaches that are all important for completing a thorough nutritional assessment.

NUTRITIONAL HISTORY

A nutritional history is directed toward identifying underlying mechanisms that put patients at risk for nutritional depletion or excess. These mechanisms include inadequate intake, impaired absorption, decreased utilization, increased losses, and increased requirements of nutrients (Table 8-1).

Table 8-1 Nutritional history screen: a systematic approach to the detection of deficiency syndromes

Mechanism of deficiency	History	Deficiency to suspect
Inadequate intake	Alcoholism	Calories, protein, thiamin, niacin, folate, pyridoxine, riboflavin
	Avoidance of fruit, vegetables, grains	Vitamin C, thiamin, niacin, folate
	Avoidance of meat, dairy products, eggs	Protein, vitamin B$_{12}$
	Constipation, hemorrhoids, diverticulosis	Dietary fiber
	Isolation, poverty, dental disease, food idiosyncrasies	Various nutrients
	Weight loss	Calories, other nutrients
	Drugs (especially antacids, anticonvulsants, cholestyramine, laxatives, neomycin, alcohol)	See Chapter 14
Inadequate absorption	Malabsorption (diarrhea, weight loss, steatorrhea)	Vitamins A, D, K, calories, protein, calcium, magensium, zinc

Continued

TABLE 8-1   Nutritional history screen: a systematic approach to the detection of deficiency syndromes—cont'd

Mechanism of deficiency	History	Deficiency to suspect
Inadequate absorption—cont'd		
	Parasites	Iron, vitamin B_{12} (fish tapeworm)
	Pernicious anemia	Vitamin B_{12}
	Surgery	
	Gastrectomy	Vitamin B_{12}, iron, folate
	Intestinal resection	Vitamin B_{12} (if distal ileum), iron, others as in malabsorption
		See Chapter 14
Decreased utilization	Drugs (especially anticonvulsants, antimetabolites, oral contraceptives, isoniazid, alcohol)	
	Inborn errors of metabolism (by family history)	Various nutrients

Increased losses	Alcohol abuse	Magnesium, zinc
	Blood loss	Iron
	Centesis (ascitic, pleural taps)	Protein
	Diabetes, uncontrolled	Calories
	Diarrhea	Protein, zinc, electrolytes
	Draining abscesses, wounds	Protein, zinc
	Nephrotic syndrome	Protein, zinc
	Peritoneal dialysis or hemodialysis	Protein, water-soluble vitamins, zinc
Increased requirements	Fever	Calories
	Hyperthyroidism	Calories
	Physiologic demands (infancy, adolescence, pregnancy, lactation)	Various nutrients
	Surgery, trauma, burns, infection	Calories, protein, vitamin C, zinc
	Tissue hypoxia	Calories (inefficient utilization)
	Cigarette smoking	Vitamin C, folic acid

THE HIGH-RISK PATIENT

Underweight (weight-for-height < 80% of standard) and/or recent loss of 10% or more of usual body weight

Poor intake: anorexia, food avoidance (e.g., psychiatric condition), "nothing allowed by mouth" (NPO) status for more than about 5 days

Protracted nutrient losses: malabsorption, enteric fistulae, draining abscesses or wounds, renal dialysis

Hypermetabolic states: sepsis, protracted fever, extensive trauma or burns

Chronic use of alcohol or drugs with antinutrient or catabolic properties: steroids, antimetabolites (e.g., methotrexate), immunosuppressants, antitumor agents

Impoverishment, isolation, advanced age

Individuals with the characteristics listed in the box are at high risk for nutritional deficiencies.

Although there are many types, the major diet histories used are the following: dietary recalls generally covering 24 hours; food records in which patients write down everything eaten during a 1- to 7-day period; and food frequency questionnaires in which patients estimate how often they eat the foods identified on a list. A variety of computer programs permit rapid estimation of nutrient intake from these questionnaires or records. Each method has advantages and disadvantages, such as labor intensity, cost, and accuracy. For instance, a 24-hour dietary recall may significantly underestimate usual intakes but can easily be elicited from most patients. Three-day food records provide a reasonable way to obtain a qualitative estimate of nutrient intakes, but food choices often change during recording periods and may not be accurately represented. Sometimes combinations of the various methods work best. For a routine nutritional assessment in the hospital or clinic setting a 24-hour dietary recall provides an overview of the patient's dietary pattern that is adequate enough to determine if further detailed evaluation is necessary. However, in the course of the entire medical history it is important to obtain information about all of the areas noted in Table 8-1 (e.g., presence of alcoholism, dental disease, drug use, malabsorption) to identify potential nutrient deficiencies not included in the dietary recall.

PHYSICAL EXAMINATION

Physical findings that suggest vitamin, mineral, and protein-energy deficiencies and excesses are outlined in Table 8-2. Most of the physical findings are not specific for individual nutrient deficiencies and must be integrated with the historical, anthropometric, and laboratory findings to make a diagnosis. For example, the finding of follicular hyperkeratosis isolated to the back of the arms is a fairly common, normal finding. On the other hand, if it is widespread on a person who consumes little fruit and vegetables and smokes regularly (increasing ascorbic acid requirements), vitamin C deficiency is a very possible cause. Similarly, easily pluckable hair may be a consequence of recent chemotherapy. On the other hand, in a hospitalized patient who has poorly healing surgical wounds and hypoalbuminemia, easily pluckable hair is strongly suggestive of kwashiorkor.

It is noteworthy that tissues with the fastest turnover rates are those most likely to show signs of nutrient deficiencies or excesses. Thus the hair, skin, and lingual papillae (an indirect reflection of the status of the villae of the gastrointestinal tract) are particularly likely to reveal nutritional problems and should be examined closely. Table 8-3 outlines causes of various nutrient deficiencies and methods for preventing their recurrence.

Anthropometrics

Anthropometrics provide information on body muscle mass and fat reserves. The most practical and commonly used measurements are body weight, height, triceps skinfold, and midarm muscle circumference.

Text continued on p. 194.

TABLE 8-2 Clinical nutrition examination

Clinical findings	Deficiency to consider*	Excess to consider	Frequency†
Hair, nails			
Flag sign (transverse depigmentation of hair)	Protein		Rare
Easily pluckable hair	Protein		Common
Sparse hair	Protein, biotin, zinc	Vitamin A	Occasional
Corkscrew hairs and unemerged coiled hairs	Vitamin C		Common
Transverse ridging of nails	Protein		Occasional
Skin			
Scaling	Vitamin A, zinc, essential fatty acids	Vitamin A	Occasional
Cellophane appearance	Protein		Occasional
Cracking (flaky paint or crazy pavement) dermatosis	Protein		Rare
Follicular hyperkeratosis	Vitamins A, C		Occasional
Petechiae (especially perifollicular)	Vitamin C		Occasional
Purpura	Vitamins C, K		Common

Physical finding	Nutrient		Frequency
Pigmentation, desquamation of sun-exposed areas	Niacin		Rare
Yellow pigmentation sparing sclerae (benign)		Carotene	Common
Eyes			
Papilledema		Vitamin A	Rare
Night blindness	Vitamin A		Rare
Perioral			
Angular stomatitis	Riboflavin, pyridoxine, niacin		Occasional
Cheilosis (dry, cracking, ulcerated lips)	Riboflavin, pyridoxine, niacin		Rare
Oral			
Atrophic lingual papillae (slick tongue)	Riboflavin, niacin, folate, vitamin B_{12} protein, iron		Common
Glossitis (scarlet, raw tongue)	Riboflavin, niacin, pyridoxine, folate, vitamin B_{12}		Occasional
Hypogeusesthesia, hyposmia	Zinc		Occasional

Continued

TABLE 8-2 Clinical nutrition examination—cont'd

Clinical findings	Deficiency to consider*	Excess to consider	Frequency†
Oral—cont'd			
Swollen, retracted, bleeding gums (if teeth are present)	Vitamin C		Occasional
Bones, joint			
Beading of ribs, epiphyseal swelling, bowlegs	Vitamin D		Rare
Tenderness (subperiosteal hemorrhage in child)	Vitamin C		Rare
Neurologic			
Headache		Vitamin A	Rare
Drowsiness, lethargy, vomiting		Vitamins A, D	Rare
Dementia	Niacin, vitamin B_{12}, folate		Rare
Confabulation, disorientation	Thiamin (**Korsakoff's psychosis**)		Occasional
Ophthalmoplegia	Thiamin, phosphorus		Occasional

Peripheral neuropathy (e.g., weakness, footdrop, paresthesias, ataxia, and decreased tendon reflexes, fine tactile sense, vibratory sense, and position sense)	Thiamin, pyridoxine, vitamin B_{12}	Pyridoxine	Occasional
Tetany	Calcium, magnesium		Occasional
Other			
Parotid enlargement	Protein (consider also bulimia)		Occasional
Heart failure	Thiamin ("wet" beriberi), phosphorus		Occasional
Sudden heart failure, death	Vitamin C		Rare
Hepatomegaly	Protein	Vitamin A	Rare
Edema	Protein, thiamin		Common
Poor wound healing, decubitus ulcers	Protein, vitamin C, zinc		Common

° In this table, "protein deficiency" is used to signify kwashiorkor.

† These frequencies are an attempt to reflect the authors' experience in the setting of a U.S. medical practice. Findings common in other countries but virtually unseen in usual medical practice settings in the United States (e.g., xerophthalmia and endemic goiter) are not listed.

TABLE 8-3 Common causes of nutrient deficiencies

Deficiency (evidence of)	History to suspect
Vitamin A	Fat malabsorption; use of cholestyramine, mineral oil
Carotene	Fat malabsorption; avoidance of fruit and vegetables, use of cholestyramine, mineral oil, neomycin
Thiamin	Alcoholism; use of antacids, cyclophosphamide
Pyridoxine	Alcoholism; use of cycloserine, ethionamide, isoniazid, oral contraceptive agents, para-aminosalicylic acid (PAS), penicillamine, tetracycline
Riboflavin	Alcoholism, use of tetracycline
Niacin	Alcoholism; carcinoid syndrome
Folic acid	Alcoholism; sprue; avoidance of fruit and vegetables; cigarette smoking; use of anticonvulsants, cycloserine, methotrexate, nitrofurantoin, oral contraceptive agents, PAS, trimethoprim
Vitamin B_{12}	Pernicious anemia, resection of terminal ileum, total gastrectomy, intestinal bacterial overgrowth, sprue; avoidance of all animal and dairy foods; use of anticonvulsants, methotrexate, PAS, tetracycline
Vitamin C	Avoidance of fruits and vegetables; cigarette smoking
Vitamin D	Fat malabsorption, renal insufficiency; use of anticonvulsants, cholestyramine, mineral oil
Vitamin E	Dietary deficiency unusual; fat malabsorption and premature infancy are predisposing factors

Vitamin K	Fat malabsorption, sterilization of gut; use of anticonvulsants, cholestyramine, warfarin, mineral oil
Calcium	Fat malabsorption, vitamin D deficiency (dietary deficiency of calcium per se unlikely); use of actinomycin D, antacids, anticonvulsants, cholestyramine, mithramycin, neomycin
Iron	Bleeding, gastrectomy, pregnancies; poor intake of meat, fruit, and vegetables; use of cholestyramine, chloramphenicol, neomycin
Magnesium	Fat malabsorption, alcoholism; use of amphotericin
Phosphorus	Alcoholism, dextrose infusions chronic acidosis, hyperparathyroidism, vitamin D deficiency; use of antacids
Zinc	Alcoholism, fat malabsorption, sickle-cell disease, acute hepatitis, burns, diabetes mellitus, nephrotic syndrome, dialysis; use of diuretics, penicillamine; chronic losses or drainage of upper intestinal fluid or exudative material

Commonly used reference standards for normal body weight are based on weight-for-height tables (see Table 15-1). Regardless of body frame type, adult patients who are 20% or more above reference standards are likely to be obese and at increased risk of comorbid conditions. Those who are 20% or more below standard weight are likely to be severely underweight and at high risk for nutritional deficiencies. Body weight is one of the most useful nutritional parameters to follow in patients who are acutely or chronically ill. Weight loss often reflects loss of lean body mass (muscle and organ tissue), especially if rapid and not associated with diuresis. This can be an ominous sign because it indicates use of vital body proteins as a metabolic fuel. Underfeeding a hypermetabolic obese patient in particular can result in protein-energy malnutrition (PEM) although the patient remains overweight and appears well fed. By contrast, weight maintenance or weight gain in a seriously ill patient may not be a favorable sign if it reflects edema and masks loss of lean body mass.

Measurement of skinfold thickness is the easiest method to estimate body fat stores, because about 50% of body fat is normally located in the subcutaneous region. The triceps skinfold (TSF) is a convenient site that is generally representative of the entire body's fat level. The TSF measurement is taken with calipers on the upper arm at the midpoint between the acromion and olecranon processes with the arm relaxed and the elbow flexed at 90° (Figure 8-1). A fold of skin on the posterior aspect of the arm is grasped and pulled away from the underlying muscle. Calipers are applied and the fold is still held to release skin tension from the calipers. The reading is taken after about 3 seconds. Clinically useful values for TSFs are listed in Table 8-4. A thickness of less than 3 mm (equivalent to about three dimes) suggests severe depletion of energy reserves. Age-adjusted anthropometric values reflecting the adult U.S. population reflect the prevalence of obesity in the population and are less useful to the clinician in detecting malnutrition.[1]

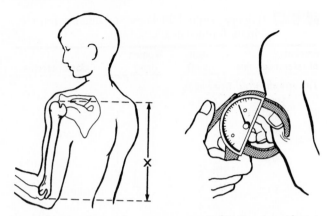

Figure 8-1 Technique for measurement of TSF. Use the midpoint of the upper arm halfway between the acromion process of the scapula and the olecranon process of the ulna.

The midarm muscle circumference (MAMC) is often used to estimate skeletal muscle mass. A tape measure is used to determine the upper arm circumference of a relaxed, extended arm at the same midpoint used for the TSF. The MAMC is calculated using the following equation and compared with reference values in Table 8-4.

MAMC (cm) = Upper arm circumference (cm) −
$$[0.314 \times TSF \ (mm)]$$

As with body weight, there is a wide variation in values of TSF and MAMC among healthy people. Persons who exercise avidly may be healthy and have TSF measurements in the low-adequate or borderline categories. Also, average values vary according to age. For these reasons, TSF and MAMC are often more useful for tracking body composition changes in patients over a period of time than as single measurements. These measurements will not be accurate in patients with edema of the upper extremities.

TABLE 8-4   Triceps skinfold thickness and midarm muscle circumference in adults

Percent of reference value	Men (mm)	Women (mm)	Calorie reserves
Triceps skinfold thickness			
100	12.5	16.5	
90	11	15	
80	10	13	Adequate
70	9	11.5	
60	7.5	10	
50	6	8	
40	5	6.5	Borderline
30	4	5	
20	2.5	3	Severely depleted

Percent of reference value	Men (cm)	Women (cm)	Muscle mass
Midarm muscle circumference			
100	25.5	23	Adequate
90	23	21	
80	20	18.5	Borderline
70	18	16	
60	15	14	
50	12.5	11.5	Severely depleted
40	10	9	

LABORATORY STUDIES

A number of laboratory tests used routinely in clinical medicine can yield valuable information about a patient's nutritional status if a slightly different approach to the interpretation of laboratory results is used. For example, abnormally low levels of serum albumin, a low total iron-binding capacity, and anergy may each have separate explanations. However, collectively they very likely represent a kwashiorkor state. In the clinical setting with a hypermetabolic, acutely ill patient who is edematous, has easily pluckable hair, and has inadequate protein intake, the diagnosis of kwashiorkor is clear-cut. Commonly used laboratory tests for assessment of nutritional status are outlined in Table 8-5. Because none of them are specific for a nutritional problem, tips are provided in the table to help avoid assigning nutritional significance to tests that may be abnormal for other than nutritional reasons.

Assessment of Body Composition

The serum creatinine level reflects muscle mass to a certain extent; a value of less than 0.6 suggests muscle wasting. The creatinine-height index—a better measure for estimating and tracking skeletal muscle mass—is determined by comparing a patient's 24-hour urinary creatinine excretion with reference values from persons of the same height. Because the rate of formation of creatinine from creatine phosphate in skeletal muscle is constant, the amount of creatinine excreted in the urine every 24 hours reflects skeletal muscle mass. Women excrete approximately 18 mg/kg per day, and men excrete approximately 23 mg/kg per day. Table 8-6 shows more detailed predicted urinary creatinine values for men and women. Values of 80% to 100% of those predicted indicate adequate muscle mass, values of 60% to 80% indicate a moderate deficit, and values less than 60% indicate a severe deficit of muscle mass. Although not readily available at most institutions, more sophisticated procedures for assessing body composition include dual-energy x-ray absorptiometry (DEXA) and underwater weighing (hydrodensitometry).

Assessment of Circulating (Visceral) Proteins

The visceral compartment is composed of proteins that act as carriers, binders, and immunologically active proteins. The serum proteins that may be used to assess nutritional status include albumin, total iron-binding capacity (or transferrin), thyroxine-binding prealbumin (or transthyretin), and retinol-binding protein. Because they have differing synthesis rates and half-lives—the half-life of albumin is about 21 days whereas that of retinol-

Text continued on p. 204.

TABLE 8-5 Routine laboratory tests used in nutritional assessment

Test (normal values)	Nutritional use	Causes of normal value despite malnutrition	Other causes of abnormal value
Serum albumin (3.5 to 5.5 g/dl)	2.8 to 3.5—compromised protein status <2.8—Possible kwashiorkor Increasing value reflects positive nitrogen balance	Dehydration Infusion of albumin, fresh frozen plasma or whole blood	LOW Common— Infection and other stress, especially with poor protein intake Burns, trauma Congestive heart failure Fluid overload Severe hepatic insufficiency Uncommon— Nephrotic syndrome Zinc deficiency Bacterial overgrowth of small bowel

Test / Normal range			
Total iron-binding capacity (TIBC) 270–400 µg/dl	<200—compromised protein status, possible kwashiorkor. Positive nitrogen balance reflected by increasing value. More labile than albumin	Iron deficiency	LOW. Similar to albumin. HIGH. Iron deficiency
Prothrombin time <2 sec beyond "control" or 70% to 100% "control" activity	Prolongation—vitamin K deficiency		PROLONGED. Anticoagulant therapy—Warfarin (Coumadin). Severe liver disease
Serum creatinine 0.6–1.6 mg/dl	<0.6—muscle wasting due to calorie deficiency. Reflects muscle mass		HIGH. Despite muscle wasting—. Renal failure. Severe dehydration

Continued

TABLE 8-5 Routine laboratory tests used in nutritional assessment—cont'd

Test (normal values)	Nutritional use	Causes of normal value despite malnutrition	Other causes of abnormal value
24 hour urinary creatinine 500-1200 mg/day (standardized for height and sex)	Low value—muscle wasting due to calorie deficiency	>24 hour collection Decreasing serum creatinine	LOW Incomplete urine collection Increasing serum creatinine Muscle wasting resulting from paralytic atrophy
24-hour urinary urea nitrogen (UUN) <5 g/day—depends on level of protein intake	Determine level of catabolism (as long as protein intake is ≥ 10 g below calculated protein loss or <20 g total, but at least 100 g carbohydrate is provided) 5-10 g/day = mild catabolism (e.g., after elective surgery); or normal-fed state		LOW Active fluid retention Increasing BUN Incomplete urine collection HIGH High protein intake Corticosteroid therapy Active diuresis Decreasing BUN

>24-hour urine collection

Gastrointestinal bleeding

10-15 g/day = moderate catabolism (e.g., in infection, major surgery)

>15 g/day = severe catabolism (e.g., in severe sepsis, major burns, head trauma)

Estimate protein balance

Protein balance = Protein intake − Protein loss

where

Protein loss (or protein catabolic rate) = [24-hour UUN (g) + 4] × 6.25

Exception—adjustment required in burn patients

Continued

TABLE 8-5 Routine laboratory tests used in nutritional assessment—cont'd

Test (normal values)	Nutritional use	Causes of normal value despite malnutrition	Other causes of abnormal value
24-hour (UUN)—cont'd	(see Chapter 21) and others with large nonurinary nitrogen losses		
Blood urea nitrogen (BUN) 8-23 mg/dl	<8—possibly inadequate protein intake >12—possibly adequate, even excessive, protein intake If serum creatinine normal, use BUN If serum creatinine elevated, use BUN/creatinine ratio		LOW Severe liver disease Anabolic state HIGH Despite poor protein intake— Renal failure (use BUN/serum creatinine ratio) Congestive heart failure Gastrointestinal hemorrhage

| Total lymphocyte count (TLC)[*] >1500/mm³ | <1500—possible immuno-compromise associated with protein-calorie malnutrition, especially kwashiorkor

Significant limitation—marked day-to-day fluctuation | Corticosteroid therapy Dehydration Shock

LOW
Severe stress, e.g., infections, with "left shift" Corticosteroid therapy Renal failure Cancer, e.g., colon

HIGH
Despite malnutrition—
Infections Leukemia, myeloma Cancer (e.g., stomach, breast) Adrenal insufficiency |

[*]TLC, White blood cell count × % lymphocytes.

TABLE 8-6 Predicted urinary creatinine values—adults[2]

Men*		Women†	
Height	Predicted creatinine‡ (mg/24 hr)	Height	Predicted creatinine‡ (mg/24 hr)
5' 2" (157.5 cm)	1288	4'10" (147.3 cm)	830
5' 3" (160 cm)	1325	4'11" (149.9 cm)	851
5' 4" (162.6 cm)	1359	5' 0" (152.4 cm)	875
5' 5" (165.1 cm)	1386	5' 1" (154.9 cm)	900
5' 6" (167.6 cm)	1426	5' 2" (157.5 cm)	925
5' 7" (170.2 cm)	1467	5' 3" (160 cm)	949
5' 8" (172.7 cm)	1513	5' 4" (162.6 cm)	977
5' 9" (175.3 cm)	1555	5' 5" (165.1 cm)	1006
5'10" (177.8 cm)	1596	5' 6" (167.6 cm)	1044
5'11" (180.3 cm)	1642	5' 7" (170.2 cm)	1076
6' 0" (182.9 cm)	1691	5' 8" (172.7 cm)	1109
6' 1" (185.4 cm)	1739	5' 9" (175.3 cm)	1141
6' 2" (188 cm)	1785	5'10" (177.8 cm)	1174
6' 3" (190.5 cm)	1831	5'11" (180.3 cm)	1206
6' 4" (193 cm)	1891	6' 0" (182.9 cm)	1240

*Creatinine coefficient (men) = 23 mg/kg of ideal body weight/24 hours.
†Creatinine coefficient (women) = 18 mg/kg of ideal body weight/24 hours.
‡80% to 100% of predicted = acceptable; 60% to 80% = moderate depletion; <60% = severe depletion.

binding protein is closer to 12 hours—some of these parameters reflect changes in nutritional status more quickly than others. The general availability and stability of albumin levels from day to day make it one of the most useful tests.

Levels of circulating proteins are influenced by their rates of synthesis and catabolism, "third spacing" (loss into interstitial spaces), and in some cases external loss. Although an adequate intake of calories and protein is necessary to achieve optimal circulating protein levels, the levels do not sensitively reflect protein intake. For example, a drop in the serum level of albumin or transferrin often accompanies significant physiologic stress (e.g., from infection or injury) and is not necessarily an indication of malnutrition or poor intake. A low serum albumin level in a burned patient with both hypermetabolism and increased dermal losses of protein may not indicate malnutrition. On the other hand, adequate nutritional support of the patient's calorie and protein needs is critical for returning circulating proteins to normal levels as stress resolves. Thus low values alone do not define malnutrition but often point toward an increased risk of malnutrition because of the hypermetabolic stress state. It is not unusual for protein levels to remain low despite aggressive nutritional support as long as significant physiologic stress persists; if the levels do not rise after the underlying illness has resolved, the patient's protein and calorie requirements should be reassessed to ensure that intake is sufficient.

Assessment of Protein Catabolic Rate Using Urinary Urea Nitrogen

Because urea is a major by-product of protein catabolism, the amount of urea nitrogen excreted each day can be used to estimate the rate of protein catabolism and determine if protein intake is adequate to offset it. Total protein loss and protein balance can be calculated from the urinary urea nitrogen (UUN) as follows:

Protein catabolic rate (g/day) =
$$[\text{24-hour UUN (g)} + 4] \times 6.25$$

The value of 4 g added to the UUN represents a liberal estimate of the unmeasured nitrogen lost in the urine (e.g., creatinine and uric acid), sweat, hair, skin, and feces. The factor 6.25 estimates the amount of protein represented by the nitrogen excreted because on average nitrogen accounts for about one sixth the weight of dietary protein. When protein intake is small (e.g., less than about 20 g per day), the equation indicates both the patient's protein requirement and the severity of the catabolic state (see Table 8-5). More substantial protein intakes can raise the UUN because some of the ingested (or infused) protein is catabolized and converted to UUN. Thus at lower protein intakes the equation is useful for estimating *requirements*, and at higher protein intakes it is useful for assessing protein *balance* (the difference between intake and catabolism; see Chapter 9).

Protein balance (g/day) =
Protein intake − Protein catabolic rate

As noted in Table 8-5, changes in the concentration of blood urea nitrogen (BUN) or body-water content during the 24-hour period of urine collection can confound interpretation of the UUN. Misleading results are particularly likely in patients who are receiving intermittent renal dialysis and have rapid changes in BUN during the UUN collection and in those undergoing rapid diuresis. If changes in BUN and body weight (as a reflection of changes in fluid status) are determined from measurements taken at the beginning and end of the urine collection, the UUN can be corrected with the calculation that follows. This calculation yields a more accurate estimation of the protein catabolic rate or urinary nitrogen appearance (UNA).

$$\text{UNA (g)} = \text{UUN (g)} + \frac{(\Delta \text{BUN} \times 10)(W_m)(BW) + (\text{BUN}_m \times 10)(\Delta W)}{1000}$$

where

ΔBUN = Change in BUN (mg/dl) during the urine collection (Final BUN − Initial BUN)

BUN_m = Mean BUN (mg/dl) during the urine collection [(Final BUN + Initial BUN)/2]

ΔW = Change in weight (kg) during the urine collection (Final weight − Initial weight)

W_m = Mean weight (kg) during the urine collection [(Final weight + Initial weight)/2]

BW = Assumed body water as a proportion of body weight (normal value = 0.5 for women and 0.6 for men; 0.05 subtracted for marked obesity or dehydration; 0.05 added for leanness or edema)

To make a corrected calculation of a patient's rate of protein breakdown, the value for UNA is substituted for UUN in the protein catabolic rate equation provided previously. In most situations the standard UUN calculation is reliable as long as both BUN and body-water content are stable during the urine collection (even if they are abnormal). Under these circumstances, ΔBUN and ΔW equal zero and UNA equals UUN.

Another common cause of a spuriously high UUN is a gastrointestinal hemorrhage. There is no accurate way to correct for this in calculating the protein catabolic rate; it should simply be taken into account qualitatively when the results of the UUN are interpreted.

Assessment of Protein Intake Using Blood Urea Nitrogen

As dietary protein intake increases, the BUN level generally rises unless the patient is unusually anabolic and using all available amino acids for protein synthesis. The converse is also true; BUN levels generally fall when protein intake is reduced. Thus in instances in which the BUN is high and there are no other causes, such as renal insufficiency, dehydration, or gastrointestinal bleeding, dietary protein intake is likely to be excessive. If the BUN is low (e.g., less than 8 mg/dl), it suggests a low and possibly inadequate protein intake. Nondietary causes of low and high BUN levels are outlined in Table 8-5.

Assessment of Immune Status Using Total Lymphocyte Count

The immunocompromise associated with kwashiorkor can be reflected by the total lymphocyte count (TLC), which is derived mathematically from the total white blood cell (WBC) and differential counts (TLC = WBC $\times$ % lymphocytes). However, it is of little use in tracking the course of nutritional status because it is affected by many medical conditions, and there is significant fluctuation in both total WBC and differential counts from day to day.

Assessment of Vitamin and Mineral Status

The use of laboratory tests to confirm suspected micronutrient deficiencies is desirable because the physical findings for these are often equivocal and nonspecific. Low blood-micronutrient levels can predate more serious clinical manifestations and may also indicate drug-nutrient interactions. Assays typically used for micronutrient assessment (with normal values) are outlined in Table 2-4. There are three general approaches to measuring vitamin levels:

1. Direct measurement of the vitamin or its derivative in body fluids by chemical or biologic means (e.g., plasma ascorbic acid level); same method used for measurement of many trace elements
2. Indirect assessment of vitamin function as reflected in enzymatic reactions under controlled conditions (e.g., erythrocyte activity coefficients for thiamin, riboflavin, and pyridoxine)
3. Measurement of abnormal metabolic end products that occur as a result of deficiency (e.g., homocysteine for folic acid or methylmalonic acid for vitamin B_{12})

References

1. Frisancho AR: New standards of weight and body composition by frame size and height for assessment of nutritional status of adults and the elderly, *Am J Clin Nutr* 40:808, 1984.
2. Blackburn GL et al: Nutritional and metabolic assessment of the hospitalized patient, *JPEN* 1:11, 1977.

Suggested Readings

Shils ME, Olson JA, Shike M, eds: *Modern nutrition in health and disease,* ed 8, Philadelphia, 1994, Lea & Febiger.
Torosian MH, ed: *Nutrition for the hospitalized patient,* New York, 1995, Marcel Dekker.

Nutritional Support: General Approach and Complications

FEEDING APPROACHES

There are four approaches to supplying nutrients using two major routes (Figure 9-1). The enteral route includes oral and tube feeding, and the parenteral route includes peripheral venous alimentation (PVA) and central venous alimentation (CVA). Every patient can be nourished by at least one of these approaches. Because they are not mutually exclusive, in many cases two or more complementary approaches can be used. Patients should not be completely unfed for more than 5 to 7 days before tube feeding or total parenteral nutrition (TPN) is instituted. Clinical judgment regarding when to intervene must be exercised if there is food intake but it is insufficient to meet the patient's needs.

The most physiologic feeding approach feasible should always be used. This means that enteral feeding whether oral or by tube is always preferred over parenteral feeding unless a contraindication is present. (i.e., If the gut works, *use* it.) The reasons for preferring the enteral route (box) go beyond the obvious fact that it is the "normal" way to ingest nutrients. The physiologic responses to enteral feeding differ significantly from those of parenteral nutrition because the latter bypasses the intestinal tract and portal circulation through the liver. Among other things, enteral feeding stimulates gut hormones, subjects nutrients to the absorptive and metabolic controls of the intestinal tract and liver, and produces less hyperglycemia, which allows for better immune function and decreases the risk of systemic infection. The buffering capacity of

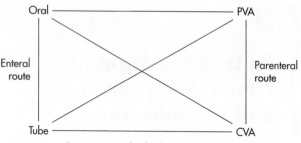

FIGURE 9-1 The feeding quadrangle.

ADVANTAGES OF ENTERAL FEEDING OVER PARENTERAL FEEDING

Physiologic superiority (e.g., gut hormones, blood glucose levels, buffering capacity)

Maintenance of intestinal structure and function

Protection against sepsis and multiple organ system failure

Gastric acid buffering

Low cost (one tenth to one third that of parenteral nutrition)

Safety (e.g., lower risk of sepsis and other central venous catheter complications)

enteral feeding can improve resistance against stress ulcers. The cost of enteral feeding is only a fraction of that of parenteral. Finally, there is evidence that the intestinal mucosa undergoes atrophy during parenteral nutrition, whereas enteral feeding maintains a more healthy mucosa. Although not firmly established in humans, this may enhance mucosal resistance to the translocation of bacteria and endotoxins and reduce the risk of sepsis, multiple organ system failure, and gastrointestinal bleeding. Although it is sometimes tempting to feed a patient parenterally when a central venous catheter is already present, convenience alone does not justify this route. Because of the recognized benefits of enteral feeding, physicians have become more aggressive in devising ways to gain enteral access for feeding (see Chapter 12).

Of the enteral options, oral feeding is preferred over tube feeding. Nasogastric tube feeding is effective in many patients who have inadequate nutrient intake as a result of a depressed appetite or an inability to eat. However, if the gastrointestinal tract is not able to be used or is unreliable for more than 5 to 7 days, use parenteral nutrition.

ENERGY REQUIREMENTS

Goals for feeding patients are derived from estimates or measurements of their energy expenditure and protein utilization.

Calculating Energy Expenditure

Basal energy expenditure (BEE [kcal per day]) can be estimated from a patient's height, weight, age, and gender using the Harris-Benedict equations:

Men: BEE = 66.47 + 13.75W + 5H − 6.76A
Women: BEE = 655.1 + 9.56W + 1.85H − 4.68A

where

W = Weight in kg
H = Height in cm
A = Age in years

These equations can be solved with a calculator or the nomograms in Figure 9-2. Actual energy requirements are then estimated by multiplying the BEE by a factor that accounts for the stress of illness. Multiplying by 1.2 to 1.5 yields a range (20% to 50% above basal) that estimates the actual energy expenditure of the majority of hospitalized patients. The lower value is used for patients without evidence of significant physiologic stress; the higher value is used for patients with marked stress such as sepsis or trauma. The result is used as a goal for feeding.

Exceptions to the "1.2 to 1.5" rule are patients with severe body burns (ones that cover more than 40% of the

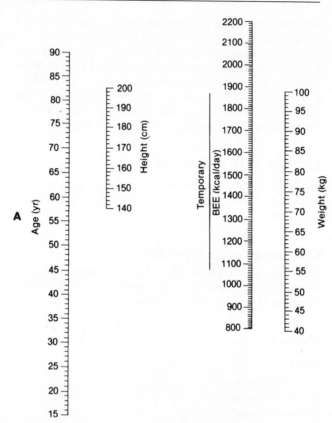

FIGURE 9-2 Nomograms for calculating BEE for (**A**) men and (**B**) women.

body surface); often calories up to 2 times the BEE are needed. For unstressed patients in whom weight gain rather than weight maintenance is desired, the BEE may also be multiplied by two. It is generally not appropriate to provide an *excessive* calorie load to stressed patients because this may aggravate the hypermetabolic state and result in increased catecholamine production, greater cardiorespiratory demand, and increased energy

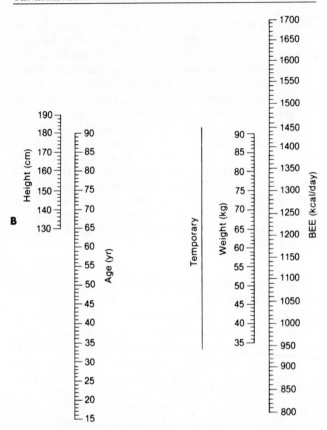

FIGURE 9-2 For legend see opposite page.

expenditure. By contrast, such high calorie levels are appropriate for weight gain in stable, unstressed cachectic patients who have become *well adapted* to feeding. (See section on Complications of Nutritional Support that follows.)

When calculating the BEE in a hospitalized patient, it is virtually always appropriate to use current rather than ideal body weight. In a markedly underweight patient the BEE is very low but nevertheless reflects the patient's adaptation to starvation (see Chapter 7). Using the patient's actual body weight also assists in avoiding the complications of rapid refeeding, which will be discussed. The greatest potential for error when using the Harris-Benedict equations is probably with morbidly obese patients because the equations assume a linear increase in energy expenditure as body weight increases. This assumption is only correct within reasonable ranges of body weight but is less accurate as weight increases above about 120 kg. In this higher range there is a lesser increase in energy expenditure with additional weight. Therefore it is probably best simply to use 120 kg in the equation when patients' body weights are greater than 120 kg so that their energy needs will not be exceeded. Calculating energy requirements in this way should meet the needs of most acutely ill obese patients.

Measuring Energy Expenditure: Indirect Calorimetry

When it is important to have a more accurate assessment of energy needs, indirect calorimetry can be used to measure them at the bedside. This technique is useful in patients who are believed to be hypermetabolic from sepsis or trauma and whose body weights cannot be obtained accurately or patients having difficulty weaning from a ventilator whose energy needs should not be exceeded to avoid excessive CO_2 production. Patients at the extremes of weight and/or age are good candidates as well, because the Harris-Benedict equations were developed in adults with roughly normal body weights.

Indirect calorimetry is based on the principle that energy expenditure is proportional to O_2 consumption and CO_2 production and the proportion of fuels being utilized is reflected in their ratio, the respiratory quotient (RQ). The test involves using a mobile metabolic cart with a clear plastic hood that is placed over the patient's head or tubing that is connected to the patient's ventilator to measure respiratory gas exchange for 20 to 30 minutes. The protocol for indirect calorimetry is provided in the box. Avoid interruptions during the test.

PREPARATION FOR INDIRECT CALORIMETRY

Thirty hours before test

24-hour urine urea nitrogen (UUN) collection (with sufficient time to receive result) if determination of carbohydrate, fat, and protein utilization desired

Ten hours before test

Patient fasting if measurement of energy *requirement* desired; may continue enteral or parenteral feeding, recognizing that results will reflect the patients energy expenditure in response to feeding and may be spuriously high if the patient is being overfed

Four hours before test

Patient resting and avoiding physical activity, physical therapy, dressing changes

Two hours before test

Endotracheal tube suctioned for the last time before test; further ventilator changes or suctioning avoided

One hour before test

Supine position, complete rest; analgesic or sedative administered if needed

If the patient is not agitated and a steady state of gas exchange can be achieved (even for as short a period as 5 minutes) during which the patient is not hyperventilating or hypoventilating, the results are likely to be a valid reflection of resting energy expenditure when extrapolated to 24 hours. If the patient is being chronically overfed, the measured energy expenditure may be falsely high. For example, if a patient has been regularly receiving 3000 kcal per day before and during the procedure and the measured energy expenditure is 2000 kcal per day, the calorie load can be reduced to the 2000 kcal level to better meet the patient's needs. To "fine-tune" treatment and more accurately estimate the patient's true energy requirements the test can be repeated. Conversely, starving or underfeeding a patient who is without significant physiologic stress may give a spuriously low estimate (by about 7% to 15%) of the patient's true energy needs. The opposite of the overfed patient approach can be used to obtain a more accurate assessment of the true energy needs.

The RQ (the ratio of CO_2 produced over O_2 consumed) provides information on substrate utilization. Each of the three major substrates has a unique RQ (0.7 for fat, 0.8 for protein, and 1 for carbohydrate), and the RQ obtained from the test reflects the proportions being utilized. For example, an RQ of 0.75 suggests that the patient is relying heavily on fat as a fuel (e.g., when energy intake is insufficient), whereas 0.9 indicates significant carbohydrate oxidation. However, each of the three substrates is inevitably being used to some extent. A value of greater than 1 suggests that the patient is receiving excess calories and synthesizing fat from carbohydrates. Measurement of the UUN allows an estimation of the amount of protein being catabolized; combining it with the RQ allows relatively accurate estimates of the amount of each of the fuels the patient is utilizing. See Chapter 13 for a discussion of the relative merits of the two forms of nonprotein calories (carbohydrate and fat) in the hospitalized patient. In patients who have pulmonary artery (Swan-Ganz) catheters, circulatory indirect calorimetry can also estimate resting energy expenditure.

PROTEIN REQUIREMENTS

Because the stress of illness usually increases protein catabolism and thereby protein requirements, the Recommended Dietary Allowance (RDA) of 0.8 g/kg per day is generally insufficient for acutely ill hospitalized patients. Protein requirements are frequently elevated twofold or more above usual levels—1.5 g/kg per day and sometimes as high as 3 g/kg per day is required.

The 24-hour UUN measurement is the most practical method for estimating a patient's protein catabolic rate, which is related to protein requirements (see Chapter 8).

An estimate of protein intake provided by a dietitian or calculated from enteral and parenteral feeding is compared with the protein catabolic rate to calculate protein balance:

Protein balance (g/day) = Protein intake −
Protein catabolic rate

A cushion of about 10 g per day above the estimated level of protein catabolism is useful to increase the certainty of a positive protein balance.

It is sometimes helpful to relate a patient's protein and energy requirements to each other. Healthy individuals need about 10% to 12% of energy as protein, but as physiologic stress increases the body derives an increasing proportion (15%, 20%, or even 25%) of its energy from protein. Therefore to avoid negative protein balance, hypermetabolic patients need a commensurate increase in protein intake.

Other groups that may benefit from relative protein intakes of 20% or greater are cachectic patients who accrue lean body mass more rapidly at these levels and elderly patients, especially those suffering from infections and other illnesses. However, when high protein intakes are used, the patient should be monitored for progressive azotemia (an increasing BUN level). When this occurs, it may be necessary to reduce the protein intake.

The relative protein content of a diet or feeding regimen is calculated as follows:

Relative protein content (% of kcal) =
$$\frac{\text{Protein content (g)} \times 4 \text{ kcal/g} \times 100}{\text{Energy content}}$$

For example,

$$\frac{100 \text{ g} \times 4 \text{ kcal/g} \times 100}{2000 \text{ kcal}} = 20\% \text{ protein}$$

Relating the energy and protein requirements calculated separately from BEE and UUN provides a cross-check to ensure that the relative protein content is in the desired range. When a UUN is not available, the equation can be rearranged to arrive at a desired protein intake:

Desired protein intake (g) =

$$\frac{\text{Energy requirement} \times \% \text{ protein desired}}{4 \text{ kcal/g} \times 100}$$

For example,

$$\frac{2000 \text{ kcal} \times 20\%}{4 \text{ kcal/g} \times 100} = 100 \text{ g}$$

Although adequate protein intake is required to support protein synthesis and prevent unnecessary wastage of muscle mass, it does not ensure that proteins (such as albumin) or muscle tissue will be synthesized. Inactive muscle cannot make full use of available amino acids, so exercise should be encouraged to to maintain and possibly build muscle mass.

Serum proteins such as albumin do not reflect changes in protein intake sensitively enough to be used to guide intake (see Chapter 8). However, if the serum albumin level falls during aggressive nutritional support, the protein balance should be reassessed to ensure that it is positive.

VITAMIN AND MINERAL ALLOWANCES

The micronutrient needs of many ill patients are higher than those listed in the RDAs (see Tables 2-1 and 2-2), but there are few clear guidelines for appropriate doses of micronutrients in individual patients. The principles discussed in previous chapters (see Chapters 1, 2, and 8) are helpful, but blood levels of vitamins, minerals, and trace elements must sometimes be measured to verify that doses are adequate. Even though blood levels are generally the best measures available, they do not always indicate sufficient levels in target tissues. Additional amounts of vitamins and minerals can be admixed with parenteral nutrition solutions, but supplements in enterally fed patients should be provided separately from the formula via an oral, tube, or intravenous route.

COMPLICATIONS OF NUTRITIONAL SUPPORT

The general complications of nutritional support are examined in this chapter. The specific complications of enteral and parenteral nutrition will be dealt with in Chapters 12 and 13.

The Hypometabolic, Starved Patient

Because chronically starved but otherwise unstressed patients are relatively well adapted to energy-deprived states, they are generally at greater immediate risk of death from inappropriate refeeding than from continued semistarvation. Hypophosphatemia and repletion heart failure are two consequences of refeeding that deserve special attention. Their pathophysiologic components are outlined in Table 9-1.

Hypophosphatemia

Potentially the most serious complication of refeeding, hypophosphatemia usually results from aggressive feeding using carbohydrate as the predominant energy source; this is especially true in parenteral nutrition. Because the metabolic rate and glucose oxidation are low during starvation, the need for phosphorus (used in glycolysis and ATP production) is relatively low. When glucose is infused, the demand for phosphorus increases dramatically and can exceed the body's ability to mobilize it from bone. When phosphate levels fall below 1 mg/dl, the risk of adverse clinical effects is high, especially (in the authors' experience) if there is concurrent hyperglycemia, which may reflect intracellular phosphate depletion. The complications of severe hypophosphatemia include weakness, muscle paralysis, decreased cardiac output, respiratory failure, decreased oxygen release from red blood cells, and decreased white blood cell bactericidal activity. Refeeding hypophosphatemia has caused cardiorespiratory failure and death within several days in patients who were chronically starved but otherwise stable.[1]

TABLE 9-1 Components of heart failure in the refeeding syndrome in cachectic patients

Underlying low cardiac output	+	Superimposed demand for increased cardiac output	→ Heart failure
Cardiac atrophy Low stroke volume		Fluid challenge ↑ plasma volume	Fluid overload
Low metabolic rate Low O_2 consumption Bradycardia		↑ catecholamines ↑ metabolic rate ↑ O_2 consumption	Cardiac and respiratory decompensation
Low blood pressure Low afterload		↑ blood pressure ↑ afterload	
Predominantly fatty acid utilization Low phosphorus requirement		Glucose challenge ↑ insulin Sodium retention ↓ phosphorus levels ↓ glycolysis ↑ blood glucose ↓ ATP production ↓ cardiac contractility ↓ minute ventilation	

Repletion Heart Failure

Repletion heart failure is another avoidable complication of refeeding starved patients. As stated by Ancel Keys, "The heart is closer to failure during early recovery than during starvation." During starvation, the metabolic rate and oxygen requirements fall as do cardiac output, blood pressure, and heart rate. During repletion, the metabolic rate rises, demand for cardiac output increases, plasma volume expands, and blood pressure rises—all potentially leading to repletion heart failure (see Table 9-1).

The Hypermetabolic, Stressed Patient

As noted in Chapter 8, energy requirements are increased in physiologically stressed patients. However, if these patients' energy needs are exceeded, especially through the use of glucose, the already elevated resting energy expenditure and oxygen consumption may be further increased, perhaps through increased catecholamine production. In essence, excessive glucose calories seem to stoke an already hot furnace. This increases demand for cardiac output, which may have consequences in patients with cardiac instability. Excessive energy loads increase the demand for oxygen—a detriment in patients with hypoxic lung disease. In addition, excessive calories can increase carbon dioxide production significantly, possibly requiring a significant increase in minute ventilation. In this setting, patients with ventilatory compromise such as chronic lung disease or those on fixed-rate ventilators can develop carbon dioxide retention and respiratory acidosis. Overfeeding, especially from TPN, may also promote fat deposition in the liver and cause abnormal liver function tests. Thus in hypermetabolic patients the aim of nutritional support should be to meet but not exceed energy needs.

THE SELECTIVE APPROACH TO NUTRITIONAL SUPPORT

Formulating an appropriate feeding approach requires distinguishing whether the patient is hypometabolic or hypermetabolic (Table 9-2).

The Hypometabolic, Starved Patient

The absence of significant physiologic stress in the hypometabolic, starved patient can be documented with a 24-hour UUN, which should show that 5 g or less of nitrogen is being excreted per day if protein intake is low. Because the major risk in this situation is excessively rapid refeeding, nutritional support of these patients should be initiated and increased cautiously, taking up to a week to

TABLE 9-2 Selective approaches to nutritional support

Patient type	Aim	Nutritional support	Precautions	Error likely
Hypometabolic, starved	Rebuild	Cautious with portion of fuel as fat	Hypophosphatemia, repletion heart failure	Commission (overzealous support)
Hypermetabolic, stressed	Replace	Aggressive but not excessive	Excessive O_2 consumption and CO_2 production	Omission (inadequate support)

TABLE 9-3	Energy goals in refeeding a hypometabolic, starved patient

Days	Energy goal
1-2	BEE × 0.8
3-4	BEE × 1
4-6	BEE × 1.2-1.5
6+	BEE × 2 if weight gain desired

reach the final energy goal (Table 9-3). This is the main means of preventing both hypophosphatemia and heart failure because it allows the patient time to adapt to new energy and glucose loads.

The enteral feeding route should be used whenever possible, and the diet or formula should be relatively high in protein as discussed previously. If the intravenous route is required, initially a third or more of the energy should be provided as lipids to minimize the glucose load. With either type of feeding, normal phosphorus levels should be documented before repletion and monitored daily during the initial period of refeeding. When parenteral feeding is used, the need for fairly high doses of phosphorus (up to 1 mmol/kg per day) should be anticipated, and phosphorus should be included in the first few bags or bottles of parenteral solution.

The Hypermetabolic, Stressed Patient

The clinical judgment of the level of physiologic stress in critically ill patients is supported by measurements of the metabolic rate and/or 24-hour UUN excretion. A UUN value greater than approximately 10 g per day when protein intake is relatively low suggests significant stress. Underfeeding a hypermetabolic patient creates a high risk for developing kwashiorkor. In these situations, nutritional support should be approached aggressively to meet but not *exceed* the patient's requirements. It is often possible to reach the goal for energy and protein intake within 24 to 36 hours of initiating enteral or parenteral support. Even if the patient is cachetic, documentation of a hypermetabolic state should prompt aggressive nutritional support that reaches the energy and protein goals within 2 to 3 days.

EFFECTS OF NUTRITIONAL SUPPORT ON PATIENT OUTCOME

Documenting the effects of nutritional support on the outcome of patient care has been difficult and controversial. In part, the difficulty relates to ethical problems in randomizing patients to feeding and nonfeeding groups. Therefore most randomized trials have enrolled patients in whom aggressive nutritional support is discretionary, especially those facing elective surgery. Nearly all of these trials have used parenteral nutrition as the study treatment. Some studies have shown less mortality and intraabdominal abscesses, peritonitis, anastomotic leaks, and ileus in patients treated with parenteral nutrition.[2] However, others have documented significantly higher rates of sepsis in these patients. In a cooperative study conducted in Veterans Affairs hospitals, preoperative TPN only benefited patients with significant protein-energy malnutrition (PEM); the types of PEM were not distinguished.[3] In the less severely malnourished patients, TPN was associated with *net harm* in the form of higher sepsis rates.

Using these results, some observers have argued that parenteral feeding should be avoided, even if it means that patients go unfed for up to 3 weeks.[4] However, a more reasonable response is to assume that enteral feeding will produce better outcomes (although few trials have directly addressed this issue[5]) and make aggressive efforts to access the gastrointestinal tract for feeding after 5 to 7 days of insufficient intake. The indications for using TPN should be fairly restrictive (see Chapter 13) but not avoided when the only alternative is protracted inadequate nutrient intake.

References

1. Weinsier RL, Krumdieck CL: Death resulting from overzealous total parenteral nutrition: the refeeding syndrome revisited, *Am J Clin Nutr* 34:393, 1981.
2. Muller JM et al: Preoperative parenteral feeding in patients with gastrointestinal carcinoma, *Lancet* 1:68, 1982.
3. Veterans Affairs Total Parenteral Nutrition Cooperative Study Group: Perioperative total parenteral nutrition in surgical patients, *N Engl J Med* 325:525, 1991.
4. Koretz RL: Nutritional supplementation in the ICU: how critical is nutrition for the critically ill? *Am J Resp Crit Care Med* 151:570, 1995.
5. Moore FA et al: Early enteral feeding, compared with parenteral, reduces postoperative septic complications: the results of a meta-analysis, *Ann Surg* 216:172, 1992.

Suggested Readings

Aspen: Guidelines for the use of parenteral and enteral nutrition in adult and pediatric patients, *JPEN* 17(S4):1SA, 1993.

Rombeau JL, Caldwell MD, eds: *Clinical nutrition: parenteral feeding,* ed 2, Philadelphia, 1992, WB Saunders.

Rombeau JL, Caldwell MD, eds: *Clinical nutrition: enteral and tube feeding,* ed 2, Philadelphia, 1990, WB Saunders.

Torosian MH, ed: *Nutrition for the hospitalized patient,* New York, 1995, Marcel Dekker.

10

The Nutrition Support Team

When instituting nutritional support such as enteral or parenteral nutrition, it is important to perform a nutritional assessment, develop and implement a nutrition care plan, monitor for tolerance and complications, and decide when to terminate the support or transition to other modes of feeding. This is a complex process and requires specialized training, knowledge, and expertise in nutritional support. For this reason, nutrition support teams (NSTs) or services have emerged to provide a coordinated and systematic approach to the various facets of nutrition support. Although NSTs first appeared over 20 years ago and their numbers are rising, the majority of hospitals do not have NSTs. In a 1991 survey of all hospitals with more than 150 beds, only 30% had NSTs and 17% planned to establish one within 2 years.

COMPOSITION AND FUNCTIONS
OF A NUTRITION SUPPORT TEAM

An NST typically consists of a dietitian, nurse, pharmacist, and physician. It may also include a social worker, respiratory therapist, PhD with nutrition expertise, and trainees from any of these disciplines who are on a nutrition rotation. Often the team is directed by a physician with expertise in nutrition, but other members of the team may serve as directors as well. There are few programs that provide formal training for nutritional support (except for those programs for dietitians and physicians), so most team members must obtain their expertise on the job. NST members may take examinations sponsored by the American Society for Parenteral and Enteral Nutrition (ASPEN) to be recognized as specialists in nutritional support. The American Board of Nutrition certifies physicians and individuals with PhDs who have broad training and experience in clinical nutrition.

Each member has a valuable role to contribute to the overall mission of the NST, which is to ensure that nutrition services are delivered in an appropriate, a safe, an efficient, and a cost-effective manner. The box on p. 228 outlines typical duties of each member of the NST. To a limited degree, members may perform some of the duties listed for other members. For the NST to be successful, it is important for the members to work together well. Team-building activities may help to improve this process.

In some institutions the NST automatically evaluates and tracks all patients on involuntary nutritional support, especially TPN. In others the team only provides consultation on request from the primary physicians. Some NSTs write the nutritional support orders themselves, and others make recommendations to the patient's primary physicians who are responsible for writing the orders. Having the NST write the orders is likely to maintain greater consistency in patient care and perhaps the lowest rate of metabolic complications. However, the consultative approach has the advantage of keeping the primary physicians in charge of patient management and promotes the teaching of nutritional support principles to the primary care team, which often includes medical students and residents. An optimal approach takes local institutional factors into consideration.

BENEFITS OF A NUTRITION SUPPORT TEAM

The potential benefits of NSTs are listed in the box on p. 230. Having an NST can result in decreased infectious and metabolic complications because of the close monitoring and TPN expertise used. By using appropriate amounts of parenteral nutrition only when indicated, an NST might

TYPICAL DUTIES OF NUTRITION SUPPORT TEAM MEMBERS

Physician

Provides leadership and directs the NST

Interprets medical information relative to nutritional support

Performs nutritional assessment—confirms history, performs physical examination, reviews laboratory data

Integrates information from other team members to develop a management plan

Assumes final responsibility for recommendations and patient care

Dietitian

Performs nutrition screening and identifies high-risk patients

Performs nutritional assessment

Determines energy and protein needs

Translates dietary prescriptions into food and/or tube feeding selections

Monitors and records energy and protein intakes

Monitors transitions in feeding

Serves as a resource for dietary issues including enteral nutrition products and costs and enteral feeding formulary

Nurse

Monitors nursing issues related to administration of nutritional support

Monitors care of feeding-access devices (catheters, feeding tubes, etc.)

Teaches and serves as a resource for patients, families, and other nurses

Pharmacist

Participates in formulating and compounding TPN solutions

Monitors quality control of TPN solutions

TYPICAL DUTIES OF NUTRITION SUPPORT TEAM MEMBERS—CONT'D

Pharmacist—cont'd

Acts as a resource for drug-related issues (drug-nutrient interactions, appropriateness of medications, compatibility of medications with TPN or enteral feedings)

Monitors TPN data

Participates in developing and maintaining a cost-effective nutritional support formulary

Any member of the NST

Ensures Joint Commission on Accreditation of Healthcare Organizations (JCAHO) standards are met

Conducts research

Provides educational programs

Deals with administrative issues

Participates in designing, implementing, and managing nutrition care plans

Provides discharge planning and outpatient management of nutritional care plans

Monitors laboratory data

Collects continuous quality improvement data

Develops materials for patient instruction and institutional procedures/guidelines

Serves as NST liaison with own or other departments

Writes procedural guidelines related to nutritional support for own department

---

reduce the costs of nutritional support. Members of an NST can participate in research studies or the education of residents, physicians, and other health care professionals. These factors may translate into improved outcomes in patient care. Although some studies have demonstrated these benefits, others have not; there is no doubt this is partly a result of the difficulties of conducting research in this area. Comparative studies that examined the effects of NSTs were generally conducted during the 1970s and

POTENTIAL BENEFITS OF A NUTRITION SUPPORT TEAM

Decreased complications

Septic
Metabolic
Mechanical (catheter related)
Drug-nutrient interactions

Decreased costs

Use of enteral feeding instead of TPN whenever possible
Decreased number of days on TPN
Use of individualized goals to avoid overfeeding
Restricted use of expensive nonstandard TPN and enteral
    formulas unless clear indications
Decreased errors in ordering and decreased waste of TPN
Potential decrease in length of hospital stay

Research
Education
Improved patient care, nutritional status, and other
    outcomes

early 1980s when two major changes—the initiation of
NSTs and development of standard hospital TPN protocols—were occurring simultaneously. Therefore it is difficult to distinguish the independent effects of these two
variables.

The main drawback of an NST is the cost of its members' salaries. However, in most cases only a portion of
each member's time and salary is devoted to nutritional
support activities. Although not conclusively shown, it is
quite likely that savings in nutritional support costs generated by an NST can offset its financial overhead.

REIMBURSEMENT FOR SERVICES

In addition to cost savings, NSTs can recoup some of
their costs by increasing the hospital's compensation for
patient care and/or obtaining direct reimbursement for

| Table 10-1 | ICD-9 codes for nutritional comorbidities or complications |

Nutritional diagnosis	ICD-9 code
Kwashiorkor	260
Marasmus	261
Marasmic kwashiorkor	262
Other protein-calorie malnutrition	
Moderate (60%-75% ideal body weight)	263
Mild (75%-90% ideal body weight)	263.1

their services. Diagnosis-related groups (DRGs) have become the standard method of reimbursement for hospital care. In addition to the primary diagnosis, complications and comorbid conditions such as malnutrition can contribute to the patient's DRG and thus to the total reimbursement. Table 10-1 lists the nutritional diagnostic codes that may impact reimbursement. In the official ICD-9-CM coding booklet the terms *marasmus, kwashiorkor,* and *marasmic kwashiorkor* are imprecisely defined and for coding purposes can be applied more loosely than indicated in Chapter 7.

In addition, other diagnoses such as specific vitamin deficiencies or toxicities may be coded. Full reimbursement will not be received unless all applicable diagnoses are appropriately coded. As discussed in Chapter 7, the prevalence of hospital-associated malnutrition is high enough that the reimbursement resulting from these diagnoses could theoretically be significant. However, a mitigating factor is that many patients requiring nutritional support are critically ill and already qualify for a maximum DRG. In this case, coding for nutritional diagnoses may not increase reimbursement. Nevertheless, having an NST with experts in nutritional assessment and diagnosis can help to ensure that all patients are properly diagnosed and treated and that sufficient information is recorded in their charts to maximize reimbursement.

Other services that may provide financial support for an NST include indirect calorimetry and placement of peripherally inserted central catheters (PICCs), both of which can be carried out by members who are not physicians. Placement of centrally inserted venous catheters or percutaneous endoscopic gastrostomy (PEG) tubes may also provide reimbursements if the physicians on the NST have the expertise to provide these services. To continue to justify the presence of an NST in the current economic environment, it is important to attempt to document cost savings and revenues as much as possible.

STANDARDS FOR NUTRITIONAL CARE

For hospitals to maintain accreditation they must meet standards of quality in patient care set by the JCAHO. These standards, including those that pertain to nutrition, have undergone substantial revisions over the past few years. They emphasize interdisciplinary delivery of care and focus on outcome measures of performance (e.g., complications and mortality).

JCAHO standards require that all hospital patients be screened to identify those who are nutritionally at risk; these patients must have nutritional assessments performed. A plan for nutritional therapy must be developed for all hospitalized patients, particularly those at risk. Ongoing monitoring for the effectiveness of the nutritional therapy must be in place. Because of the emphasis on an interdisciplinary approach (i.e., all medical personnel being responsible for ensuring that the standards are met), NSTs are ideal for designing and implementing programs to meet JCAHO standards.

OTHER SETTINGS FOR NUTRITION SUPPORT TEAMS

The NST model can also be applied to an out-of-hospital nutrition practice. Maintaining continuity in the transition to posthospital care is important. A patient leaving the hospital who needs home parenteral nutrition is a good example of a case in which a smooth transition is critical. By utilizing a team approach to issues related to home TPN, such as catheter care, medication administration, education of patients and their families, and dietary allowances, the NST can help ease the transition from the hospital to the home.

Ambulatory care in a nutrition clinic also lends itself to a team approach. In this setting, nursing and pharmacy may not occupy roles that are as visible as they are in the inpatient setting, but the combined input of physicians and dietitians are central to outpatient nutrition care. A clinical psychologist must also be included if the clinic treats patients with eating disorders. It is important to have one member, usually a physician, with expertise in nutrition who is responsible for overall direction and coordination of care.

STARTING A NUTRITION SUPPORT TEAM

The positive effects of NST consultations, particularly automatic ones, depend largely on local institutional factors. Before assuming that automatic consultations or the writing of orders are needed from an NST, the nature and severity of the local problems should be evaluated. Less costly approaches, such as changes in standard order forms or reducing the number of people involved in monitoring (especially of catheter insertion and care) from a multidisciplinary group to a single person, may furnish some of the benefits of an NST. On the other hand, in hospitals where inexperienced physicians write TPN orders only occasionally, where complication rates are unacceptable, and/or where TPN is used inappropriately in place of enteral feeding, central management by an NST may be required.

Starting an NST can be a large undertaking but is easier if certain steps are followed. Initially, individuals from dietetics, nursing, pharmacy, and the medical staff who have an interest in nutritional support should be identified. Physicians from different divisions including gastroenterology, surgery, critical care, and nutrition (if a department exists) should represent the medical staff. Key leaders who can offer support should be identified in each area and should be involved in the development process. Specific local needs and objectives such as refining TPN ordering or improving compliance with JCAHO standards should be addressed. Consideration could be given to collecting data on quality or cost savings to help justify an NST.

Once an NST is established, it can have a number of functions. Continuous quality-improvement programs related to screening and assessment, complications, and appropriate energy and protein goals can be developed. Protocols can be established for administering nutritional support that follow practice guidelines established by AS-PEN. It is important to continue collecting data on complications, cost savings, and attainment of JCAHO standards. Programs for educating other medical personnel can also be developed, such as nutrition support rotations for trainees in all the disciplines represented by the NST.

Suggested Readings

Clemmer TP: Nutrition support teams: role in the new health care environment, *Nutr Clin Pract* 9:217, 1994.

Gales BJ, Gales MJ: Nutritional support teams: a review of comparative trials, *Ann Pharmacother* 28:227, 1994.

Special reports: focus on nutrition support teams: a review of comparative trials, *Ann Pharmacother* 28:227, 1994.

Special reports: health care in transition. Charting a course for nutrition support professionals, *Nutr Clin Practice* 10:1S-82S, 1995.

Wesley JR: Nutrition support teams: past, present, and future, *Nutr Clin Prac* 10:219, 1995.

11

Therapeutic Diets

Diet is the most important aspect of therapy in the treatment of many disease states, complementing and even replacing drugs in some cases. Therapeutic diets represent permutations of the general dietary guidelines described in Chapter 1. A useful schema of therapeutic diets has a breakdown of the general diet into its basic components (water, carbohydrate, fiber, protein, fat, vitamins, minerals, and other substances such as alcohol) and consistencies (liquid, soft, or solid). It is possible to alter (restrict or increase) each of these to form therapeutic diets as shown by the following examples:

- Fluid-modified diet: restricted fluid for treating heart or renal failure
- Carbohydrate-modified diet: for treating diabetes and/or hypertriglyceridemia
- Protein-modified diet: low protein for treating unstressed patients with chronic renal failure; high protein for treating stressed patients
- Fat-modified diet: low total and saturated fat for treating hypercholesterolemia; low total fat for treating malabsorption syndromes
- Mineral-modified diet: low sodium, potassium, and phosphorus for treating renal failure
- Other substances diet: restricted alcohol for treating hypertriglyceridemia
- Modified-consistency diet: soft diets for treating patients without teeth; high fiber for treating constipation

MODIFIED DIETS: CONSISTENCY

Clear-liquid diet (nutritionally incomplete)

This diet consists of clear fluids that leave little residue and are absorbed with minimum digestive activity; it includes only broth, gelatin, strained fruit juice, clear beverages, and low-residue supplements. Because some of these liquids have high osmolalities, they may not be well tolerated by some patients. Clear liquids generally do not provide the Recommended Dietary Allowances (RDAs) for any nutrients, except perhaps vitamin C. They should not be used for more than 2 to 3 days without supplementation.

Full-liquid diet

This diet includes food that is liquid at room temperature. Many foods such as whole milk, custard, pudding, strained cream soups, eggnog, and ice cream contain fat and lactose, which some patients tolerate poorly. Complete enteral supplements may be preferred in such cases or may be added to increase calories and protein (see Chapter 12). This diet can meet the RDA for all nutrients except iron for women of childbearing age. Modifications of the full-liquid diet can be made, such as creating one that is high in protein/calories or low in fat. To minimize lactose intake, lactose-free, oral-feeding supplements and lactase-treated dairy products may be used.

A consultation with a registered or licensed dietitian is invaluable for assistance in prescribing and monitoring therapeutic diets. Tables 11-1 to 11-6 outline diets for specific medical conditions and with particular modifications. Consistency-modified diets are described in the box. The rationales for many of the therapeutic diet are explained in subsequent chapters.

Text continued on p. 262.

MODIFIED DIETS: CONSISTENCY—CONT'D

Soft diet

A soft diet consists of food that is tender but not ground or pureed. Whole meat, cooked vegetables, and fruit of moderate fiber content (e.g., canned) are allowed. This diet generally excludes fried food, most raw fruit and vegetables, and very coarse bread and cereal and is fairly low in fiber and residue. The gastrointestinal soft diet omits highly seasoned, spicy food and food that is high in fiber.

Pureed or ground diet

This diet includes food that is especially easy to masticate and swallow. It is useful for patients who have dysphagia or dental problems.

Low-fiber, low-residue diet

This diet is intended to reduce fecal bulk and restricts intake of milk, whole-grain bread and cereal, fruit, and certain vegetables.

High-fiber diet

This diet includes unrefined starch (whole-grain bread, brown rice, potatoes, corn, beans), raw fruit, and vegetables. Bran and other fibers may be added if desired.

TABLE 11-1 Diets according to diagnosis

Diagnostic category	Diet order	Comments
Cardiovascular diseases, hyperlipidemias		
Congestive heart failure (CHF)	Sodium-restricted Fat restricted (see hypercholesterolemia)	Specify grams of sodium. Initially 1-2 g are suggested for acute CHF. A more severe restriction such as 0.5-1 g is occasionally required.
Hypertension	Sodium-restricted	Specify grams of sodium (usually 2-3 g).
Myocardial infarction	Sodium- and fat-restricted	Specify grams of sodium and fat. In some cases, caffeine may be restricted.
Hypercholesterolemia (see Chapter 18)	Low-fat, low-cholesterol	Specify percent calories as fat and milligrams cholesterol. The *step I diet* is as follows: <300 mg cholesterol, <30% calories as fat, <10% of calories as saturated fat, 10%-15% of calories as monounsaturated fats, ≤10% of calories as polyunsaturated fatty acids daily. The *step II diet* is as follows: <200 mg cholesterol, <30% of calories as fat, <7% of calories as saturated fat, 10%-15% of calories as monounsaturated fats, and ≤10% of calories as polyunsaturated fatty acids daily.

Hypertriglyc-eridemia	Moderate restriction in total fat; sucrose and alcohol-restricted; calories to achieve or maintain ideal body weight	Specify % calories as fat (generally <30% of calories from fat with increased servings of complex carbohydrates, such as fruit and vegetables, and starches). Concentrated sweets are restricted.
Endocrine and metabolic disorders		
Diabetes mellitus, Type I, insulin-dependent (see Chapter 16 for more details)	Low-fat, low-cholesterol, high fiber, appropriately-timed	Coordinate meals with insulin regimen and blood glucose monitoring schedule. Fat and cholesterol are the same as for Step I or II diet, depending on LDL cholesterol levels. The remainder of calories are from monounsaturated fats and carbohydrates. Individualize intake of carbohydrates based on caloric needs, eating habits, and glucose and lipid control. Sucrose, fructose, and sucrose-containing foods may be substituted for other carbohydrates in the meal plan. Use nonnutritive sweeteners in moderation. Fiber intake should be 20-35 g/day.

Continued

TABLE 11-1 Diets according to diagnosis—cont'd

Diagnostic category	Diet order	Comments
Endocrine and metabolic disorders—cont'd		
Diabetes mellitus, Type II, non–insulin-dependent (see Chapter 16)	Low-fat, low-cholesterol, high-fiber	This has the same considerations as Type I diabetes, with emphasis on achieving glucose, lipid, and blood pressure goals. Weight reduction is beneficial even if ideal body weight is not achieved.
Hypoglycemia, postprandial	Restricted in refined sugars; six small meals daily	Low in refined carbohydrates and high in complex carbohydrates and protein. The diabetic exchange system can be used to optimize the diet. Diagnosis of hypoglycemia is often questionable.
Gout	Purine-restricted	Follow the general dietary guidelines. Control weight. Avoid fasts or severe calorie- and carbohydrate-restricted diets that elevate uric acid levels. Use alcohol and purine-rich foods (organ meats, anchovies, sardines, meat extracts) only in moderation.

Obesity (see Chapter 15)	Weight reduction	Specify calories to achieve 1-2 lb of weight loss per week. Less than 1000 kcal/day is generally not recommended because of difficulty in achieving nutritional adequacy. Low-fat, high-fiber diets are optimal for long-term weight reduction.
Gastrointestinal conditions		
Esophageal stricture	Either high-protein-high-calorie full liquid diet, enteral formulas, or pureed diet; may progress to soft diet with small, frequent feedings	Use tube feeding if oral intake is insufficient and enteral access can be established.
Hiatal hernia with esophagitis, gastroesophageal reflux, peptic ulcer disease	Individualized, eliminating symptom-causing foods	Foods may be irritating via 3 mechanisms: 1. Direct irritation because of osmolality, astringency, or acidity (e.g., citrus juice, spicy food) 2. Increased gastric secretions (e.g., coffee, alcohol) 3. Relaxed lower esophageal sphincter (chocolate)

Continued

TABLE 11-1 Diets according to diagnosis—cont'd

Diagnostic category	Diet order	Comments
Gastrointestinal conditions—cont'd		
Postgastrectomy	Postgastrectomy	Postgastrectomy patients are at risk for weight loss, anemia (vitamin B_{12}, folate, and iron deficiencies), dumping syndrome, diarrhea, and reactive hypoglycemia.
		Frequency and volume of feedings should be individualized to patient tolerance.
		Fluid and meals should initially be separated and fluid intake adjusted to tolerance.
		Simple sugars should be omitted initially but can often be included later.
		Lactose intolerance may be present.
		A low-fiber diet is often helpful initially, and fiber may be added as the patient progresses.
Gastric reduction/ gastroplasty	Gastric reduction	Individualize to the patient and the postoperative interval as follows:
		Provide a clear liquid diet for the first several postoperative days. Use small, frequent feedings. A clear liquid supplement can be useful.

		When tolerated, advance to six small meals of pureed foods, and then to solid foods.
		Liquids should generally be separated from solid foods.
		Monitor the patient to ensure nutritional adequacy; vitamin and mineral supplements may be needed.
		Monitor the patient's rate of weight loss closely.
Celiac disease (gluten enteropathy, nontropical sprue)	Gluten-free	Celiac disease is hypersensitivity to the protein gliadin.
		Wheat, rye, oats, barley, and food containing these grains should be omitted from the diet.
		Corn, rice, tapioca, soybeans, arrowroot, and potato flours can be used as substitutes.
Constipation, diverticulosis, hemorrhoids	High-fiber (20 to 35 g/day)	Soluble fibers include gums, mucilages, pectins, and hemicelluloses. Food sources include fruit and vegetables, barley, oats, oat bran, and legumes (dried beans and peas).
		Insoluble fibers include cellulose, lignin, and some hemicelluloses. Food sources include fruit, vegetables, cereal, whole-wheat products, and wheat bran.
		An excessive intakes of fiber may reduce the absorption of calcium, copper, iron, magnesium, selenium, and zinc.
		Try dietary sources of fiber before using fiber supplements.

Continued

TABLE 11-1 Diets according to diagnosis—cont'd

Diagnostic category	Diet order	Comments
Gastrointestinal conditions—cont'd		
Acute inflammatory bowel disease	Individualized	A soft, low-fiber diet may be tolerated.
		Bowel rest with total parenteral nutrition may be useful if oral intake is not tolerated (e.g., because of strictures).
Chronic inflammatory bowel disease, regional enteritis (Crohn's disease of the small intestine)	Individualized	Many patients have no food intolerances (i.e., no clear links between food and symptoms) and should not be restricted.
		However, some patients may benefit from avoiding lactose, highly osmotic fruit juice, alcohol, and caffeine.
		Patients with significant bowel narrowing benefit from a low-fiber diet that includes beans, nuts, and seeds.
		Malabsorption may be present, especially after bowel resection. A low-fat diet with medium-chain triglyceride (MCT) supplementation may be beneficial. Home parenteral nutrition is helpful or lifesaving in severe malabsorption.
		Pay careful attention to fat-soluble vitamins, folic acid, and vitamin B_{12} status (especially if there is ileal involvement).

Ulcerative colitis	Individualized	Patients with extensive or acute colitis may benefit from avoiding high-fiber foods, but fiber restriction is not recommended or required for all patients. Lactose intolerance should be suspected. Avoiding highly spiced foods, highly osmotic fruit juice, caffeine, and alcohol may be useful for some patients.
Irritable bowel syndrome	High-fiber	High-fiber diets may be useful. Consider a trial of restrictions of lactose, caffeine, and spicy foods. Remove restrictions that provide no benefits.
Milk/lactose intolerance	Lactose-restricted	Lactose is a disaccharide of glucose and galactose and is found in milk products. Lactase deficiency may be congenital or acquired and occurs in degrees. Some lactase-deficient individuals can tolerate small amounts of lactose, such as milk used in preparing food. Those individuals with the most severe lactase deficiencies must avoid all milk-containing products (including products prepared with milk or milk powder as a component).

Continued

TABLE 11-1 Diets according to diagnosis—cont'd

Diagnostic category	Diet order	Comments
Gastrointestinal conditions—cont'd		
Milk/lactose intolerance—cont'd		Those individuals with less severe deficiencies often tolerate cultured dairy products (buttermilk, acidophilus milk, yogurt, cottage cheese) in which bacteria have largely digested the lactose.
		Lactase enzyme is available for addition to foods or consumption before eating lactose-containing foods.
		Nondairy supplements can be used as milk substitutes.
		Lactalbumin, lactate, and calcium compounds do not contain lactose.
Malabsorption (see Chapter 20)	Low-fat, individualized	Fat restriction is indicated if there is symptomatic steatorrhea or if there is divalent cation deficiency (i.e., Ca, Mg, Zn). A suggested restriction is 40-50 g fat/day.
	MCTs	MCT and MCT-containing products can be used to add a readily absorbed source of calories.
		MCTs, which are comprised of fattty acids only 8 to 10 carbons long, are readily absorbed with minimal digestion; the majority enter the portal system rather than the lymphatic system.

Acute pancreatitis	Progress from nothing by mouth to oral intake as tolerated	MCTs can replace long-chain triglycerides in the diet for energy purposes but do not satisfy essential fatty acid requirements. MCTs are available as an oil, a powdered formula, and in complete oral feeding formulas (e.g., Lipisorb). MCTs can be combined in a blender with beverages, used in fried and sautéed foods, and added to cereal, vegetables, and potatoes. MCTs are usually added to a 25-50 g total fat diet Parenteral nutrition is indicated for severe cases.
Pancreatic insufficiency	Low-fat	The suggested restriction is 40-50 g fat/day usually with pancreatic enzyme replacement. MCT supplementation is useful if additional calories are needed. Monitor fat-soluble vitamin status; vitamin and mineral supplementation is usually indicated.

Continued

TABLE 11-1 Diets according to diagnosis—cont'd

Diagnostic category	Diet order	Comments
Gastrointestinal conditions—cont'd		
Hepatic insufficiency without encephalopathy (see Chapter 20)	Regular ± sodium-restricted	Use high-calorie, high-protein diet if weight gain is desired. Fat restriction is unnecessary unless fat malabsorption is symptomatic. Assess vitamin and mineral statuses and use supplementation if indicated. Restrict sodium to 1-3 g/day if ascites or edema is present.
Hepatic encephalopathy (see Chapter 20)	Protein- and sodium-restricted vs. branched-chain amino acid modified	With history or likelihood of encephalopathy, restrict protein to 0.5-0.7 g/kg dry body weight. This may be increased according to tolerance or as encephalopathy improves. Restrict sodium and fluid intake if edema or ascites is present. Branched-chain amino acid products (Hepatamine, HepaticAid, etc.) are useful if encephalopathy does not respond to other therapies. Generally 1.2-1.5 g/kg are prescribed (i.e., protein restriction is removed).

Gallbladder disease	Individualized; calories for desirable weight, restriction of fat and alcohol	Consult dietitian to obtain patient tolerances. Provide small, frequent meals. If the patient has chronic cholecystitis and dyspepsia, restrict to 40-50 g fat/day. If the patient has acute cholecystitis, restrict to 25-30 g fat/day while in hospital only.
Renal disorders Chronic renal insufficiency (pre-end-stage, see Chapter 23)	Individualized for degree of renal impairment; consideration of protein, sodium, potassim, and fluid restrictions	Tailor energy intake to the patient. Generally, 25-40 kcal/kg ideal body weight is recommended. If weight loss is a problem, caloric intake should be increased. If hypertension and edema are problems, restrict sodium (1-3 g/day) and fluid. Consider protein restriction if dialysis is avoided. However, prolonged protein restriction will cause negative nitrogen balance. In advanced renal insufficiency, potassium, magnesium, and phosphorus are restricted. Phosphorus intake should generally be around 8-12 mg/kg ideal body weight, and phosphorus binders (antacids) should be used.

Continued

TABLE 11-1 Diets according to diagnosis—cont'd

Diagnostic category	Diet order	Comments
Renal disorders—cont'd		
Chronic renal insufficiency—cont'd		Calcium intake should be around 1200-1600 mg/day; supplements are often required.
		1,25-dihydroxy vitamin D (Rocaltrol) may be required.
		Avoid large doses of vitamin A because patients with renal insufficiency are at risk for vitamin A toxicity.
		Assess trace element needs (e.g., iron, zinc).
		Rule out hyperlipidemias.
		If diabetes is present, see previous diabetic guidelines, and chapter 16.
End-stage renal disease (ESRD) with dialysis (see Chapter 23)	Individualized	Adjust energy for activity level and body weight: *Hemodialysis:* 30-35 kcal/kg ideal body weight/day *Peritoneal dialysis:* 25-35 kcal/kg ideal body weight/day Protein: *Hemodialysis:* 1.1-1.4 g/kg ideal body weight/day *Peritoneal dialysis:* 1.2-1.5 g/kg ideal body weight/day

Phosphorus:

Both hemodialysis and peritoneal dialysis: ≤17 mg/kg ideal body weight/day

Sodium:

Hemodialysis: 2-3 g/day

Peritoneal dialysis: 2-4 g/day

Potassium:

Hemodialysis: about 40 mg/kg ideal body weight/day

Peritoneal dialysis: typically unrestricted

Fluid restriction needs vary according to urine output and the patient's condition:

Hemodialysis: generally 500-750 ml + urine output or 1000 ml/day if the patient is anuric.

Peritoneal dialysis: generally around 2000 ml/day

Calcium supplementation in hemodialysis and peritoneal dialysis depends on serum level.

Adjust energy intake to promote weight loss or weight gain as needed.

Posttransplant (see chapter 28) — Individualized

Continued

TABLE 11-1 Diets according to diagnosis—cont'd

Diagnostic category	Diet order	Comments
Renal disorders— cont'd		
Posttransplant —cont'd		Protein needs are determined by degree of catabolism and interval posttransplant:
		First month: 1.3-2 g/kg ideal body weight/day, thereafter 1 g/kg ideal body weight/day
		Restrict sodium initially to between 500 mg and 2 g/day.
Miscellaneous disorders		
Corticosteroid therapy	Low-sodium, high-protein	Steroid therapy can cause proteolysis, sodium retention, and glucose intolerance.
		Note recommendations for diabetics, above.
Dental impairment	Ground, pureed, or full liquid	See previous box on modified diets (consistency).
		A patient should not use a straw with fresh dental sutures.
Diets for diagnostic tests		
72-hour stool fat	100 g fat or regular	The diet should contain 80-100 g fat/day and should be consumed for 3 days before and during the stool collection.
		Daily fecal fat should be <6% of intake.
		Intake should be monitored to document adequate fat intake.

Glucose tolerance test	Regular	At least 150 g/day of carbohydrates for several days before the test, because carbohydrate restriction can give a falsely abnormal glucose tolerance test. No food or beverages except water should be consumed for 10-14 hours prior to the test.
5-hydroxyindole-acetic acid (5-HIAA) test	5-HIAA or low serotonin	This test is used to detect carcinoid tumors. The diet is consumed for 3 days followed by a 24-hr urine sample to measure 5-HIAA. Avoid bananas, tomatoes, tomato juice, pineapple, pineapple juice, avocados, eggplant, plums, kiwi, walnuts, and pecans.
Urine hydroxyproline test	Hydroxyproline test or collagen-free	This test is used in the diagnosis of metabolic bone diseases. The diet is consumed for 1-2 days followed by a 24-hr urine sample to measure hydroxyproline. Food to avoid includes all meats; animal bones, skin, cartilage; fish; gelatin and gelatin-containing foods; turkey rolls; ham; other meats with gelatin; broth; bouillon; gravy; and ice creams made with gelatin stabilizers. Urinary tests for collagen crosslinks (pyridinoline and deoxypyridinoline) avoid the need for a special test diet.

TABLE 11-2   Modified diets: fat

Daily fat intake	Food limitation	Practicality
90-110 g (35%-40% of calories*)	—	Average American diet
65-80 g (25%-30% of calories)	Meat is limited to 8-9 oz/day. (One egg = 1 oz meat.) Fat is limited to 3-7 tsp butter, mayonnaise, salad dressing, or oil. Whole milk intake is in limited amounts. All products prepared with fat (biscuits, cornbread, cakes, pastries, fried food) are excluded unless fat in these products is counted as a part of the total fat allowance.	Very practical for home use and recommended for all; easily manipulated according to patient preferences

40-50 g† (15%-20% of calories*)	All fried foods are excluded from the diet. Meat and eggs are limited to 6 oz of lean meat, poultry, fish, or eggs if 3 tsp of margarine or equivalent is used daily. 8-9 oz of meat and eggs may be used daily if no extra fat such as that in whole milk, margarine, butter, mayonnaise, salad dressing, nuts, and gravies is used.	Fairly practical for home use
20-25 g† (8%-10% of calories*)	Meat and eggs are limited to 5 to 6 oz/day. All other above restrictions apply.	Generally for hospital use only
Fat-free (about 2 g/day)	No meat or eggs are allowed. Starch, vegetables, and fruit are consumed in unlimited amounts if prepared without fat. Skim milk is allowed.	For hospital use only

* Based on 2400 calories/day.

† MCT oil may be added to these diets. Generally, start by adding 1 tsp/meal and gradually increase to 2-4 tsp/meal.

TABLE 11-3 Modified diets: protein

Daily protein intake	Food limitations*	Practicality
150-200 g	Meat, cheese, eggs: >10 oz/day (one egg = 1 oz meat); starch: 5 or more servings/day; vegetables: 4 or more servings/day; fruits: 3 or more servings/day Milk, shakes, eggnog, protein supplements added	High-protein, high-fat diet; dietitian supervision preferable.
100-140 g	Meat, cheese: 10 oz/day; starch: 5-6 servings/day; vegetables: 4-5 servings/day; fruits 3-4 servings/day; milk included	Average American diet; relatively high in fat
60 g (10% of calories)†	Meat, cheese: 6 oz/day; starch: 5 servings/day; vegetables: 4 servings/day; fruits: 3 servings/day; milk in limited amounts; calories increased with sugar and fat	Generally acceptable for home use; diet fairly easily manipulated according to patient preferences

40 g (6% of calories)†	Meat, cheese: 4 oz/day; starch: 3 servings/day; vegetables: 4 servings/day; fruits: 3 servings/day; calories increased with sugar and fat	Difficult to follow at home unless patient is unusually cooperative
20 g (3% of calories)†	Meat cheese: essentially none; eggs: 2/day; starch: 2 servings/day; fruits: 2 servings/day; vegetables: 2 servings/day; calories increased with sugar and fat	Should be limited to hospital use
8-10 g (trace)	Meat, cheese, eggs, milk: essentially none; starch, vegetables: severely limited; (low-protein bread only); calories mostly from fruit, juice, sugar, and fat	For hospital use only

° Serving sizes: most vegetables, ½ cup; most fruits, 1 piece or ½ cup; starch, 1 slice bread or ⅓ to ½ cup of cooked starch.
† Based on 2400 calories/day.

TABLE 11-4 A Modified diets: potassium

Potassium level	Food limitations	Practicality
3 g (80 mEq)	—	Average American diet
1.5 g (40 mEq)	Limited meat, vegetables, fruit; milk, potatoes, tea, coffee, chocolate only in minimal amounts	Most common level used for renal diets; not practical to prescribe a low-potassium, high-protein diet

TABLE 11-4 B Foods with low or high potassium contents°

Amount per 120 ml (½ cup)	
Low (<2.5 mEq [100 mg])	**High (>5 mEq [200 mg])**
Bean sprouts	Asparagus
Beets	Bran and whole-grain cereals
Cabbage, cooked or raw	Broccoli
Carrots	Brussels sprouts
Cauliflower, cooked	Collards
Corn	Dried beans and peas (including lima beans), cooked
Cucumber	
Eggplant	
Fruit: apples and applesauce; blueberries; cherries; cranberries; lemons; pears, canned; pineapple, fresh or canned; plums, fresh or canned; raspberries; tangerines	Fruit, dried or cocktail
	Fruit, fresh: apricots, bananas, grapefruit, oranges, peaches, pears, strawberries
	Melons: cantaloupe, honeydew, watermelon
	Mushrooms
Green beans and peas, cooked	Potatoes, cooked
Lettuce	Rhubarb
Onions, cooked	Some salt substitutes (read labels)
Radishes	Spinach, cooked
Summer squash, cooked	Sweet potatoes, cooked
	Tomatoes
	Winter squash, cooked

°The primary sources of potassium in the diet are fruit, vegetables, and milk. See Table 2-25 for further description of the potassium content of foods.

TABLE 11-5 Modified diets: sodium[*]

Daily sodium (Na) intake	Food limitations	Practicality
5-6 g Na$^+$ (12.5-15 g salt)	Includes table salt, heavily or visibly salted items	Average American diet
4 g Na$^+$ (10 g salt)	No additional salt on tray or at table	Practical for home use
3 g Na$^+$ (7.5 g salt)	Food only lightly salted in preparation; heavily or visibly salted items restricted (potato chips, pretzels, crackers, pickles, olives, relishes, sauces, more commercially prepared soups); no salt on tray	Practical for home use
2 g Na$^+$ (5 g salt)	Above limitations plus no salt in food preparation; most processed foods avoided (canned food, luncheon meat, bacon, ham, cheese) unless calculated into diet; regular bread, butter, and milk in limited amounts	Fairly practical for home use with cooperative patients
1 g Na$^+$ (2.5 g salt)	Above limitations plus use of only salt-free bread	Practical for home use with only unusually cooperative patients
0.5 g Na$^+$ (1.25 g salt)	Above limitations plus limitation of meat (4 oz/day), eggs, some vegetables; milk (1 pt/day) and salt-free butter allowed	Not practical for home use

[*]Also see box on following page.

HIGH-SODIUM FOODS TO OMIT IN SODIUM-RESTRICTED DIETS

Condiments

Pickles, olives, relish, salted nuts, meat tenderizer, commercial salad dressings, monosodium glutamate (Accent, others), steak sauce, ketchup, soy sauce, Worcestershire sauce, horseradish sauce, chili sauce, commercial mustard, onion salt, garlic salt, celery salt, butter salt, seasoned salts. (NOTE: Salt substitutes often contain substantial amounts of sodium; read labels. Many salt substitutes contain potassium and should be avoided by patients taking spironolactone or ACE inhibitors.)

Bread

Salted bread and crackers

Meat, fish, poultry, cheese, and substitutes

Cured, smoked, and processed meat such as ham, bacon, corned beef, chipped beef, wieners, luncheon meat, bologna, salt pork, regular canned salmon and tuna; all cheese except low-sodium cheese and cottage cheese; TV dinners, pizza, frozen Italian entrées, imitation sausage; and bacon

HIGH-SODIUM FOODS TO OMIT IN SODIUM-RESTRICTED DIETS—CONT'D

Beverages

Commercial buttermilk, instant hot cocoa mix

Soups

Commercial canned and dehydrated soup (except low-sodium soup), bouillon, consommé

Vegetables

Sauerkraut, hominy, pork and beans, canned tomato and vegetable juice

Fats

Gravy, regular peanut butter

Potato or potato substitutes

Potato chips, corn chips, salted popcorn, pretzels, frozen potato casseroles, commercially packaged rice and noodle mixes, dehydrated potatoes and potato mixes, bread stuffing

TABLE 11-6	Foods with low or high phosphorus contents*

Low	High
Most fruit	Bran
Most vegetables	Carbonated beverages (phosphoric acid added)
	Dried beans and peas
	Meat (including chicken), fish
	Milk, dairy products*

*See Table 2-24 for further description of the phosphorus content of foods.

REFEEDING AFTER BRIEF BOWEL REST

Patients who have been without enteral feeding for less than 1 or 2 weeks can usually gradually resume a full diet within several days. The commonly used regimen of advancing from clear liquids to full liquids to soft or solid food has two inherent drawbacks: (1) some clear liquids are high in osmolality, and (2) full liquids are often high in fat and lactose. Clear liquids may be most appropriate for testing a patient's swallowing mechanism, but the high osmolalities may not be well tolerated and juice often forms gas. The fat and lactose content of full liquids can complicate the refeeding of a patient with an impaired intestinal tract; the guidelines in the box on the following page are generally satisfactory.

Because tube feeding helps maintain the bowel's fully functional state, it is not necessary for tube-fed patients to follow this regimen. Their adaptation to oral intake is usually determined by their ability to chew and swallow or the underlying bowel disease when present.

REFEEDING AFTER PROLONGED BOWEL REST OR BOWEL RESECTION

Patients who have been without enteral feeding for 3 weeks or more or recently had a substantial part of their small intestine removed (short bowel syndrome) usually experience digestive dysfunction and malabsorption when

REFEEDING AFTER BRIEF BOWEL REST

Day 1

Clear liquids to check swallowing followed by low-lactose full liquids, e.g., oral-feeding formulas (see Chapter 12)

Days 2 to 3

Lactose-free, oral-feeding formulas or six small feedings of a 30 to 40 g fat, low-lactose, soft diet

Days 4 to 5

50-g fat diet, progressing to regular diet as tolerated

they begin to ingest food orally; refeeding should therefore be approached slowly. If patients have diarrhea at the outset, they may need to be on "nothing by mouth" (NPO) status for 1 or 2 days until the stooling stops; then refeeding can be started. If diarrhea persists after 2 days of NPO status, secretory or inflammatory processes should be ruled out.

General Guidelines

Initially, meals should be small and consist of soft, nonfibrous, bland foods. Salt should be used only in small amounts if at all in meal preparation, and fat (e.g., butter, margarine, cooking oil) should be avoided. As refeeding progresses, salt may be added to food at the table, and a medium-chain triglyceride (MCT) oil supplement may be used as needed for calories. Patients should only have minimal amounts of liquid with meals to minimize the transit rate and dilution of gastric juices; the major portion of liquids should be consumed between meals.

The patient should start by eating only two different foods at each meal to determine which foods can be tolerated. Six small meals per day should be eaten according to the guidelines and food groups listed in the boxes on pp. 264-265.

REFEEDING AFTER PROLONGED BOWEL REST OR BOWEL RESECTION

Days 1 to 5

Eat two foods at each meal, with the total amount being no more than ½ cup.

Combine one half of a serving from group A with one half of a serving from group B or combine one half of a serving from group C with 1 serving from group D.

Days 6 to 10

Eat three foods at each meal. Combine 1 serving *each* from groups A, B, and E *or* groups B, C, and D.

Days 11 to 15

If extra calories are needed, add 1 to 2 tsp of MCT oil to each meal by cooking vegetables and meat in the oil or adding it to vegetables, starch, and meat at the table.

Eat four foods at each meal. Combine 1 serving *each* from groups A, B, C, and D *or* groups A, B, C, and E.

If desired, small amounts of salt may be used at the table.

The duration of each of the three phases can be adjusted according to patient tolerance. After the third phase, new foods can be added to the diet about every 2 days to monitor the tolerance of each new food. Tailor the dietary regimen to each patient's needs. See the discussion of the management of malabsorption in Chapter 20.

PREFERRED FOODS FOR REFEEDING

Group A—starch (serving size: ½ cup)

Potatoes° (boiled, baked, mashed), white rice,° canned pumpkin,° sweet potatoes, acorn squash, enriched noodles or spaghetti, instant oatmeal, cream of wheat, puffed rice cereal, crisped rice cereal, corn flakes, white bread, graham crackers

Group B—vegetables (serving size: ½ cup; well cooked)

Carrots,° yellow squash or zucchini,° beets, asparagus tips, green beans

Group C—fruit (serving size: ½ cup)

Applesauce,° stewed apples or pears without skin,° bananas, canned peaches or pears

Group D—dairy products (serving size as shown)

Buttermilk° (skim only): 4 to 6 oz
Low-fat cottage cheese: ⅓ cup
Plain low-fat yogurt: 4 oz

Group E—meat (serving size: 2 oz; boiled, baked, or broiled with no added fat)

Skinned poultry, fish

Beverages

Tea, water, tomato juice, homemade vegetable broth (low salt, not from bouillon)

°Preferred selections for days 1 to 5.

Suggested Readings

American Dietetic Association and National Kidney Foundation Council on Renal Nutrition—Renal Dietitians Dietetic Practice Group: *National renal diet: professional guide,* 1993, The Association.

American Heart Association: *Dietary treatment for hypercholesterolemia. A handbook for counselors,* Dallas, 1988, The Association.

Cerda JJ: Diet and gastrointestinal disease, *Med Clin North Am* 77:881, 1993.

Department of Food and Nutrition Services, UAB Hospital: *Manual for nutritional management,* 1993, University of Alabama at Birmingham.

Dietary Department, University of Iowa Hospitals and Clinics: *Recent advances in therapeutic diets,* ed 4, Ames, Iowa, 1989, Iowa State University Press.

Franz MJ et al: Nutrition principles for the management of diabetes and related complications, *Diabetes Care* 17:490, 1994.

Marulendra S, Kirby DF: Nutrition support in pancreatitis, *Nutr Clin Pract* 10:45, 1995.

Position statement: nutrition recommendations and principles for people with diabetes mellitus, *Diabetes Care* 17:519, 1994.

Signore J: *Handbook of clinical dietetics,* ed 2, Hanover, Mass, Yale University Press, 1992.

12

Enteral Nutrition

Although enteral nutrition is technically any nutrient delivery system that uses the gastrointestinal tract, the term is generally used to refer to tube feeding. Tube feeding is indicated when the oral intake of nutrients is insufficient to meet requirements for more than 5 to 7 days, provided the gastrointestinal tract is functional. The advantages of enteral nutrition over parenteral nutrition are reviewed in Chapter 9.

GASTROINTESTINAL ACCESS

The selection of tubes and pumps specifically designed for feeding is quite broad. Because of their pliability and long-term tolerance, small-gauge feeding tubes should virtually always be used for enteral feeding. However, gastric contents cannot be reliably aspirated through these tubes, so the need for frequent gastric aspiration in selected patients remains the only justification for using larger, more rigid nasogastric tubes for feeding.

Although many tubes have weighted tips that are intended to prevent retrograde migration or facilitate nasoduodenal intubation, such weights may actually impede passage of the tip through the gastric pylorus. When transpyloric feeding is necessary (e.g., to reduce the risk of aspiration or bypass a gastric ileus) nasoduodenal intubation can be carried by several techniques. A conservative method involves administering 10 mg of metoclopramide intravenously (IV) and inserting an ample length of an *un-*

weighted tube into the stomach.[1] If this fails, the use of various fluoroscopic and endoscopic methods can be considered.

Although soft nasogastric tubes have been used safely for years in some patients, long-term tube feeding is usually best accomplished through a percutaneous endoscopic gastrostomy (PEG). This method of gastrostomy placement has supplanted surgical gastrostomies because of lower morbidity and cost. However, the risk of tube-feeding aspiration is not appreciably lower with gastrostomies than with nasogastric tubes, so in patients at high risk for aspiration, duodenal intubation through the nose, a PEG, or placement of a jejunostomy tube is advisable. Jejunostomy tubes can sometimes be placed using a laparoscope, obviating the need for a laparotomy.

It is not always necessary to confirm tube placement radiographically before beginning to feed patients who are not at high risk for aspiration (i.e., alert with a normal gag reflex). Simple insufflation of air and auscultation of the stomach often suffice and allow earlier institution of feeding. However, radiographic confirmation of tube placement is required in patients who are at risk for aspiration.

FORMULA SELECTION

Enteral feeding formula choices have increased phenomenally in the last decade. Although many new formulas have been designed to meet the needs of specific patient groups, special benefits of these formulas have not always been demonstrated in controlled trials, and their costs are virtually always higher than those of standard formulas. Specialized formulas are therefore sometimes promoted for features that have little physiologic significance and no proven clinical superiority. For this reason, in selecting feeding formulas features that are major (important in all cases) must be distinguished from those that are minor (important only in selected cases) or inconsequential (virtually never important). The box stratifies the compositional parameters of feeding formulas in this manner. Table 12-1 contains information on the contents and

CRITERIA FOR EVALUATING ENTERAL FEEDING FORMULAS

Major criteria

Energy density (1, 1.5, or 2 kcal/ml)
Protein content (less than or greater than 20% of total energy)
Route of administration (tube/oral vs. tube only)
Cost (per 1000 kcal)

Minor criteria

Complexity (polymeric vs. oligomeric)
Osmolality
Protein source (e.g., casein, soy, peptides, amino acids)
Fat content
Fat source (long- vs. medium-chain triglycerides [MCTs])
Residue content
Electrolyte and mineral content
Form (liquid vs. powder)
Vitamin content
Lactose content

Inconsequential criteria

Carbohydrate source (e.g., corn starch or syrup, sucrose)
Method of preparation (compounded vs. blenderized)

Specialized or "disease-specific" formulas

Results of clinical studies (needed to substantiate claims)

prices of many commercially available adult feeding formulas, which are arranged by major criteria and selected minor criteria. It also lists a number of specialized or "disease-specific" formulas.

Major Criteria

Appropriate choices can usually be made by considering only the major criteria. Energy density determines the amounts of most nutrients delivered per liter, including

Text continued on p. 280.

TABLE 12-1 Enteral feeding formulas

Category and product	Manufacturer[a]	kcal/ml	mOsm/ kg water	Price per 1000 kcal[b]	Protein g/L	Protein % kcal
Nutritionally complete, lactose-free formulas (1 kcal/ml)						
Standard protein						
TUBE/ORAL						
Ensure	Ross	1.06	470	$6.28	37	14
Ensure HN	Ross	1.06	470	$6.72	44	17
Glucerna	Ross	1	375	$11.50	42	16
Isosource	Sandoz	1.2	360	$5.35	43	14
Isosource HN	Sandoz	1.2	330	$5.78	53	17
Nutren 1.0 (14)[c]	Clintec	1	300–350	$6.04	40	16
TUBE ONLY						
Attain	Sherwood	1	300	$4.02	40	16
Isocal	Mead Johnson	1.06	270	$5.96	34	13
Isocal HN	Mead Johnson	1.06	270	$6.27	44	16
Osmolite	Ross	1.06	300	$6.96	37	14
Osmolite HN	Ross	1.06	300	$7.23	44	17

TABLE 12-1 Enteral feeding formulas—cont'd

Category and product	Fat		Carbohydrate		NA⁺ (mg/1000 kcal)	K⁺ (mEq/1000 kcal)	kcal to meet adult vitamin RDA
	g/L	% kcal	g/L	% kcal			
Nutritionally complete, lactose-free formulas (1 kcal/ml)							
Standard protein							
TUBE/ORAL							
Ensure	37	32	145	54	800	38	2000
Ensure HN	36	30	141	53	755	38	1400
Glucerna	56	48	94	36	930	40	1400
Isosource	41	30	170	56	1000	37	1800
Isosource HN	41	30	160	53	920	37	1800
Nutren 1.0 (14)ᶜ	38	33	127	51	876	32	1500
TUBE ONLY							
Attain	35	30	135	54	800	41	1250
Isocal	44	37	135	50	500	32	2000
Isocal HN	45	38	124	46	877	39	1250
Osmolite	38	31	145	55	600	25	2000
Osmolite HN	37	30	141	53	877	38	1400

Continued

TABLE 12-1 Enteral feeding formulas—cont'd

Category and product	Manufacturer[a]	kcal/ml	mOsm/ kg water	Price per 1000 kcal[b]	Protein g/L	Protein % kcal
Nutritionally complete, lactose-free formulas—cont'd						
Fiber-containing (g fiber/1000 kcal)[d]						
Ensure/fiber (13)	Ross	1.1	480	$6.05	40	14
Jevity (14)	Ross	1.06	310	$7.78	44	17
Profiber (12)	Sherwood	1	300	$5.31	40	16
Sustacal/fiber (6)	Mead Johnson	1.06	480	$6.21	46	17
Ultracal (14)	Mead Johnson	1.06	310	$6.76	44	16
High protein						
Promote (14)[c]	Ross	1	340	$8.05	63	25
Replete (14)[c]	Clintec	1	300-350	$6.80	62	25
Sustacal	Mead Johnson	1	650	$5.98	61	24
Milk-based (lactose-containing) oral supplement						
Carnation Instant Breakfast w/ whole milk	Clintec	0.93	661-747	$2.00	45	19

TABLE 12-1 Enteral feeding formulas—cont'd

Category and product	Fat g/L	Fat % kcal	Carbohydrate g/L	Carbohydrate % kcal	Na⁺ (mg/1000 kcal)	K⁺ (mEq/1000 kcal)	kcal to meet adult vitamin RDA
Nutritionally complete, lactose-free formulas—cont'd							
Fiber-containing (g fiber/1000 kcal)ᵈ							
Ensure/fiber (13)	37	29	162	57	770	39	1530
Jevity (14)	37	30	152	53	877	38	1400
Profiber (12)	35	30	147	55	800	38	1250
Sustacal/fiber (6)	35	30	140	53	680	34	1500
Ultracal (14)	45	38	123	46	880	39	1250
High protein							
Promote (14)ᶜ	26	23	130	52	930	51	1000
Replete (14)ᶜ	34	30	113	45	876	39	1000
Sustacal	23	21	140	55	920	53	1070
Milk-based (lactose-containing) oral supplement							
Carnation Instant Breakfast w/ whole milk	18	18	143	63	1030	73	1000

Continued

TABLE 12-1 Enteral feeding formulas—cont'd

Category and product	Manufacturer[a]	kcal/ml	mOsm/ kg water	Price per 1000 kcal[b]	Protein g/L	% kcal
1.5 kcal/ml						
Standard protein						
Comply	Sherwood	1.5	410	$2.85	60	16
Ensure Plus	Ross	1.5	690	$4.92	55	15
Ensure Plus HN	Ross	1.5	650	$5.28	63	17
Nutren 1.5	Clintec	1.5	430–530	$4.48	60	16
Sustacal Plus	Mead Johnson	1.5	670	$4.31	61	16
Standard protein, high fat						
Nutrivent	Clintec	1.5	330–465	$5.87	68	18
Pulmocare	Ross	1.5	520	$6.10	63	17
Respalor	Mead Johnson	1.5	580	$6.46	76	20
High protein						
Traumacal	Mead Johnson	1.5	560	$6.46	82	22

TABLE 12-1 Enteral feeding formulas—cont'd

Category and product	Fat g/L	Fat % kcal	Carbohydrate g/L	Carbohydrate % kcal	NA+ (mg/1000 kcal)	K+ (mEq/1000 kcal)	kcal to meet adult vitamin RDA
1.5 kcal/ml							
Standard protein							
Comply	60	36	180	48	730	32	1500
Ensure Plus	53	32	200	53	700	33	2130
Ensure Plus HN	50	30	200	53	790	31	1425
Nutren 1.5	68	40	170	44	780	32	1500
Sustacal Plus	58	34	190	50	560	25	1800
Standard protein, high fat							
Nutrivent	95	55	101	27	520	21	1500
Pulmocare	92	55	106	28	873	29	1420
Respalor	71	42	148	38	835	25	2150
High protein							
Traumacal	68	40	142	38	800	24	3000

Continued

TABLE 12-1 Enteral feeding formulas—cont'd

Category and product	Manufacturer[a]	kcal/ml	mOsm/ kg water	Price per 1000 kcal[b]	Protein g/L	Protein % kcal
2 kcal/ml						
Standard protein						
Deliver	Mead Johnson	2	640	$3.63	75	15
Magnacal	Sherwood	2	590	$2.51	70	14
Nepro	Ross	2	635	$7.00	70	14
Nutren 2.0	Clintec	2	720	$3.74	80	16
Two Cal HN	Ross	2	690	$4.25	84	17
Specialized or "disease-specific" formulas						
Malabsorption						
Lipisorb	Mead Johnson	1.35	630	$8.83	57	16
Critical care						
Crucial	Clintec	1.5	490	$22.67	94	25
Immun-Aid	McGaw	1	460	$15.00	80	32
Impact (10)[c]	Sandoz	1	375	$26.38	56	23
Perative	Ross	1.3	425	$10.42	67	21

TABLE 12-1 Enteral feeding formulas—cont'd

Category and product	Fat g/L	Fat % kcal	Carbohydrate g/L	Carbohydrate % kcal	NA⁺ (mg/1000 kcal)	K⁺ (mEq/1000 kcal)	kcal to meet adult vit-amin RDA
2 kcal/ml							
Standard protein							
Deliver	102	45	200	40	400	22	2000
Magnacal	80	36	250	50	500	16	2000
Nepro	96	43	215	43	415	13.5	1900
Nutren 2.0	106	45	196	39	650	25	1500
Two Cal HN	91	40	220	43	655	32	1900
Specialized or "disease-specific" formulas							
Malabsorption							
Lipisorb	57	37	161	47	1000	32	1600
Critical care							
Crucial	68	39	135	36	780	32	1500
Immun-Aid	22	20	120	48	575	27	2000
Impact (10)ᶜ	28	25	130	52	1100	33	1500
Perative	38	25	177	54	800	34	1500

Continued

TABLE 12-1 Enteral feeding formulas—cont'd

Category and product	Manufacturer[a]	kcal/ml	mOsm/ kg water	Price per 1000 kcal[b]	Protein g/L	Protein % kcal
Specialized or "disease-specific" formulas—cont'd						
Hepatic encephalopathy (high in branched-chain amino acids, low in aromatic amino acids)						
Hepatic Aid II	McGaw	1.2	560	$34.31	46	15
NutriHep	Clintec	1.5	690	$34.56	40	11
Small-peptide formulas						
Alitraq	Ross	1	575	$42.12	53	21
Criticare HN	Mead Johnson	1.06	650	$25.06	38	14
Peptamen	Clintec	1	270–380	$27.80	40	16
Peptamen VHP	Clintec	1	300–430	$31.28	63	25
Reabilan HN	Clintec	1.33	490	$22.36	59	17
Vital HN	Ross	1	500	$29.16	42	17

[a]Clintec Nutrition Co, Deerfield, IL; McGaw, Irvine, CA; Mead Johnson & Co., Evansville, IN; Ross Laboratories, Columbus, OH; Sandoz Nutrition, Minneapolis, MN; Sherwood Medical, St. Louis, MO.

[b]1995 institutional list prices for minimum orders are given for comparison. The price may decrease significantly when ordered in large quantities. The price charged to patients is generally higher than the institutional price.

[c]The fiber content of the same product with added fiber (when available) is given in parentheses. The nutrient compositions of these products are otherwise virtually identical.

TABLE 12-1 Enteral feeding formulas—cont'd

Category and product	Fat		Carbohydrate		Na⁺ (mg/1000 kcal)	K⁺ (mEq/1000 kcal)	kcal to meet adult vitamin RDA
	g/L	% kcal	g/L	% kcal			
Specialized or "disease-specific" formulas—cont'd							
Hepatic encephalopathy (high in branched-chain amino acids, low in aromatic amino acids)							
Hepatic Aid II	37	28	173	57	<240	<4	NP[e]
NutriHep	21	12	290	77	142	15	1500
Small-peptide formulas							
Alitraq	16	13	165	66	1000	31	1500
Criticare HN	5.3	4	220	82	600	32	2000
Peptamen	39	33	127	51	500	32	1500
Peptamen VHP	39	33	105	42	560	38	1500
Reabilan HN	54	35	158	48	750	32	2000
Vital HN	11	9	185	74	570	36	1500

[d]Sustacal With Fiber and Ensure With Fiber differ from Sustacal and Ensure, respectively, in their contents of other nutrients. For fiber-containing supplements that are otherwise virtually identical to nonfiber products having the same names, see the previous footnote (c).

[e]Not possible (product is devoid of some or all vitamins).

not only calories but protein, water, and others as well. Higher energy-density formulas (1.5 to 2 kcal/ml) are very useful for delivering high calorie loads or restricting fluid intake but can result in dehydration in patients who are unable to consume additional water as needed or have high water requirements. The fluid status of these patients should be carefully monitored.

Once the energy density has been selected, the formula of choice is usually determined by the protein content, route of administration (oral or tube), and cost. Protein content should be considered not only in absolute terms but also relative to total energy (as percent of calories). As shown in Table 12-1, the term *high nitrogen* (HN) is unreliable. Some formulas designated as HN have protein contents as low as 16% of energy, so the term should be disregarded.

Minor Criteria

Among the minor criteria for formula selection, protein complexity has received much attention. Oligomeric formulas that contain peptides (from hydrolyzed proteins) or free amino acids, often referred to by the misnomer "elemental," have previously been thought to be more efficiently absorbed in patients with impaired gastrointestinal functioning. However, clinical trials have concluded peptides confer minimal advantage if any over whole proteins (polymeric formulas) and that free amino acids are inferior to both. These formulas are also considerably more expensive than standard formulas (see Table 12-1).

Osmolality was once thought by many clinicians to have a major effect on the tolerance of enteral formulas, particularly with regard to diarrhea. However, several controlled clinical trials have now established that osmolality does not independently influence formula tolerance. The practice of diluting formulas to half or quarter strength or choosing prediluted "starter" formulas is still somewhat widespread in spite of evidence that doing so only delays adequate intake. Feedings should be started with formulas that are full strength and diluted only to provide supplemental water when other routes are not adequate.

Specialized Formulas

Many new specialized or "disease-specific" enteral feeding formulas have been marketed in the last decade for patients with critical illnesses (e.g., trauma and sepsis), malabsorption, diabetes, pulmonary disease, hepatic encephalopathy, renal failure, or AIDS. Because these formulas are classified as food by the U.S. Food and Drug Administration, they can be released on the market without undergoing the extensive clinical testing required for drugs. Although their compositions have most often been based on plausible ideas generated from basic or clinical research, these formulas still require clinical testing to substantiate special therapeutic properties and justify their inevitably higher costs. Such tests have not been conducted on all the formulas, and when they have the results have often been negative. Therefore it is important not to choose an enteral formula simply because a diagnosis is embedded in its name or it has an unusual compositional feature. Although certain formulas are listed as specialized in Table 12-1, this is not intended to suggest that they are truly disease specific. Other formulas with disease-oriented names are listed among the general formulas because their features are not particularly unique, but this does not mean they are totally comparable to the others in the category. For more information, see the chapters devoted to the specific illnesses in question.

Hospital Formularies

Within each category of Table 12-1, the listed formulas are therapeutically equivalent for most applications. This stratification aids clinicians in choosing appropriate formulas and developing hospital enteral feeding formularies. At the University of Alabama Hospital the categories are submitted to vendors every other year for competitive bidding, and the product with the lowest price per 1000 kcal in each category is included in the hospital formulary for 2 years. When a nonformulary product is ordered, its formulary equivalent is substituted. The use of certain specialized formulas is limited to specific clinical situations or requires the approval of the hospital's nutrition support service. These measures help to confine the use of expensive formulas to situations in which they have proven therapeutic superiority.

INFUSION METHODS

The continuous-drip method with a closed, aseptic system is generally preferred. A pump should always be used to avoid accidental infusions of dangerously large volumes. Continuous feeding assures more reliable nutrient delivery and may reduce the risks of gastric distention and pulmonary aspiration during feeding. The initial infusion rate and rapidity of its increase should vary depending on the overall condition of the patient. A patient who has an impaired mental status or has not used the gastrointestinal tract for a prolonged time (i.e., greater than 2 weeks) should have feedings introduced and increased more slowly than in alert patients whose intestines have been used recently.

The bolus method is most useful for long-term feeding in stable patients. It allows more mobility and reduces cost because a pump and infusion set are not required. The guidelines listed in the box on the following pages apply to adults.

COMPLICATIONS
Diarrhea

Diarrhea, which has been blamed on many factors, commonly complicates enteral feeding. However, most of the proposed causes have only been *associated* with diarrhea in tube-fed patients and there is little or no objective evidence for causal relationships. Unproven factors include hypertonic feeding formulas, hypoalbuminemia, bacterial contamination of the feeding and/or dysentery, inadequate fiber in feeding formulas, certain infusion

GUIDELINES FOR INITIATING ENTERAL FEEDING

Continuous feeding

Begin feeding at a rate that is between 10 and 50 ml per hour.

Check for gastric residual (greater than 100 to 200 ml) after about 8 hours, especially in patients with impaired mental status. Reinstill the aspirated contents into the gastrointestinal tract. Discontinue the feeding temporarily, or postpone increasing the rate if residuals greater than 100 to 200 ml are present. Checking residuals is an unreliable method for detecting gastric retention when pliable feeding tubes are used, so it should be combined with questioning of the patient regarding fullness and a physical examination for distention.

Increase the rate in increments of 20 to 40 ml/hr every 8 to 24 hours to attain the final rate (calculated to meet energy and protein requirements) in as little as 1 day or as many as 5 days, depending on the state of the gastrointestinal tract. The final rate should generally not exceed 125 to 150 ml/hr; higher nutrient requirements should be met with 1.5 to 2 kcal/ml formulas.

Wean the patient to oral intake by gradually reducing the infusion rate, interrupting the infusion before meals, or infusing only at night to improve appetite during the day.

Discontinue enteral feeding only when adequate oral intake has been achieved.

Continued

methods (e.g., bolus infusions or rapid increase in the infusion rate), fecal impaction, lactose, excessive fat, or inadequate vitamin A in feeding formulas. The best-documented causal factors are medications, pseudomembranous colitis, and gastrointestinal dysfunction (box), none of which are necessarily related to tube feeding. Tube feeding itself not usually responsible for diarrhea and should not be identified as the cause until others have been ruled out.

Bolus feeding

The patient should be in the sitting position, and feedings should be limited to waking hours whenever possible.

Begin with 50 to 100 ml boluses of undiluted feeding every 2 to 4 hours. Check gastric residuals before each feeding, and delay the feeding if the residual is greater 100 to 200 ml. Increase the size of boluses every 8 to 24 hours to 100 ml, 150 ml, 200 ml, etc. until requirements are met. In alert patients, it is sometimes possible to increase the volume to as high as 400 ml per feeding. If possible, avoid feeding during the night.

Flush the line with water after each infusion and clamp or cap the tube. If water requirements are not met by the formula, additional water should be given with the flush.

Rinse the infusion syringe after each bolus; discard it daily if used in the hospital, or wash it well if used at home.

Do not allow opened formula to sit at room temperature for more than 4 hours.

Wean patients to oral intake by eliminating feedings that precede meals. Discontinue enteral feeding only when adequate oral intake has been achieved.

LIKELY CAUSES OF DIARRHEA IN TUBE-FED PATIENTS

Medications

Elixir medications containing sorbitol (acetaminophen, theophylline, cough preparations, codeine, vitamins, many others)[2]

Magnesium-containing antacids (Mylanta, Maalox etc.)

Oral antibiotics (definite), IV antibiotics (questionable)

Phosphorus supplements, cimetidine, metoclopramide, lactulose, other assorted medications

Pseudomembranous colitis
Gastrointestinal disorders

Surprisingly, the medication that most commonly causes diarrhea in tube-fed patients is one that clinicians do not often request, so they are unaware that it is being administered. It is sorbitol, present in many liquid medications as a vehicle and sweetener. It is listed as an inactive ingredient and its quantity is not required on medication package inserts, so it was not suspected as a cause of diarrhea until a well-controlled study ruled out other causes.[3] Because they are easy to deliver, elixirs are commonly administered to patients with feeding tubes. Medications previously administered orally or IV are often replaced by elixirs when a feeding tube is placed. Patients who receive more than one liquid medication or several doses of a single one may thus receive substantial amounts of sorbitol—commonly more than 20 g per day—which causes diarrhea in virtually all persons. Thus there is a common scenario that is played out when a sorbitol-containing medication is started at the same time enteral nutrition begins—diarrhea develops, the tube feeding is unjustly identified as the cause, and tube feeding is stopped, resulting in inadequate intake.

Any form of magnesium given in sufficient quantities can cause diarrhea. Thus when magnesium-containing antacids are used in tube-fed patients (e.g., to prevent stress ulcers), the patients may develop diarrhea. Antacids based on aluminum alone or an aluminum-magnesium combination are practical alternatives. Some but not all oral antibiotics cause diarrhea by altering the intestinal flora. Although antibiotics administered IV have been implicated as well, confirmatory data are less firm, especially in critically ill patients who have multiple confounding factors. Additional medications that can have diarrhea as a direct side-effect are listed in the box. Many other medications may cause diarrhea, so product inserts and pharmaceutical references should be consulted whenever the cause for diarrhea is not obvious.

The box on the following page lists measures to take and avoid when a tube-fed patient develops diarrhea. The most important step is to consider all medications, particularly liquid ones, as possible causes. See Table 14-3 and

Managing Diarrhea in Tube-Fed Patients

Do's

- Carefully review all medications.

  Eliminate all elixirs containing sorbitol. If in doubt about the sorbitol content of any medication, discontinue it or change it to another form.

  Eliminate magnesium-containing antacids.

  Eliminate any other potential causes.

- Measure stool *C. difficile* titer.

- Consider measuring the stool osmotic gap to help distinguish between osmotic and secretory diarrhea by using the following equation:

$$\text{Stool osmotic gap} = \text{Stool osmolality} - 2\,(\text{Stool sodium} + \text{Stool potassium})$$

  >140: osmotic diarrhea, likely a result of medications or possibly tube feeding.

  <100: secretory diarrhea, possibly a result of pseudomembranous colitis or nonosmotic medications.

- Consider giving psyllium or pectin (30 ml up to t.i.d.).

Dont's

- Don't give antidiarrheal agents before a cause for the diarrhea is determined; use them only as a last resort.
- Don't infuse albumin IV with the assumption that it will remedy the diarrhea.
- Don't stop a feeding any longer than is necessary to determine whether it is causing diarrhea.
- Don't change the feeding formula with the assumption that doing so will relieve the diarrhea.

the second reference at the end of this chapter for sorbitol contents of several medications. These lists are not exhaustive, and because sorbitol concentrations are not listed on package inserts, pharmaceutical manufacturers may change them without notification. Therefore all liquid medications should be suspected as causes of diarrhea and if possible discontinued or changed to other forms until the diarrhea has resolved.

When medications are clearly not responsible for the diarrhea, determine whether pseudomembranous colitis is the cause by measuring the stool *Clostridium difficile* titer. If this is negative, gastrointestinal dysfunction is a probable cause. The stool osmotic gap (see box) can help establish a secretory cause if it is low or direct a further search for exogenous osmotic substances if it is high. The enteral feeding can be stopped to determine its role, but it should be resumed once a determination is made unless the diarrhea is compromising the patient. Changing to an isotonic feeding formula (much less diluting one) or to a small-peptide or fiber-containing formula will *not* relieve the diarrhea. If there is still no clear cause, pectin may be administered to give substance to the stool. Antidiarrheal agents such as kaolin-pectin, loperamide, or diphenoxylate with atropine may be given as a *last* resort.

Gastric Retention and Pulmonary Aspiration

Gastric retention is variously defined as the presence of more than 100 to 200 ml of tube feeding in the stomach. Monitoring retention by periodic suctioning of stomach contents through the tube with a syringe is not reliable when soft feeding tubes are used. Therefore a combination of gastric suctioning, questioning of the patient, physical examination, and sometimes radiography should be used.[4] Although ileus (the absence of bowel activity usually because of sepsis, trauma, or surgery) is probably the most common cause of gastric retention, hypokalemia, drug side effects, and obstruction must be ruled out. Parenteral nutrition is required in cases of unremitting retention.

The most serious and potentially lethal complication of tube feeding—pulmonary aspiration of gastric contents—is most common in patients with impaired mental status and intestinal ileus. In these patients, aspiration can usually be prevented by elevating the head during feeding (to avoid gastroesophageal reflux) and careful monitoring for distention. In patients at especially high risk, inserting the tube into the duodenum is advisable.

Metabolic Complications

Enteral nutrition results in far fewer metabolic complications than does parenteral nutrition. The most common metabolic complication of enteral feeding is probably hyperglycemia, particularly in patients with preexisting glucose intolerance. This can be handled through tighter diabetes control. Hyperglycemia rarely necessitates reduction of the feeding.

Tube feeding formulas with high energy density or protein content do not contain enough water for some patients to handle the renal solute load. Patients receiving these formulas who are unable to regulate their fluid needs voluntarily and do not have adequate intravenous fluid intake may become dehydrated, hyperosmolar, and hyperglycemic. The osmolality of the formula is not related to these problems because carbohydrates (the major osmotic component) are ordinarily metabolized and do not contribute to the renal solute load except when glycosuria occurs. The fluid status and blood glucose levels of patients at risk should be closely monitored.

References

1. Lord LM et al: Comparison of weighted vs. unweighted enteral feeding tubes for efficacy of transpyloric intubation, *JPEN* 17:271, 1993.
2. Johnston KR, Govel LA, Andritz MH: Gastrointestinal effects of sorbitol as an additive in liquid medications, *Am J Med* 97:185, 1994.

3. Edes TE, Walk BE, Austin JL: Diarrhea in tube-fed patients: feeding formula not necessarily the cause, *Am J Med* 88:91, 1990.
4. McClave SA et al: Use of residual volume as a marker for enteral feeding intolerance: prospective blinded comparison with physical examination and radiographic findings, *JPEN* 16:99, 1992.

Suggested Readings

Rombeau JL, Caldwell MD, eds: *Clinical nutrition: Enteral and tube feeding*, ed 2, Philadelphia, 1990, WB Saunders.

13

Parenteral Nutrition

Parenteral nutrition or intravenous feeding has many different names; probably the most common are total parenteral nutrition (TPN) and hyperalimentation (or hyperal). The latter is not preferred because it implies that parenteral nutrition gives patients more nutrition than they require, which is rarely the case. More specific terms are central parenteral nutrition (CPN), central venous alimentation (CVA), peripheral parenteral nutrition (PPN), and peripheral venous alimentation (PVA).

Parenteral nutrition can be used to satisfy all of a patient's nutritional requirements or supplement an insufficient oral or enteral intake. In doing this, energy is supplied by dextrose and vegetable oil-derived lipid emulsions; protein by crystalline amino acids; and vitamins, minerals, and trace elements in pure forms. When necessary, it is possible to add certain medications such as insulin.

INDICATIONS FOR PARENTERAL NUTRITION

Parenteral nutrition is indicated when a patient's gastrointestinal tract is either unavailable for use or unreliable for more than 5 to 7 days or when extended bowel rest is desired for therapeutic reasons. Specific indications and contraindications are listed in the box.

Because there are no situations in which a person should absolutely not be fed, the contraindications are all relative. Surprisingly, some clinicians still tend to resort to

INDICATIONS AND CONTRAINDICATIONS FOR PARENTERAL NUTRITION

Prolonged unavailability or unreliability of the gastrointestinal tract

Conditions obviating enteral access
    Perioperative (bowel resection or other gastrointestinal surgery; head and neck surgery)
    Trauma to the abdomen or head and neck
Intestinal obstruction
Intestinal ileus not amenable to duodenal feeding
Severe malabsorption (e.g., short bowel syndrome)
Intractable intolerance of enteral feeding

Intentional bowel rest

Enteric fistulae
Crohn's disease unresponsive to other therapy
Intractable diarrhea
Unremitting pancreatitis

Relative contraindications

Functional gastrointestinal tract
Intended use for less than about 5 days
Imminent death from underlying disease

TPN when enteral feeding can be used; this should be strongly discouraged.

As in any therapeutic feeding situation, before parenteral nutrition has begun, definitive objectives must be set. The patient's energy and protein requirements should be estimated or measured as described in Chapter 9, and a goal for weight maintenance or weight gain should be clear.

ROUTES OF ADMINISTRATION
Central Parenteral Nutrition

To help patients attain sufficient energy intakes without giving them an excessive volume of fluid, the nonprotein energy must be concentrated. Using final concentrations of up to 35% dextrose results in a fluid osmolality of roughly 1800 mOsm/kg of water (before being admixed with lipids), which is very irritating to the venous endothelium. Therefore these solutions must be infused into central veins where they are rapidly diluted by high blood-flow rates. The catheter tip is introduced into the superior vena cava or right atrium through the subclavian or internal jugular vein or by using a peripherally inserted central (PIC) line.

Peripheral Parenteral Nutrition

When central venous catheterization is undesirable or unavailable, more dilute solutions can be infused into peripheral veins. Even with final dextrose concentrations of only 10%, the osmolality of the dextrose/amino acid solution is 900 to 1100 mOsm/kg of water, resulting in phlebitis and fairly short periods of vein patency. To meet energy requirements and reduce osmolality, IV lipid emulsions must be admixed in the solution or infused as a "piggyback." Total volumes of more than 3 L must be often used, exceeding the tolerance of some patients. For these reasons, PPN is only feasible for very short periods of time, making its benefits questionable and requiring that careful consideration be given as to whether it is appropriate for each patient. PIC lines provide a welcome alternative, allowing CPN to be infused through a peripherally inserted catheter.

MACRONUTRIENTS
Dextrose Monohydrate

The major source of nonprotein energy in TPN is dextrose (D-glucose). It is provided in the monohydrous form for intravenous use, which reduces its energy yield to 3.4 kcal/g rather than the 4 kcal/g of enteral glucose and other carbohydrates. Dextrose contributes the majority of the osmolality of the TPN solution. It is supplied by manufacturers in concentrations of up to 70%.

Lipid Emulsions

Intravenous lipid emulsions, generally derived from safflower oil, soybean oil, or a combination of the two, are available in 10% or 20% concentrations, yielding 1.1 kcal/ml and 2 kcal/ml, respectively. The only advantage of the latter is its lower fluid volume for a given energy yield. They can be admixed with dextrose and amino acids in 3-in-1 or total nutrient admixtures (TNAs) in a variety of concentrations if certain guidelines are observed. The lipids reduce the osmolality and hence the caustic nature of the high concentrations of dextrose used in parenteral nutrition.

In CPN, lipid emulsions must be used at least once or twice weekly to prevent essential fatty acid deficiencies. The continuous infusion of concentrated dextrose and the consequent steady elevation of insulin levels can prevent mobilization of endogenous adipose tissue stores of EFAs, resulting in biochemical evidence of an EFA deficiency within 1 or 2 weeks. Lipid emulsions prevent this. When a clear contraindication to the use of lipid emulsions exists (which is extremely rare), a tablespoon of a vegetable oil such as safflower oil rubbed on the skin daily can prevent an EFA deficiency but may not be sufficient to correct a preexisting deficiency.

Daily lipid intake is mandatory when PPN is used because it is virtually impossible to meet energy requirements with the more dilute glucose solutions required in PPN. Without adequate nonprotein calories, the infused amino acids will be oxidized to provide energy. This defeats one of the major purposes of parenteral nutrition, which is to meet all metabolic requirements. In addition, parenteral nutrition is more physiologic if lipids are provided daily as a source of nonprotein energy, as shown in the box on the following page.

In some patients the inclusion of lipids as a daily energy source is particularly beneficial. Glucose-intolerant patients can achieve better glucose control and lower insulin requirements when less dextrose is infused. Cachectic patients accrue lean body mass more efficiently and

ADVANTAGES OF INCLUDING LIPIDS AS A DAILY ENERGY SOURCE IN TOTAL PARENTERAL NUTRITION

Improves glucose tolerance
Lowers insulin levels
Reduces the risk of refeeding complications
Facilitates nitrogen balance
Promotes synthesis of proteins such as albumin in the liver
Readily used as an energy source by hypermetabolic, stressed patients
Less CO_2 generated by lipid oxidation than glucose oxidation

run less risk of developing the glucose-induced complications of refeeding such as hypophosphatemia (see Chapter 9). Patients with ventilatory failure and CO_2 retention can benefit from the fact that less CO_2 production is associated with lipid oxidation than glucose oxidation (see Chapter 22).

For these reasons and because the cost per kilocalorie of lipid emulsions is comparable to that of dextrose, total nutrient admixtures are the preferred form of parenteral nutrition. TNAs require only one large bag of parenteral nutrition per day and are therefore cost-efficient because they decrease the number of syringes, intravenous containers, and other pharmacy supplies used and reduce the time required by pharmacists and nurses for compounding and administering TPN. It is possible to package 2-in-1 dextrose-amino acid formulas in large bags as well. The use of one TPN container per day can reduce physician error and inadequate nutrient delivery resulting from time gaps between TPN infusions. Only one physician order is required each day, and nurses can begin each day's TPN bag at the same hour. In hospitals in which pharmacies are not set up to formulate TNAs, it is possible to use lipids daily by piggybacking a 500-ml bottle of 10% lipid emulsion daily into the TPN, preferably over 24 hours.

IV lipid emulsions have very few adverse effects, and documentation of adverse effects often consists of only one or two reports of single cases. Although potentially serious, hypersensitivity (reported as dyspnea, flushing, chest pain, back pain, and urticaria) is rare enough not to warrant the use of small test doses before lipid infusion. Severe hypoxemia can be aggravated by rapid infusion of lipids if the clearance of circulating triglycerides is delayed. However, this complication can nearly always be prevented by infusing the lipids over 12 to 24 hours. Serum triglyceride levels greater than 500 mg/dl can cause pancreatitis, so it is prudent to document acceptable levels at least once during lipid infusion. Some patients have carbohydrate-induced hypertriglyceridemia, which may not be aggravated by the lipid infusion.

The common assumption that standard doses of lipid emulsions (e.g., 500 ml of 10% lipids per day) cause or aggravate liver enzyme abnormalities or fatty deposits in the liver is not well founded. When associated with TPN, these abnormalities are generally a result of constant and sometimes excessive glucose delivery, which lipid emulsions can relieve. (See discussion of complications in this chapter.)

Amino Acids

The crystalline amino acids used in TPN are available in concentrations between 3.5% and 15% (3.5 and 15 g/100 ml, respectively) and yield 4 kcal/g. Their energy content should be counted as part of the patient's total energy intake, despite the intent that they be used for protein synthesis. The reason for this is that most patients on TPN have at best in only a slightly positive nitrogen balance, and the infused amino acids are used primarily to replace protein that is catabolized (and hence used as fuel).

Among the specialized amino acid formulas available for use in patients with specific disease states, efficacy has been documented only for those enriched with branched-chain amino acids for treating hepatic encephalopathy (see Chapter 20).

MICRONUTRIENTS
Vitamins

The U.S. Recommended Dietary Allowances (RDAs) for micronutrients do not apply to parenteral nutrition because the absorptive process is bypassed. The American Medical Association (AMA) Nutrition Advisory Group's guidelines (box below) for maintenance parenteral vitamin requirements are reflected in the commercial multivitamin preparations most commonly used in TPN.

These levels have been shown to maintain already normal circulating vitamin levels but cannot be assumed to be sufficient to correct preexisting vitamin deficiencies or cover the needs of hypermetabolic, stressed patients. Consider whether the patient's vitamin intake has been adequate in the weeks preceding TPN and whether signs

---

PARENTERAL MULTIVITAMIN COMPOSITION*

Vitamin A: 3300 IU (990 µg)

Thiamin (vitamin B_1): 3 mg

Riboflavin (vitamin B_2): 3.6 mg

Niacin: 40 mg

Pyridoxine (vitamin B_6): 4 mg

Pantothenic acid: 15 mg

Vitamin B_{12}: 5 µg

Vitamin C: 100 mg

Vitamin D: 200 IU (5 µg)

Vitamin E: 10 mg (10 IU)

Folic acid: 400 µg

Biotin: 60 µg

*Recommended for daily use in parenteral nutrition by the AMA Nutrition Advisory Group.[1] These amounts are contained in the standard dose of most preparations designed for parenteral nutrition.

of a vitamin deficiency are present. If a deficiency is likely, parenteral vitamin intake should exceed maintenance levels for at least several days. This can be achieved by using single vitamin preparations such as vitamin C in added doses or by using multiple vials of multivitamin preparations, although the latter approach may still result in a low intake of some vitamins. In addition, because vitamin C requirements may be increased in the stress state, it is often advisable to use additional amounts (e.g., 500 to 1000 mg per day).

Vitamin K, the only vitamin missing from the maintenance vitamin preparations, is generally provided in the form of 10 mg of phytonadione once weekly. This dose may need to be reduced or eliminated if the patient is on anticoagulants or has a thrombotic tendency; it may need to be increased if the prothrombin time is prolonged because of vitamin K deficiency.

Minerals

The major minerals provided in parenteral nutrition are shown in the box below and paired with the salts with which they are most commonly used.

It is usually possible to make precise changes in the patient's mineral and acid-base status by altering the levels of the minerals (except for calcium, which has levels that are tightly regulated by parathormone). By substituting acetate for chloride with or without changes in sodium and potassium intake, it is usually possible to correct metabolic acidosis. It is also acceptable to use bicarbonate

---

MINERALS PROVIDED IN PARENTERAL NUTRITION

Cations and associated anions

Sodium: acetate, chloride, phosphate, bicarbonate
Potassium: acetate, chloride, phosphate
Calcium: gluceptate, gluconate, chloride
Magnesium: sulfate

DAILY MINERAL ALLOWANCES IN TPN

Phosphate: 20 to 40 mmol per day
Sodium: 60 or more mEq per day
Potassium: 60 or more mEq per day
Calcium: 10 to 15 mg per day
Magnesium: 16 to 24 mEq day

for this purpose, but acetate is preferred because buffering capacity can be lost if bicarbonate spontaneously converts to CO_2. Bicarbonate raises the pH of TPN, possibly precipitating with calcium or magnesium.

Although the amounts of minerals provided to patients in TPN must be individualized, there are suggested ranges for daily maintenance intake (box above).

When a patient needs more phosphorus, it can be provided in the sodium or potassium salt form. The solubility of admixtures of calcium, magnesium, and phosphorus is limited, and restrictions vary according to the amino acid preparation used (particularly its pH), so hospital pharmacies should have strict guidelines governing admixtures based on the products they use. The relative amounts of phosphorus, sodium, and potassium patients receive from sodium phosphate and potassium phosphate depend on the pH of the solution and how it is ordered. Most commercial potassium phosphate preparations provide 4.4 mEq potassium and 3 mmol phosphorus per ml. Therefore if an order is written for "20 mEq K^+ as K^+Phos," the patient will receive 20 mEq of potassium and about 14 mmol of phosphorus; if the order is written as "20 mmol of P as K^+Phos," the patient will receive 20 mmol of phosphorus and about 29 mEq of potassium. The latter is preferred.

Trace Elements

As with vitamins, multiple trace-element solutions that satisfy the maintenance requirements of most patients are available. The composition of a representative solution is shown in the box on the following page.

MULTIPLE TRACE-ELEMENT SOLUTION FOR TPN

Zinc (as sulfate): 4 mg
Copper (as sulfate): 0.8 to 1 mg
Chromium (as chloride): 10 to 12.5 µg
Manganese (as the sodium salt): 0.4 to 0.8 mg

Patients who have losses or increased requirements for zinc should be given additional doses—5 to 10 mg elemental zinc per day in patients who are stressed, postoperative, or have draining wounds and up to 12 to 17 mg for each liter of upper intestinal fluid lost through diarrhea or fistulae.

Iron dextran can be added to parenteral nutrition when needed to support iron status or correct deficiency. However, because most patients do not receive TPN long enough for poor intake to deplete their body iron stores, this is rarely necessary. When needed, it should be used cautiously in patients with autoimmune conditions because they have higher rates of hypersensitivity. Even then, a maximum daily dose of 50 mg of elemental iron generally prevents reactions and is better assimilated by the hematopoietic system than are higher doses. Intravenous selenium and molybdenum are available but are generally reserved for patients on long-term home parenteral nutrition with no other source.

DRUGS

Hyperglycemia is common in patients receiving TPN not only because of the large dextrose load but because most of the patients are in metabolic stress and some are diabetic. Therefore regular human insulin is added to the parenteral nutrition when necessary to control hyperglycemia. When insulin is used, a minimum dose of 15 U per bag or bottle should be provided to allow for adsorption to the container and tubing. However, before doing so be certain that the hyperglycemia is not simply a transient effect of TPN initiation and is not caused by hypophosphatemia. In the latter case, treatment should be directed toward repleting phosphorus, which in turn should relieve the hyperglycemia.

A number of other drugs such as cimetidine, ranitidine, heparin, and hydrocortisone are stable in certain parenteral nutrition admixtures. However, with some TNA formulations the drugs can disrupt the lipid emulsion, so seek advice on the specific drug and TPN formulation to be admixed (see Suggested Readings).

MANAGEMENT OF PARENTERAL NUTRITION
Inserting the Catheter

The method for inserting a subclavian central venous line is shown in Figure 13-1. For alternative methods using the internal jugular or PIC-line approach, see the Suggested Readings. Careful sterile technique is vital. Proper placement should be documented radiographically before parenteral nutrition is begun. Appropriate standing orders for catheter care are shown in the box on the following page. The catheter port designated for TPN can be changed

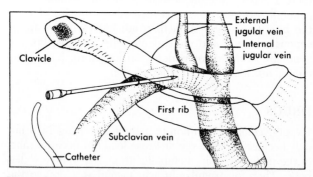

FIGURE 13-1   Subclavian line insertion. To insert the catheter needle into the right subclavian vein, the index finger of the left hand should be placed in the sternal notch and the thumb along the clavicle. A point is selected just inside the middle third of the clavicle. The needle is inserted with the bevel pointed upward through the pectoralis major muscle. The needle should hug the undersurface of the clavicle and should be aimed toward the index finger.

later if necessary, but the TPN port should not be used simultaneously for anything else. If the infusion is suddenly interrupted, it is prudent to infuse $D_{10}W$ to prevent hypoglycemia, although hypoglycemia is rare in hospitalized TPN patients.

Ordering Solutions

Before parenteral nutrition is ordered, a few basic decisions must be made. First, energy and protein requirements should be calculated (see Chapter 9). Calculation of the relative protein requirement (percent of energy as protein; see Chapter 9) helps in choosing the relative amounts of amino acids and nonprotein calories to include in the TPN regimen. Decide whether to use intravenous lipids daily or twice weekly as previously discussed. (If TNAs are available, they should generally be used.)

TPN order sheets used at the University of Alabama Hospital for 3-in-1 and 2-in-1 mixtures are shown in Figures 13-2 and 13-3, respectively. For the former, the concentrations and volumes of dextrose and amino acids de-

---

NURSING GUIDELINES FOR TPN PATIENTS

Obtain routine vital signs.

Record intake and output.

If a double- or triple-lumen catheter is used, label one lumen for TPN use exclusively.

Use an intravenous pump to maintain a constant infusion rate. If the infusion falls behind schedule, the rate can be increased by up to 20% in order to achieve the energy goal.

If the infusion is interrupted for any reason, infuse $D_{10}W$ at 50 to 75 ml/hr through a central or peripheral line. Notify the physician.

Change the intravenous administration set and tubing daily when hanging a new bag or bottle.

Maintain an aseptic, occlusive dressing, and change it at least twice weekly.

University of Alabama Hospital

ADULT PARENTERAL NUTRITION ORDER FORM

Date due _____   Time due _____   Bag # _____

The following information is required before the first bag of TPN will be formulated. Indicate with an asterisk if either height or weight is estimated. See instructions on back of form.

Nutritional diagnosis (circle any that apply): kwashiorkor (260); marasmus (261); other protein-calorie malnutrition—severe (262), moderate (263), mild (263.1)

Problem requiring TPN use _____

Height _____   Weight _____ lb/kg   Age ____   Sex ____   BEE[1] ____

Stress factor used[2] _____   Total calories per 24 hours (rounded to multiple of 200) _____

| Check one | Formula | Percent of calories from | | | Approximate volume per 1000 kcal |
		Dextrose	Amino acids[3]	Fat	
	Central vein use only				
	Regular protein	60	15	25	760
	Intermediate protein	60	19	21	840
	High protein	60	24	16	930
	Restricted protein	60	10	30	650
	Reduced carbohydrate, high fat	45	15	40	770
	Regular protein, fat-free	85	15	0	740
	Special formula				
	Peripheral vein	32	16	52	1410

Additives	Quantity ordered	Suggested adult daily guidelines
Sodium acetate[4]	mEq	60+ mEq sodium
Sodium chloride	mEq	
Potassium acetate[4]	mEq	60+ mEq potassium
Potassium chloride	mEq	
Phosphorus as potassium[5,6]	mmol	30-40 mmol phosphorus (*Note:* max 15 mmol/L solution)
Phosphorus as sodium[6]	mmol	
Calcium gluceptate[6]	mEq	10-15 mEq (*Note:* max 10 mEq/L solution)
Magnesium sulfate[6]	mEq	16-24 mEq
MVI-12	ml	10 ml
Trace elements[7]	ml	4 ml
Vitamin K	mg	10 mg once weekly
Optional additives		
Extra ascorbic acid	mg	
Extra zinc	mg	
Insulin, regular human	U	

Date ordered _____   Time ordered _____   Physician signature _____

FIGURE 13-2   **Front,** Example of a TNA order form.

Instructions

A. Please use one of the listed formulas if possible. Special formulas may require the approval of Pharmacy. For assistance, page the Unit Dietitian, Pharmacist, or Nutrition Fellow.

B. These mixtures may require up to 4 hours of preparation time; please allow for this. Orders received between 6:00 AM and 4:00 PM will be filled the same day.

C. Central vein formulas utilize 70% dextrose, 10% amino acids, and 20% fat emulsion to provide maximally concentrated solutions. Sterile water may be requested as an additive. The peripheral vein formula utilizes 20% dextrose, 8.5% amino acids, and 10% fat emulsion. In either case the final total volume is determined by the formula, number of calories, and additives ordered. The approximate final volume and hourly infusion rate will be noted on each bag. The infusion rate may require adjustment by the nurse so that the entire volume is infused within 24 hours.

Footnotes

1. Basal energy expenditure (BEE) is calculated as:

   Women $BEE = 655.10 + 9.56W + 1.85H - 4.68A$
   Men $BEE = 66.47 + 13.75W + 5.00H - 6.76A$

   where:
   W = weight (kg)
   H = height (cm)
   A = age (yrs)
   "Dry" weight should be used in edematous patients, and a moderately obese weight such as 100 kg should be used in severely obese patients.

2. Commonly used stress factors by which the BEE is multiplied to estimate total calorie requirements include: unstressed or minor surgery, 1.2; trauma, 1.34; sepsis, 1.6; major burns, 1.5-2. A general range of 1.2 to 1.5 times BEE is also acceptable. However, this amount should usually not be given on the first day of TPN. Rather, begin with about half the desired calories on the first day and increase to the desired calorie level as tolerated (usually on the second day for stressed patients but not before 4-6 days in severely cachectic patients).

3. Determine protein needs, preferably from a 24-hour urinary urea nitrogen (UUN) measurement, which can be used to calculate protein balance as long as the BUN and fluid status are stable:

   Protein loss (g/day) = (24-hour UUN [g] + 4) × 6.25
   Protein balance = Protein intake − Protein loss

   The Recommended Dietary Allowance for protein is 0.75 g/kg/day, but stress increases protein requirements, often to 1-1.5 g/kg/day. For healthy people, 10%-12% of calories should be protein; in stressed patients, 15%-24% of calories should be protein. Protein provides 4 kcal/g.

4. Either acetate or chloride is acceptable for most patients, but acetate is often preferable because it assists in correcting metabolic acidosis.

5. Use some phosphorus in each bag of TPN, particularly the *first* bag unless specifically contraindicated. Each 3 mmol of phosphorus contains approximately 4 mEq of cation (sodium or potassium).

6. Safe limits of compatible electrolyte concentrations *per 1000 ml final volume*, in addition to the phosphorus present in the amino acid base solution are:

Formula	Central vein	Peripheral vein
Calcium, mEq	10	5
Magnesium, mEq	20	20
Phosphorus, mmol	15	10

7. Each milliliter of trace elements contains 1 mg zinc, 0.2 mg copper, 0.1 mg manganese, 0.028 mg iodine, and 3.125 μg chromium.

FIGURE 13-2   **Back,** Example of a TNA order form.

University of Alabama Hospital

DAILY PARENTERAL NUTRITION ORDER FORM
(1) TPN orders may utilize either standard formulas (A, B, C) or individualized ingredients (amino acids, dextrose, water).
(2) Number bottles sequentially.
(3) Orders should be for 24 hours.
(4) Orders for initial bottle should be written at least 1 hour prior to planned START TIME.
(5) For further information refer to the *Handbook of Clinical Nutrition.* | Addressograph

Bottle =				
Begin: Date/hr				
Infusion time or rate[1]				
Optional Formula code (A, B, or C below)				
Amino acid sol'n _____ %	ml	ml	ml	ml
Dextrose _____ %	ml	ml	ml	ml
Water for injection	ml	ml	ml	ml
ELECTROLYTES (Suggested adult guidelines)				
Sodium as chloride (60+ mEq/Day)	mEq	mEq	mEq	mEq
as bicarbonate[2]	mEq	mEq	mEq	mEq
Potassium as chloride (60+ mEq/day)	mEq	mEq	mEq	mEq
Phosphate as K buffer[3] (20-40 mM/day)	mM	mM	mM	mM
Calcium as gluceptate (10-15 mEq/day)	mEq	mEq	mEq	mEq
Magnesium as sulfate (8-20 mEq/day)	mEq	mEq	mEq	mEq
VITAMINS MVI-12[4] (10 ml QD)	ml	ml	ml	ml
Ascorbic acid (1000 mg QD)	mg	mg	mg	mg
Vitamin K[4] (10 mg/wk)	mg	mg	mg	mg
Insulin, regular	U	U	U	U
OTHER				
Trace elements (2 ml/day)	ml	ml	ml	ml
Lipid emulsion 10% (peripheral)	ml	ml	ml	ml

Physician signature

Formula A		Formula B		Formula C	
Base solution[5]	1000 ml	Base solution[5]	1000 ml	Base solution[5]	1000 ml
Ascorbic acid	1000 mg	Potassium	29.3 mEq	Magnesium as sulfate	16 mEq
[4]Multivitamin		Phosphorus	20 mM	Calcium as gluceptate	15 mEq
Potassium	29.3 mEq	Sodium	25 mEq	Sodium as chloride	40 mEq
Phosphorus	20 mM	Bicarbonate	25 mEq	Trace elements[6]	2 ml

[1]Suggested initial rate: bottle 1, 50 ml/hr; bottle 2-3, 75 ml/hr; bottle 4-6, 100 ml/hr.
[2]Poorly compatible with Ca & Mg salts.
[3]Poorly compatible with Ca salts: 20 mM of phosphate as K buffer contains 29.3 mEq of potassium.

[4]Vitamin schedule:	[5]Base solution contains:		[6]Trace elements contained per ml:	
MVI-12: daily	Calories (carbohydrate)	850 Kcal	Zinc	2 mg
Vitamin K 10 mg:	Protein	42.5g	Copper	0.4 mg
Wed.	Glucose	250g	Manganese	0.2 mg
	Nitrogen	6.7g	Iodine	0.056 mg
	Phosphorus	0	Chromium	6.25 μg
	Potassium	2.7 mEq	Sodium chloride	9 mg
	Acetate	45 mEq		
	Chloride	17.5 mEq		

N-112 (25391)
Rev. 81

FIGURE 13-3   Example of a 2-in-1 TPN order form.

sired must be indicated; for the latter, only the total calories desired must be indicated and an admixture of carbohydrate, protein, and fat chosen. In both cases the quantities of micronutrients must be specified. TPN orders must be written daily.

To facilitate ordering solutions the energy and protein content of a container of TPN can be calculated as follows:

Protein content = (ml aa)[aa conc (g/ml)]
Energy content = (Protein content)(4 kcal/g) + (ml dex)
 [Dex conc (g/ml)](3.4 kcal/g) + (ml lipids)(1.1 or 2 kcal/ml)

where

 dex = Dextrose
 aa = Amino acids
 conc = Concentration (e.g., 50% dextrose = 0.5 g/ml and
  8.5% amino acids = 0.085 g/ml)
1.1 kcal/ml applies to 10% lipids and 2 kcal/ml to 20% lipids.

As an example, a solution containing 500 ml of 10% amino acids, 500 ml of 50% dextrose, and 500 ml of 10% lipids (either admixed or separately) has the following composition:

Protein content = (500 ml)(0.1 g/ml) = 50 g
Energy content = (50 g)(4 kcal/g) +
  (500 ml)(0.5 g/ml)(3.4 kcal/g) + (500 ml)(1.1 kcal/ml)
  = 200 kcal protein + 850 kcal dextrose +
   550 kcal lipids
  = 1600 kcal total

The relative contributions of carbohydrate, protein, and fat are calculated as:

850/1600 = 53% carbohydrate
200/1600 = 13% protein
550/1600 = 34% fat

Table 13-1 lists sample CPN and PPN formulations using 2-in-1 or 3-in-1 admixtures, daily or twice-weekly lipid options, and various amounts of protein.

TABLE 13-1 Sample parenteral nutrition formulas

Formula description	Amino acids (%, ml)a	Dextrose (%, ml)a	Lipid (%, ml/day)b	Energy density (kcal/ml)c	Volume (ml/2000 kcal)d
2-in-1, separate daily lipid, standard protein (12%-14% protein, 59%-61% CHO,e 27% fat)	8.5%-10% 500	50% 500	10% 500	1.02-1.05	1950
2-in-1, separate daily lipid, standard protein (15% protein, 58% CHO, 27% fat)	10% 600	70% 400	10% 500	1.2	1700
2-in-1, separate twice-weekly lipid, standard protein (17% protein, 83% CHO)	8.5% 500	50% 500	—	1.02	2000
2-in-1, separate daily lipid, high protein (22% protein, 51% CHO, 27% fat)	10% 650	50% 350	10% 500	0.85	2200
2-in-1, separate daily lipid, high protein (19% protein, 55% CHO, 26% fat)	10% 600	50% 400	10% 500	0.9	2100
2-in-1, separate twice-weekly lipid, high protein (20% protein, 80% CHO)	10% 600	70% 400	—	1.2	1667

	Protein		CHO[e]		Lipid[b]		Energy density[c]	Total kcal
Peripheral, 2-in-1, separate daily lipid (24% protein, 48% CHO, 28% fat)	8.5%	500	20%	500	10%	500	0.51	3340
Peripheral, 3-in-1 (16% protein, 32% CHO, 52% fat)	8.5%	950	20%	940	10%	950	0.7	2840
3-in-1, standard protein (15% protein, 60% CHO, 25% fat)	10%	750	70%	500	20%	250	1.3	1500
3-in-1, high protein (20% protein, 60% CHO, 20% fat)	10%	1000	70%	500	20%	200	1.2	1700

[a] For 2-in-1 solutions, ml/1-L container; for 3-in-1 solutions, ml/day. For these illustrations, it is assumed that 2-in-1 solutions are contained in 1-L bottles or bags, and 3-in-1 solutions in 2- or 3-L bags.

[b] In 3-in-1 solutions, lipid is admixed with the dextrose and amino acids. In 2-in-1 solutions, lipid is piggybacked into the TPN IV or infused in a separate IV or lumen. When lipid is used twice weekly, the amount is not listed in this table.

[c] For 2-in-1 solutions, energy density is given only for the dextrose-amino acid mixture; 10% lipid emulsions yield 1.1 kcal/ml; 20% lipid emulsions yield 2.0 kcal/ml.

[d] For 2-in-1 solutions with separate daily lipid, includes 500 ml 10% intravenous lipid.

[e] Carbohydrate.

The initial infusion rate varies among patients (see Chapter 9). Highly stressed patients who have been receiving intravenous dextrose infusions can start receiving at about 50 ml/hr and be advanced quickly (e.g., every 8 hours) to reach their full energy requirements within 24 to 48 hours. Severely cachectic, chronically starved patients should be fed more gradually (see Table 9-3). When TNAs are used, simply order gradually increasing calorie levels on the days preceding full feeding. With 1-L containers of 2-in-1 solutions, the pertinent number of containers should be ordered each day and the infusion rate set to achieve the appropriate energy intake. It is not necessary to start with low concentrations of dextrose (e.g., 20% as opposed to 50% or 70%) when the initial rate of infusion is low.

Terminating the Infusion

Dextrose infusion stimulates insulin secretion, and insulin levels remain elevated for a short time after the dextrose infusion ceases. If the infusion is terminated abruptly, hypoglycemia occasionally ensues. Although many patients receiving TPN are protected from this by stress-induced, insulin-resistant hyperglycemia, it is wise to taper the infusion rate by 50% to 70% for 30 to 60 minutes before discontinuing parenteral nutrition. Longer tapering periods are unnecessary, and no tapering is required if the patient is being fed enterally or orally at the time TPN is discontinued.

Follow-Up

Aside from proper general medical and nursing care, laboratory monitoring is the major method required for tracking the course of TPN. Fluctuations in serum electrolytes often necessitate adjustment of the formula from day to day. However, additions should not be made to a container of TPN currently being infused, nor should TPN be used to correct major electrolyte abnormalities. In these

Laboratory Tests to Monitor Parenteral Nutrition

Measure daily until stable, then 2 to 3 times weekly:

Electrolytes (sodium, potassium, chloride, bicarbonate)
Glucose
Phosphorus

Measure 1 to 2 times weekly:

Calcium, magnesium
Liver function tests
Blood urea nitrogen (BUN), creatinine
Serum albumin

situations, it is more appropriate to use a separate intravenous line. A general outline for laboratory monitoring is given in the box.

COMPLICATIONS

Serious complications of parenteral nutrition can nearly always be avoided by careful patient management.[2] Technical complications, which relate to central venous catheter placement and are therefore not unique to parenteral nutrition, are best prevented by careful, unhurried insertion of the central line by an experienced physician. The most common complications are the development of a pneumothorax or hemothorax.

When sepsis occurs in a patient receiving TPN, it usually results from a lapse in aseptic catheter-care technique. Sepsis was common in the early 1970s when experience with parenteral nutrition was not widespread. Its prevalence decreased when nursing guidelines such as those listed were standardized, but it increased again after triple-lumen central venous catheters were introduced, probably because of frequent manipulation of the catheter ports.

The offending organisms in TPN sepsis are usually skin contaminants such as *Staphylococcus aureus, S. epidermidis,* and *Candida albicans,* but there are sometimes gram-negative bacteria such as *Pseudomonas* and *Klebsiella* organisms in hospitalized patients. Definite catheter sepsis usually requires removal of the catheter, but if the source of a fever is uncertain, the catheter can be cultured and replaced over a guidewire until the results of the catheter culture are available. If the catheter culture is positive, the replacement catheter should be removed and if necessary a new one placed in a different site; if the culture is negative, the replacement catheter does not need to be disturbed.

Infections involving tunneled Silastic catheters can usually be treated without catheter removal. In these cases, successful treatment often requires infusion of urokinase through the catheter to lyse an infected thrombus.

Metabolic complications of TPN are more common than technical and septic complications, because the metabolic requirements of individual patients cannot be fully reduced to standard guidelines. The most serious complication, as discussed in Chapter 9, is sudden, severe hypophosphatemia induced by dextrose infusion.[2,3] Although phosphorus levels drop in most patients after initiation of TPN, severely cachectic patients are the most susceptible to its potentially lethal effects. These can be prevented by putting *phosphorus* in the *first* container of TPN in all patients, unless a specific contraindication exists (mainly hyperphosphatemia in renal failure). Because the risk of transient *hyper*phosphatemia is minimal except in hypercalcemic patients (whose risk of calcium-phosphate crystallization is greater), phosphorus should be placed in the first few containers of TPN until the patient's response has been determined.

In patients receiving TPN, serum phosphorus levels below 2 mg/dl are potentially serious and should be corrected by infusing about 1 mmol/kg phosphorus over 24 hours. Levels below 1 mg/dl require immediate attention and should be treated by decreasing the rate of dextrose infusion and by giving about 1.5 mmol/kg phosphorus over

24 hours, preferably through another IV line. More rapid infusion rates (e.g., in 6 hours) can cause calcium-phosphate precipitation in the kidneys and muscles and should be avoided.

The most common but generally less serious metabolic abnormality in patients receiving TPN is hyperglycemia. After ruling out hypophosphatemia as a possible cause, it is treated by adding insulin to the TPN container, reducing the dextrose load by substituting lipids for dextrose, and/or ensuring that the total energy load is not excessive.

Hypokalemia and hyperkalemia are also common metabolic complications of TPN. They can be readily prevented and treated by using appropriate amounts of potassium in the TPN. Hyponatremia and hypernatremia require assessment of both sodium and water balances and should be treated by appropriate alterations in total sodium and water intakes.

Mild to moderate elevations in liver enzymes and bilirubin occur frequently in patients receiving parenteral nutrition. The abnormalities are associated with intrahepatic cholestasis and fatty deposition in the liver, probably induced by constant dextrose infusion. It is usually benign and self-limited, requiring no intervention. If progressive increases are seen, causes other than the TPN should first be ruled out. If the TPN energy load is excessive, it should be reduced. If dextrose is being used as the predominant energy source, it may help to substitute lipids for a portion of the dextrose calories.

If these are not the causes, cycling the TPN (i.e., infusing the same energy load in a shorter time and giving the liver a rest during part of each day) is often effective. This is done by increasing the infusion rate by 25% to 33% to deliver the daily amount over 16 to 18 hours, then tapering at an intermediate rate for 30 to 60 minutes, and capping the infusion port or infusing non–glucose-containing IV fluids during the remaining 6 to 8 hours. As an alternative, the TPN infusion can be tapered and maintained at a "keep open" rate of about 10 ml/hr for 6 to 8 hours.

References

1. American Medical Association, Department of Foods and Nutrition: Multivitamin preparations for parenteral use: a statement by the Nutrition Advisory Group, *JPEN* 3:258, 1979.
2. Weinsier RL, Bacon J, Butterworth CE, Jr: Central venous alimentation: A prospective study of the frequency of metabolic abnormalities among medical and surgical patients, *JPEN* 6:421, 1982.
3. Weinsier RL, Krumdieck CL: Death resulting from overzealous parenteral nutrition: the refeeding syndrome revisited, *Am J Clin Nutr* 34:393, 1981.

Suggested Readings

LaFrance RJ, Miyagawa CI: *Pharmaceutical considerations in total parenteral nutrition.* In Fischer JE, ed: *Total parenteral nutrition,* ed 2, Boston, 1991, Little, Brown.

Rombeau JL, Caldwell MD, eds: *Clinical nutrition: parenteral feeding,* ed 2, Philadelphia, 1992, WB Saunders.

Torosian MH, ed: *Nutrition for the hospitalized patient,* New York, 1995, Marcel Dekker.

14

Drug-Nutrient Interactions

Drug-nutrient interactions can manifest themselves in many ways. Food can increase, decrease, or delay drug absorption. Foods can also influence the rate of drug metabolism by either increasing or decreasing the production of drug-metabolizing enzymes or influencing splanchnic-hepatic blood flow. Varying the protein/carbohydrate ratio in a diet, consuming a diet high in charcoal-broiled beef or cruciferous vegetables, or consuming grapefruit juice simultaneously with certain medications have all been found to influence the metabolism of some drugs. A drug loses its therapeutic efficacy when a food substance delays or prevents it from being absorbed or accelerates the rate of its metabolism or elimination. A toxic reaction from a drug is possible when a food increases its absorption or prevents its metabolism or elimination. In general, drugs should not be taken with meals unless they would otherwise cause significant gastrointestinal upset. Table 14-1 reviews the influence of food on drugs when they are taken together and makes recommendations concerning their administration times.

Drugs that inhibit monoamine oxidase can produce a hypertensive crisis when taken in conjunction with foods that have high tyramine contents. The severity of the response is related to the dosage of the drug and the level of tyramine in the particular food. The drugs and food involved are listed in Table 14-1.

Drugs can also induce nutritional deficiencies by decreasing nutrient intake, causing malabsorption or hyper-

TABLE 14-1 Nutrient effects on drugs

Effect	Drug
Decreased absorption	
Avoid taking these drugs with food. Take at least 1 hour before or 2 hours after a meal.	Ampicillin
	Atenolol
	Captopril
	Cephalexin
	Cloxacillin
	Erythromycin stearate
	Furosemide
	Hydralazine
	Iron
	Isoniazid
	Levodopa/carbidopa
	Midazolam
	Penicillin G
	Penicillin V
	Propantheline
	Quinidine
	Methotrexate
	Tetracycline
	Zinc sulfate
Increased absorption	
Food will alter the amount of the drug absorbed, therefore the drug should be taken at the same time(s) or way each day.	Atovaquone
	Carbamazepine
	Diazepam
	Dicumarol
	Griseofulvin
	Labetalol
	Lithium
	Melphalan
	Methoxsalen
	Metoprolol
	Metronidazole
	Nitrofurantoin

TABLE 14-1 Nutrient effects on drugs—cont'd

Effect	Drug
Increased absorption—cont'd	
	Phenytoin
	Propafenone
	Propranolol
	Spironolactone
	Sulfadiazine
Delayed absorption	
Food will delay the absorption of these drugs but not the overall amount absorbed. These drugs should be taken at least 1 hour before or 2 hours after a meal.	Acetaminophen
	Aspirin
	Cimetidine
	Doxycycline
	Hydrochlorothiazide
	Hydrocortisone
	Indomethacin
	Ketoprofen
	Pentobarbital
	Pentoxifylline
	Sulfisoxazole
	Suprofen
	Tocainide
Monoamine oxidase inhibitors	
Foods to avoid or limit	
Ale, beer, Chianti and vermouth wines, hard cheeses, breads and crackers containing cheese, broad bean pods, fava beans, sauerkraut, Brewer's yeast, gravies, soups and sauces made from meat extracts, sour cream, chocolate, soy sauce, and yogurt	Isocarboxazid
	Pargyline
	Phenelzine
	Tranylcypromine

excretion of nutrients, increasing nutrient catabolism, or impairing nutrient utilization. The clinical significance of drug-induced deficiencies depends on the level of depletion reached, which is in turn influenced by the initial nutrient level and the presence of other risk factors such as poor intake, poverty, disability, alcohol abuse etc. (see Chapter 8). The dose of the drug and duration of time the drug is being taken are also very important. Table 14-2 lists drugs that can induce nutrient deficiencies, and their clinical significance.

The "active" ingredient in a drug is not always the agent involved in drug-nutrient interactions. For instance, sorbitol is used as a base in many liquid medicinal preparations because it enhances their palatability, improves solutions' stabilities, and does not crystallize like other syrup vehicles. It is not absorbed by the gastrointestinal tract and does not raise blood glucose levels. However, sorbitol is far from inactive. Osmotic diarrhea almost always results when patients receive 20 to 30 g per day of sorbitol, and some patients have diarrhea with only 10 g per day. Because liquid drug preparations are very frequently given to patients receiving enteral feedings, sorbitol is a common but often undetected cause of diarrhea in these patients (see Chapter 12). Table 14-3 lists common liquid medications and their sorbitol contents. It should be noted that drug manufacturers can change the amount of sorbitol in their products at will because it is listed among the "inactive" ingredients, the contents of which are not disclosed on the label.

Text continued on p. 335.

TABLE 14-2 Drug effects on nutrients

Drug	Nutrient effect	Mechanism	Situation	Clinical significance*
Antiinfective drugs				
Aminosalicylic acid	Decreased vitamin B12 absorption	Unknown	Dose and duration related	(+) Megaloblastic anemia reported
	Decreased fat absorption	Unknown	Dose related, demonstrated with 12 g/day in normal subjects	(?) Mild steatorrhea
Amphotericin B	Hypokalemia, hypomagnesemia, and hyperkaluria	Direct toxic effect on the distal tubular epithelium	Dose-related response	(+) Reports of severe hypokalemia and hypomagnesemia
Capreomycin	Hypokalemia, hypomagnesemia, and hypocalcemia	(?) hyperaldosteronism or direct renal toxicity	Long-term therapy	Responded to withdrawal of the drug and supplementation with electrolytes
Cycloserine	Decreased serum folate	Unknown	Dose related	(?) Reports of anemia responsive to folate and pyridoxine

Continued

*(+), Significant; (?), uncertain; (O), none known.

TABLE 14-2 Drug effects on nutrients—cont'd

Drug	Nutrient effect	Mechanism	Situation	Clinical significance*
Antiinfective drugs—cont'd				
Gentamicin, tobramycin, amikacin, and sisomicin	Hypokalemia, hypomagnesemia, hypocalcemia; increased urinary potassium and magnesium loss	Unknown	Long-term therapy	(+) Cases reported with hypocalcemia responsive to magnesium replacement, supplementation of magnesium and potassium required
Isoniazid	Pyridoxine deficiency	Isoniazid-pyridoxine hydrazone formation that inhibits pyridoxine kinase with rapid urinary excretion of the complex	Dose dependent, slow acetylators, alcoholics, and malnourished more susceptible	(+) Neuritis common, convulsions reported; pyridoxine prophylaxis recommended

Neomycin	Decreased absorption of vitamin A, amino acids, fat, xylose, sucrose, lactose, calcium, potassium, and sodium	Precipitation of bile salts and direct toxic effect to the intestinal mucosa	Demonstrated in studies in doses of 1-12 g/day	(?) Effects last 6-14 days after drug is discontinued
Pyrimethamine	Folate deficiency	Blocks dihydrofolate reductase	25 mg daily dose for 7 weeks	(+) Folic acid deficiency due to the direct effect of the drug
Sulfasalazine	Decreased serum folic acid	Inhibition of intestinal transport system responsible for folate absorption	Demonstrated in normal patients and in patients with inflammatory bowel disease	(?) May promote the development of a folate deficiency in patients with inflammatory bowel disease, which may increase the risk for colon cancer in patients with ulcerative colitis

Continued

°+, Significant; ?, uncertain; O, none known.

TABLE 14-2 Drug effects on nutrients—cont'd

Drug	Nutrient effect	Mechanism	Situation	Clinical significance*
Cardiovascular drugs				
Hydralazine	Pyridoxine deficiency	(?) Binds to pyridoxal phosphate to form a hydrazone with increased urinary excretion of the complex	Risk factors include slow acetylators, high dose therapy, and limited B_6 intake	(+) Case reports responsive to supplemental B_6 and withdrawal of the drug
Sodium nitroprusside	Decreased levels of serum B_{12}	Unknown	Hypotensive anesthesia and in post MI patients	(?) Rebound of serum cobalamin levels 24 hours after infusion is discontinued
Central nervous system drugs				
Aspirin	Decreased total serum and protein bound serum folate	(?) Redistribution of serum folate	Dose dependent	(0) No reports of folate deficiency, rebounds quickly with aspirin withdrawal

Drug	Effect	Mechanism	Comments	Significance
	Decreased plasma, leukocyte, and platelet ascorbic acid levels	Increased urinary excretion and (?) competitive inhibition of ascorbic acid uptake into leukocytes	Observed in single and multiple-dose therapy	(?) Significantly lower leukocyte and platelet ascorbic acid levels with 8–12 tablets/day, variable reports of correction with vitamin C supplementation
Phenytoin, phenobarbital, primidone, and carbamazepine	Decreased serum calcium, decreased serum 25-hydroxy-cholecalciferol	Unknown, (?) induction of hepatic microsomal enzymes or direct inhibitory effect on intestinal calcium transport and bone metabolism	At-risk patients: those with dark or black skin whose diet and exposure to sunlight might be inadequate, on chronic, high-dose, multiple drug therpy with restricted physical activity;	(+) Reports of osteomalacia and rickets responding to vitamin D supplementation

*+, Significant; ?, uncertain; O, none known.

Continued

TABLE 14-2 Drug effects on nutrients—cont'd

Drug	Nutrient effect	Mechanism	Situation	Clinical significance*
Central nervous system drugs—cont'd				
Phenytoin—cont'd	Decreased serum folate	Unknown	does not appear to be dose or duration related	(+) Cases of macrocytosis reported (<1% incidence of megaloblastic anemia); responsive to folate supplementation
Phenytoin, barbiturates, and primidone	Decreased vitamin K dependent coagulation factors (II, VII, IX, and X) in neonates	Unknown, (?) enzyme induction or competitive inhibition of clotting factor production	Newborn infants whose mothers were on chronic therapy	(+)Case reports of hemorrhage generally within the first 24 hours after delivery; most respond to vitamin K supplementation

Electrolyte drugs			
Potassium chloride slow release	Changes ileal pH < 6, which inhibits activity of intrinsic factor	Long-term therapy in elderly patients	(?)Possibility of B_{12} deficiency with prolonged use
Gastrointestinal drugs			
Aluminum hydroxide	Forms insoluble complex in the gastrointestinal tract	Long-term, high-dose therapy and in those with limited phosphate intake	(+)Reports of hypophosphatemia and osteomalacia
	Hypophosphatemia		
Cholestyramine	Binds intrinsic factor and complexes bile salts	Demonstrated in normal patients and in children with hypercholesterolemia	(+)Vitamin deficiencies possible
	Decreased absorption of vitamins B_{12}, A, E, D, K, and folic acid; decreased fat absorption		
Cimetidine	(?)Decreased acid mediated release of B_{12} from food	Therapeutic doses	(?)B_{12} deficiency possible with prolonged therapy or if body stores are low
	Decreased absorption of food bound or protein-bound vitamin B_{12}		

Continued

°+, Significant; ?, uncertain; O, none known.

TABLE 14-2 Drug effects on nutrients—cont'd

Drug	Nutrient effect	Mechanism	Situation	Clinical significance*
Gastrointestinal drugs—cont'd				
Sucralfate	Decreased serum phosphate	Forms insoluble complex in the gastrointestinal tract	Documented in end-stage renal disease patients receiving 1 g 4 times/day	(+)Comparable portency of aluminum hydroxide in lowering serum phosphate levels
Hormones				
Oral contraceptives	Decreased serum folate	Unknown, (?) altered metabolism	Usually no deficiency unless diet is marginal; longer-term use and diet related	(+)Cases of megaloblastic anemia reported
	Riboflavin deficiency	Unknown		(+)Report of decreased erythrocyte glutathione reductase levels
	Pyridoxine deficiency	Unknown, (?) altered metabolism	Demonstrated with estrogen-containing products only	(+)Depression responsive to B₆ supplementation

Other agents			
Alcohol			
	Folic acid deficiency	Decreased intake, absorption, entero-hepatic recirculation, and hepatic storage	(+)Folate-deficiency anemia occurs commonly
	Thiamin deficiency	Decreased intake and active intestinal transport; defective phosphorylation and storage in liver	High frequency in alcoholism probably related to deficient intake	(+)Peripheral neuropathy, Wernicke-Korsakoff syndrome
	Pyridoxine deficiency	Decreased production of pyridoxal phosphate (active form) from pyridoxine in liver		(?)Sideroblastic anemia, neurologic dysfunction

Continued

°+, Significant; ?, uncertain; O, none known.

TABLE 14-2 Drug effects on nutrients—cont'd

Drug	Nutrient effect	Mechanism	Situation	Clinical significance*
Other agents—cont'd				
Alcohol—cont'd	Vitamin A deficiency	Decreased retinol-binding protein (RBP) production in presence of liver disease; accelerated destruction in liver	Decreased liver vitamin A content, proportional to extent of liver disease	(+)Night blindness, perhaps other manifestations
	Magnesium deficiency	Increased urinary excretion, especially with acute alcohol administration	Low serum and muscle Mg^{++} levels common in alcoholics	(+)Hypocalcemia, neuromuscular excitability
	Increased iron absorption	(?)Increased gastric acid secretion, increasing nonheme iron absorption		(+)Increased risk for iron overload and organ damage; iron deficency uncommon in alcoholics except with gastrointestinal bleeding

Decreased serum phosphorus	Increased urinary excretion	Reports of hypophosphatemia in up to 50% of alcoholics; may be involved in alcoholic myopathy	(+)Increased risk of glucose-induced hypophosphatemia
Zinc deficiency	Poor intake, increased urinary excretion, and decreased serum levels, especially in presence of liver disease	May overlap with vitamin A deficiency because zinc is needed to mobilize RBP from liver and to convert retinol to retinal	(+)May contribute, with vitamin A deficiency, to night blindness
Decreased lactose absorption	Decreased intestinal lactase	Blacks more susceptible than whites	(+)Often improved lactose intolerance on alcohol withdrawal

°+, Significant; ?, uncertain; O, none known.

Continued

TABLE 14-2 Drug effects on nutrients—cont'd

Drug	Nutrient effect	Mechanism	Situation	Clinical significance*
Other agents—cont'd				
Colchicine	Increased fecal loss of sodium, potassium, fat and nitrogen; decreased absorption of D-xylose and vitamin B_{12}	Disruption of intestinal mucosal function	Doses of 1.9-3.9 mg/d	(?)Theoretical consideration; effect reversed 4-7 days after drug is stopped

D-penicillamine	Pyridoxine deficiency	Antagonism of pyridoxal-5'-phosphate		(+)Reports of peripheral neuropathy and optic neuritis responding to pyridoxine supplementation
Methotrexate	Folate deficiency, decreased serum vitamin B_{12}, decreased D-xylose absorption	Binds to dihydrofolate reductase; (?) B_{12} impaired absorption; decreased intestinal epithelium mitotic count	Dose- and duration-related	(+)Folic acid deficiency due to direct effect of the drug; decreased B_{12} in psoriasis patients

°+, Significant; ?, uncertain; O, none known.

TABLE 14-3 Sorbitol content of selected drug preparations

Active ingredient	Dosage form	Brand name	Manufacturer	Sorbitol content (g/ml)	Sorbitol content (g/common dose)
Acetaminophen	—	—	Roxane	0.35	7.1 g/650 mg
	Elixir	Tylenol	McNeil	<0.2	<4 g/650 mg
	Solution	Tylenol	McNeil	0	0 g/650 mg
Acetaminophen with codeine	—	—	Carnick	0.06	0.9 g/15 ml
	—	—	Roxane	0	0 g/15 ml
Aluminum hydroxide and magnesium carbonate	Suspension	Gaviscon	Marion Merrell Dow	0.073	1.1 g/15 ml
Aluminum hydroxide and magnesium hydroxide	Suspension	Maalox	Rhone-Poulenc Rorer	0.045	0.675 g/15 ml
	Suspension	Maalox TC	Rhone-Poulenc Rorer	0.15	2.25 g/15 ml
		Maalox Plus Extra Strength	Rhone-Poulenc Rorer	0.1	1.5 g/15 ml
Amantadine	Solution	Symmetrel	Du Pont	0.72	7.2 g/100 mg
Aminocaproic acid	Syrup	Amicar	Lederle	0.26	5.2 g/5 g
Aminophylline	—	—	Roxane	0.136	1.3 g/200 mg
Calcium carbonate	Suspension	—	Roxane	0.28	1.4 g/500 mg

Drug	Form	Trade name	Manufacturer		
Carbamazepine	Suspension	Tegretol	Ciba-Geigy	0.17	1.7 g/200 mg
Charcoal, activated	Syrup	—	Paddock	0.4	48 g/25 g
Chloral hydrate	Syrup	—	UDL	0.4	2 g/500 mg
Chlorpromazine		—	Roxane	0.14	0.7 g/500 mg
Cimetidine	Solution	Tagamet	Roxane	0.035	0.03 g/25 mg
			Smith Kline Beecham	0.5	2.5 g/300 mg
Codeine phosphate		—	Roxane	0.28	1.4 g/15 mg
Dexamethasone		Hexadrol	Organon	0.51	3.86 g/0.75 mg
			Roxane	0.24	1.84 g/0.75 mg
Diazepam	Solution	—	Roxane	0.21	1.05 g/5 mg
Diphenoxylate and atropine	Solution	Lomotil	GD Searle	0.21	1.05 g/5 ml
Doxepin			Roxane	0.455	2.275 g/5ml
			Warner Chilcott	0.257	1.93 g/75mg
Doxycycline		Vibramycin	Pfizer	0.7	7 g/100 mg
Furosemide		Lasix	Hoechst-Roussel	0.35	1.4 g/40 mg
			Roxane	0.49	0.49 g/40 mg

Continued

TABLE 14-3 Sorbitol content of selected drug preparations—cont'd

Active ingredient	Dosage form	Brand name	Manufacturer	Sorbitol content (g/ml)	Sorbitol content (g/common dose)
Guaifenesin	Syrup	—	Roxane	0.11	0.53 g/5 ml
Hydroxyzine	—	—	Pfizer	1.16	5.8 g/25 mg
Hydromorphone	—	Dilaudid	Knoll	0.13	2.6 g/4 mg
Indomethacin	—	Indocin	Merck Sharp & Dohme	0.35	1.75 g/25 mg
Lithium	—	Cibalith-S	Ciba-Geigy	0.77	3.86 g/300 mg
	Syrup	—	Roxane	0.54	2.7 g/300 mg
Methadone	Solution	—	Roxane	0.14	0.7 g/10 mg
Metoclopramide	Syrup	—	Roxane	0.28	2.8 g/10 mg
	—	Reglan	Wyeth-Ayerst	0.35	3.5 g/10 mg
	—	—	Warner Chilcott	0.42	4.2 g/10 mg
Milk of magnesia	—	—	Roxane	0.2	6.09 g/30 ml
Milk of magnesia with cascara	—	—	Roxane	0.11	0.53 g/5 ml
Minocycline	—	Minocin	Lederle	0.1	1.03 g/100 mg
Molindone	Concentrate	Moban	DuPont	0.26	0.65 g/50 mg
Nalidixic acid	—	NegGram	Winthrop	0.7	7 g/500 mg

Drug	Form	Brand	Manufacturer		
Nortriptyline	—	Aventyl	Eli Lilly	0.64	8 g/25 mg
Oxybutynin	Syrup	Ditropan	Marion Merrell Dow	0.26	1.3 g/5 mg
Perphenazine	Solution	Trilafon	Schering	0.2	0.5 g/4 mg
Potassium chloride	Solution	—	UDL	0.18	0.45 g/10 mEq
Propranolol	—	—	Roxane	0.63	3.15 g/20 mg
Pseudoephedrine	Syrup	Sudafed	Burroughs Wellcome	0.35	1.75 g/30 mg
Pseudoephedrine and triprolidine	Syrup	Actifed	Burroughs Wellcome	0.49	2.45 g/5 ml
Pyridostigmine	Syrup	Mestinon	ICN	0.14	0.7 g/60 mg
Ranitidine	Syrup	Zantac	Glaxo	0.1	1 g/150 mg
Sodium polystyrene sulfonate	Suspension	—	Roxane	0.235	14.7 g/15 g
Sulfamethoxazole	—	Gantanol	Roche	0.143	0.72 g/500 mg
Tetracycline	Suspension	Sumycin	Bristol-Myers Squibb	0.23	2.3 g/250 mg
Theophylline	—	Slo-Phyllin 80	Rorer	0.4	3.7 g/300 mg
			Roxane	0.455	25.6 g/300 mg
		Aerolate	Fleming	0.304	9.12 g/300 mg

Continued

TABLE 14-3 Sorbitol content of selected drug preparations—cont'd

Active ingredient	Dosage form	Brand name	Manufacturer	Sorbitol content (g/ml)	Sorbitol content (g/common dose)
Thiabendazole	—	Mintezol	Merck Sharp & Dohme	0.28	1.4 g/500 mg
Thiothixene	—	Navane	Roerig	0.6	0.6 g/5 mg
			Lemmon	0.5	0.5 g/5 mg
Trihexyphenidyl	—	Artane	Lederle	0.83	4.15 g/2 mg
Valproate sodium	Syrup	Depakene	Abbott	0.15	1.5 g/250 mg
Vitamin E	Solution	Aquasol	Astra	0.2	0.04 g/10 IU

Suggested Readings

Feinman L, Lieber CS: *Nutrition and diet in alcoholism.* In Shils ME, Olson JA, Shike M, eds: *Modern nutrition in health and disease,* ed 8, Philadelphia, 1994, Lea & Febiger.

Johnston KR, Govel LA, Andritz MH: Gastrointestinal effects of sorbitol as an additive in liquid medications, *Am J Med* 97:185, 1994.

Lutomski DM et al: Sorbitol content of selected oral liquids, *Ann Pharmacother* 27:269, 1993.

Roe DA: *Diet, nutrition, and drug reactions.* In Shils ME, Olson JA, Shike M, eds: *Modern nutrition in health and disease,* ed 8, Philadelphia, 1994, Lea & Febiger.

Williams L, Davis JA, Lowenthal DT: The influence of food on the absorption and metabolism of drugs, *Med Clin N Am* 77:815, 1993.

PART III

Nutrition in Specific Clinical Situations

PART II

Nutrition in Specific Clinical Situations

15

Obesity

OBESITY AS A PUBLIC HEALTH ISSUE

Obesity is a public health problem of epidemic proportion and is probably the most significant nutritional problem in this country today. In a little over a decade, between the time periods of 1976 to 1980 and 1988 to 1991, the prevalence of significantly overweight adults in the United States increased by 33%, which is considerably different from the *decrease* of 23% targeted by the U.S. Public Health Service. Currently over 20% of adolescent children and approximately one third of adults in the United States are overweight. Minority populations, especially minority women, are disproportionately affected—nearly 50% of African-American women are overweight. It is not clear whether obesity is a direct risk to good health, but it unquestionably increases the risk of other diseases including coronary artery disease, diabetes, hypertension, and certain cancers.

It is estimated that overweight employees cost businesses more than employees who have any other health risks, including risks resulting from smoking. Health insurance claims of overweight employees are about 37% higher than those for their slimmer counterparts, and the number of days spent in hospitals for overweight employees is 143% greater. About one fourth of men and one half of women are attempting to lose weight. Thus aside from its direct adverse health effects, overweight employees represent a huge economic cost to employers and our collective productivity because of time taken away from work for health reasons. The overall economic cost of obesity is estimated to be over $100 billion per year—$70 billion in healthcare costs for obesity-related illness plus $33 billion in expenditures on weight-loss products and services. This problem has demanded that physicians focus even more in their healthcare practices on the comorbidities of obesity and their prevention. In fact, 97% of physicians indicated that avoiding excess calorie intake is one of the most important recommendations they can make to patients to promote good health.

ETIOLOGY

It is almost certain that there are different types and multiple causes of obesity. Although the mechanisms causing obesity are not completely understood, their net effect is an imbalance of energy intake and expenditure.

Genetic Factors

Discovery of the ob gene in the mouse model has raised hopes that a gene or a gene product might be found that will directly help humans. This important discovery in inbred mice has important implications for our understanding of the causation of obesity; however, to date no genetic abnormalities have been found that explain weight gain in humans.

Given the right environmental conditions, it has been clearly established in humans that certain familial traits contribute to a *predisposition* to obesity, but these traits alone do not account for the development of obesity. It is also unclear how these genetic or familial factors predispose persons to weight gain. There are currently no firm data to indicate that an individual who is lean but genetically predisposed to obesity will have specific characteristics, such as certain taste preferences, metabolically efficient muscle-fiber types, or reduced maintenance energy requirements (which will be discussed). Having a genetic predisposition for or against obesity does not preclude an overriding environmental influence. In fact, regardless of a person's familial or genetic predisposition, environmental factors such as increased requirements for routine physical activity or unavailability of energy-dense foods can prevent the development of obesity.

There are also well established racial differences in the predisposition to obesity and its complications. African-American women are more likely to be obese and have obesity-related medical complications than white women, yet some recent data suggest that black women have smaller rather than larger visceral fat stores in comparison to white women.

Neuroendocrine Syndromes

Neuroendocrine abnormalities (box on following page) cause less than 1% of obesity cases, and the abnormalities that are more likely to cause obesity (e.g., hypothyroidism, Cushing's syndrome, polycystic ovary syndrome) rarely cause severe degrees of obesity. Thus a markedly obese person is least likely to have an underlying neuroendocrine disorder.

Abnormalities of Energy Metabolism

To predispose a person to gain weight, an abnormality in energy metabolism has to cause a reduction in maintenance energy requirements. Thus assuming that energy intake and voluntary physical activity remain the same, the metabolic disorder has to reduce daily energy expenditure. There are three major components of energy expenditure: (1) resting energy expenditure, (2) thermic effect of food, and (3) activity-related energy expenditure (box on p. 343).

Resting and total daily energy expenditures are somewhat variable among individuals, even those of the same size. Nevertheless, on average, the energy requirements increase in proportion to the amount of weight gained, and heavier persons almost invariably have *higher* daily energy needs. Thus at the present time there is no consis-

NEUROENDOCRINE SYNDROMES THAT CAUSE OBESITY (RARE)

Hypothyroidism and hypopituitarism

May cause moderate obesity, but the main contributor to excess weight in these conditions is fluid and not adipose tissue

Cushing's syndrome

Rarely causes gross obesity; typically has a truncal distribution

Castration and ovarian failure

Predispose persons to obesity; usually accompanied by hot flashes and other symptoms of vasomotor instability and elevated urinary gonadotropin levels

Polycystic ovary (Stein-Leventhal) syndrome

May cause a combination of hypothalamic and endocrine obesity; characterized by reduced or absent menses, moderate hirsutism, and weight gain; usually develops in young women shortly after menarche

Insulinoma

May predispose persons to generalized obesity; need for further evaluation indicated by typical symptoms of hunger and hypoglycemia

Hypothalamic lesions

Resulting from malignancy, trauma, or infection, can in rare instances cause weight gain by affecting appetite control; may result in massive obesity

Prader-Willi, Fröhlich's, and Laurence-Moon-Biedl syndromes

Associated with childhood obesity, mental retardation, and failure of sexual development; must distinguish Fröhlich's habitus (obesity and apparently delayed genital development) from true Fröhlich's syndrome

MAJOR COMPONENTS OF ENERGY EXPENDITURE

Resting energy expenditure (REE)

Normally REE accounts for greater than 60% of the total energy expenditure and is related most directly to the amount of fat-free (lean) mass, which is more metabolically active than fat mass. Because obese persons tend to have increased amounts of fat-free mass (probably to support the increase in fat mass), they have increased REEs. Currently most studies have shown that the REE adjusted for fat-free mass is normal in obese persons and normal-weight persons who are predisposed to obesity.

Thermic effect of food (TEF)

The contribution of the TEF to the total daily energy expenditure is small—approximately 10% of energy intake. Although a number of studies have found the TEF to be blunted in obese persons, the potential energy "savings" from an abnormal TEF is probably less than 25 kcal per day, which is an insufficient amount to explain the development of obesity.

Activity-related energy expenditure (AEE)

The AEE normally represents 20% to 30% of the daily energy expenditure, depending on the amount of the person's physical activity. Although obese persons tend to be less physically active than lean persons, their AEEs are not necessarily lower because they require more energy to conduct the same amount of physical activity as lean persons. It is not known whether the reduced level of physical activity is secondary to the obese state or if it contributes to weight gain. There is no evidence that obesity-prone persons tend to perform identical physical activities more efficiently (using less energy) than normal persons.

tent, convincing evidence that reduced energy requirements contribute meaningfully to the tendency of some individuals to gain weight.

Environmental Factors

Exogenous factors that may predispose persons to obesity include dietary excesses and physical inactivity. Without question, an altered energy intake can cause weight gain or loss. Although the rate of the weight change may vary somewhat among individuals, weight gain cannot be avoided when calorie intake continually exceeds requirements, and weight loss cannot be avoided when calorie intake fails to meet requirements. As noted previously, obese persons must take in more calories to sustain their increased body masses. However, studies of eating behaviors of obese subjects have failed to identify any consistent patterns of calorie intake, eating frequency, or food preferences that account for their obese states.

Large secular-trend surveys appear to indicate that the average fat and energy intakes in the United States have actually fallen since the late 1970s, even as the prevalence of obesity has risen. The increased availability and use of low-fat and fat-free foods has obviously not produced the desired effects. Data on physical activity are harder to obtain, but it would seem that the average level of physical activity must have declined significantly to account for the divergent patterns of an increase in obesity and a decrease in fat and calorie intake. It is illogical to expect that genetic factors are to blame.

CLINICAL ASSESSMENT OF OBESE PATIENTS
Medical History

The medical history should identify factors that could potentially contribute to an individual's obesity as well as possible comorbidities of existing obesity. As noted previously, neuroendocrine causes are uncommon. Nevertheless, the symptoms listed in Table 15-1 can indicate the possibility that a secondary cause may exist. When taking a

TABLE 15-1 Historical features that suggest secondary causes for obesity

History or symptoms	Consideration
Cold intolerance, menstrual abnormalities, constipation, weakness (in adults); retarded mental and physical maturation (in children)	Hypothyroidism, hypopituitarism
Hypertension, glucose intolerance, menstrual dysfunction, weakness, back pain, compression fractures, easy bruising	Cushing's syndrome
Reduced or absent menses shortly after menarche, hirsutism	Polycystic ovary syndrome
Hypoglycemia	Insulinoma
Uncontrollable, ravenous appetite	Hypothalamic lesions
Childhood onset, mental retardation, failure of sexual development	Prader-Willi, Lawrence-Moon-Biedl, Fröhlich's syndromes
Medication use	Phenothiazines, corticosteroids

medical history, signs of medical complications (which are discussed later) should also be elicited.

Assessment of Degree of Obesity

Normative values for defining obesity are not derived from data on optimum health, but it is still important to attempt to classify individuals according to their "desirable" weights. A variety of data sets have been developed for reference weights, although none are currently considered ideal. Table 15-2 provides weight-height reference

TABLE 15-2 Weight-height reference chart (adults)

| Height (no shoes) | | Reference weight | | | |
| | | Women | | Men | |
ft/in	cm	lb	kg	lb	kg
4'10"	147	101	46	—	—
4'11"	150	104	47	—	—
5'0"	152	107	47	—	—
5'1"	155	110	50	—	—
5'2"	157	113	51	124	56
5'3"	160	116	53	127	58
5'4"	162	120	54	130	59
5'5"	165	123	56	133	60
5'6"	167	128	58	137	62
5'7"	170	132	60	141	64
5'8"	172	136	62	145	66
5'9"	175	140	63	149	68
5'10"	178	144	65	153	69
5'11"	180	148	67	158	71
6'0"	183	152	69	162	74
6'1"	185	—	—	167	76
6'2"	188	—	—	171	78
6'3"	190	—	—	176	80
6'4"	193	—	—	181	82

values for men and women derived from early Metropolitan Life Insurance Company actuarial data.[1] More recent data suggest higher reference standards. However, they do not provide a more accurate prediction of an ideal body weight because in general they fail to control for a number of confounding variables including cigarette smoking, the biologic effects of comorbidities of obesity, or weight loss resulting from subclinical disease. The most recent large studies among adult men and women control for these factors and have found that the lowest mortality occurs among individuals weighing (on average) 15% to 20% be-

| TABLE 15-3 | Guidelines for assessing health risk from obesity |

Degree of obesity	Body mass index (kg/m²)	Health risk
Grade 0	<25	Low or normal
Grade I	25-29.9	Mildly increased
Grade II	30-40	Moderately increased
Grade III	>40	Markedly increased

low the U.S. average and suggest the upward trend in recommended desirable weights is unjustified.[2,3]

The degree of obesity can be expressed as percentage overweight, with a desirable body weight of usually between 90% and 120%. A body weight-for-height of 120% or more of the value provided in Table 15-2 is considered an established health hazard. Another method for assessing degree of obesity is the body mass index (BMI):

$$BMI = \frac{Weight\ (kg)}{Height^2\ (m)}$$

Individuals with unusually large muscle masses or older adults with spinal deformities may be misclassified as obese. Regardless, the general guidelines depicted in Table 15-3 are useful.

Various methods have been developed to estimate body fat content using simple anthropometric measurements such as multiple skinfold measurements taken with calipers (see Chapter 8). In one such method the biceps, triceps, subscapular, and suprailiac skinfold thicknesses are added, and the estimated percent body fat is located on Table 15-4 with reference to the person's age and sex.[4] Normal is about 17% to 27% for women and 15% to 20% for men. For greater accuracy, average the skinfold measurements on the right and left sides of the body.

TABLE 15-4 Estimating body fat content from the sum of four skinfolds[4]

Equivalent fat content as percentage of body weight for a range of values for the sum of four skinfolds*

Skinfolds (mm)	Men (age in years)				Women (age in years)			
	17-29	30-39	40-49	50+	16-29	30-39	40-49	50+
15	4.8				10.5			
20	8.1	12.2	12.2	12.6	14.1	17.0	19.8	21.4
25	10.5	14.2	15.0	15.6	16.8	19.4	22.2	24.0
30	12.9	16.2	17.7	18.6	19.5	21.8	24.5	26.6
35	14.7	17.7	19.6	20.8	21.5	23.7	26.4	28.5
40	16.4	19.2	21.4	22.9	23.4	25.5	28.2	30.3
45	17.7	20.4	23.0	24.7	25.0	26.9	29.6	31.9
50	19.0	21.5	24.6	26.5	26.5	28.2	31.0	33.4
55	20.1	22.5	25.9	27.9	27.8	29.4	32.1	34.6
60	21.2	23.5	27.1	29.2	29.1	30.6	33.2	35.7
65	22.2	24.3	28.2	30.4	30.2	31.6	34.1	36.7
70	23.1	25.1	29.3	31.6	31.2	32.5	35.0	37.7
75	24.0	25.9	30.3	32.7	32.2	33.4	35.9	38.7

80	24.8	26.6	31.2	33.8	33.1	34.3	36.7	39.6
85	25.5	27.2	32.1	34.8	34.0	35.1	37.5	40.4
90	26.2	27.8	33.0	35.8	34.8	35.8	38.3	41.2
95	26.9	28.4	33.7	36.6	35.6	36.5	39.0	41.9
100	27.6	29.0	34.4	37.4	36.4	37.2	39.7	42.6
105	28.2	29.6	35.1	38.2	37.1	37.9	40.4	43.3
110	28.8	30.1	35.8	39.0	37.8	38.6	41.0	43.9
115	29.4	30.6	36.4	39.7	38.4	39.1	41.5	44.5
120	30.0	31.1	37.0	40.4	39.0	39.6	42.0	45.1
125	31.0	31.5	37.6	41.1	39.6	40.1	42.5	45.7
130	31.5	31.9	38.2	41.8	40.2	40.6	43.0	46.2
135	32.0	32.3	38.7	42.4	40.8	41.1	43.5	46.7
140	32.5	32.7	39.2	43.0	41.3	41.6	44.0	47.2
145	32.9	33.1	39.7	43.6	41.8	42.1	44.5	47.7
150	33.3	33.5	40.2	44.1	42.3	42.6	45.0	48.2
155	33.7	33.9	40.7	44.6	42.8	43.1	45.4	48.7

*Biceps, triceps, subscapular, and suprailiac of men and women of different ages.

Continued

TABLE 15-4 Estimating body fat content from the sum of four skinfolds—cont'd

Equivalent fat content as percentage of body weight for a range of values for the sum of four skinfolds*

Skinfolds (mm)	Men (age in years)				Women (age in years)			
	17-29	30-39	40-49	50+	16-29	30-39	40-49	50+
160	34.1	34.3	41.2	45.1	43.3	43.6	45.8	49.2
165	34.5	34.6	41.6	45.6	43.7	44.0	46.2	49.6
170	34.9	34.8	42.0	46.1	44.1	44.4	46.6	50.0
175	35.3					44.8	47.0	50.4
180	35.6					45.2	47.4	50.8
185	35.9					45.6	47.8	51.2
190						45.9	48.2	51.6
195						46.2	48.5	52.0
200						46.5	48.8	52.4
205							49.1	52.7
210							49.4	53.0

*Biceps, triceps, subscapular, and suprailiac of men and women of different ages.

Distribution of Body Fat

Body-fat distribution is also an important predictor of potential health risks, independent of the degree of obesity. The easiest way to measure body-fat distribution is with the waist/hip circumference ratio. With the patient standing, the waist circumference is taken where it is narrowest and the hip circumference is taken where it is widest. A ratio of greater than 0.8 for women and greater than 0.95 for men reflects an abdominal or android pattern ("apple" shape) that is generally associated with increased visceral fat and indicates a greater risk for hypertension, hyperinsulinemia, diabetes, and cardiovascular disease.

Physical Examination

One of the unfortunate consequences of obesity is that precise physical examinations are often difficult. An accurate blood pressure measurement, auscultation of the heart and lungs, palpation of the abdomen, detection of breast masses, and other aspects of the exam are compromised to the degree that the patient is obese. Important aspects of the physical examination that are used to identify coexisting medical disorders and rule out endocrine abnormalities are listed in the box on the following page.

Laboratory Assessment

No particular laboratory test is indicated simply because a patient is obese, and lab tests should not be allowed to replace a thorough medical history and physical examination. Rather, tests should be dictated by individual findings (Table 15-5).

Clinical Classification

Unfortunately, appropriate clinical classifications of obese patients are still based on ill-defined criteria. The categories shown in Table 15-6 are frequently used and provide information about predisposition, duration, severity, and risk of medical complications resulting from the obe-

PHYSICAL EXAMINATION OF AN OBESE PATIENT

Blood pressure

Blood pressure should be taken using a cuff size appropriate for the patient's arm circumference. (This information is shown on the cuff itself, but if in doubt use the larger cuff to avoid spuriously high readings.)

Skin

Red or purple depressed striae, hirsutism, acne, and moon facies with plethora suggest Cushing's syndrome; mild hirsutism is also seen in polycystic ovarian syndrome. Dry, coarse, cool, and pale skin suggests hypothyroidism.

Fat distribution

Truncal distribution with fat accumulation around the supraclavicular areas and dorsocervical spine (buffalo hump) suggest Cushing's syndrome.

Thyroid gland

Enlargement of the thyroid gland suggests hypothyroidism.

Edema

Boggy, nonpitting edema of the eyes, tongue, hands, and feet suggests myxedema of hypothyroidism.

Neurologic exam

A slow ankle reflex with a delayed relaxation phase suggests hypothyroidism; muscle weakness suggests Cushing's syndrome and hypothyroidism.

---

sity. For example, a patient might be classified as having adult-onset, positive family history, primary Grade II obesity with gynoid pattern and concurrent hypertension.

COMPLICATIONS

It is important to keep in mind the following points regarding medical complications of obesity: (1) not all obese

TABLE 15-5 Laboratory tests for causes or complications of obesity

Suspected condition	Diagnostic tests
Cushing's syndrome	24-hr urinary-free cortisol (abnormal: >150 µg/24 hr) *plus* Low-dose dexamethasone suppression test (0.5 mg every 6 hours for 2 days, collecting 24 hr-urinary 17-OH corticosteroids on second day [abnormal: >3.5 mg/24 hr])
Diabetes	Fasting serum glucose
Gallstones	Ultrasonography
"Hypometabolism"*	Resting energy expenditure by indirect calorimetry
Hypothyroidism	Serum TSH (normal generally <5 µU/ml)
Hyperlipidemia	Fasting total cholesterol, triglycerides, HDL cholesterol
Periodic/sleep apnea	Sleep studies for oxygen desaturation ENT exam for upper airway obstruction

* Some patients relate histories suggesting unusual energy efficiencies (i.e., inability to lose weight despite energy intakes well below their estimated requirements). However, studies conducted in clinical research center conditions provide no conclusive evidence that significant variations in efficiency of energy expenditure exist. Nevertheless, the use of indirect calorimentry may be helpful in some patients to document normal energy expenditure relative to their body size and estimate calorie needs for weight loss.

persons have medical complications, and (2) the known comorbidities of obesity are not evenly distributed among obese persons. Consequently it cannot be assumed that an obese person will have a comorbid condition. The fact that weight loss improves conditions such as hypertension and

TABLE 15-6 Clinical classification of obesity	
Category	**Clinical classification**
Age of onset	Juvenile vs. adult-onset
Familial predisposition	Positive if at least one first-degree relative has a history of obesity
Etiology	Caused by an identifiable endocrine or metabolic disorder vs. their behavioral patterns
Severity	Percent desirable weight or grade of obesity by BMI
Fat pattern	Gynoid vs. android, peripheral vs. central, or lower vs. upper body according to waist/hip ratio or other method of assessment
Comorbidities	Presence of disease associates (e.g., hypertension, glucose intolerance, respiratory complications)

hyperlipidemia does not guarantee that the obesity was the primary or sole cause of the condition. Energy restriction and a reduction in salt intake may have accounted for the changes. In fact, when an individual is stable at a reduced body weight, the blood pressure and serum lipid levels usually rebound somewhat. Only if these levels remain improved can it be assumed that they were caused by obesity. In distinguishing the individual contribution of obesity to overall mortality, a recent prospective study of intentional weight loss and mortality indicated that weight loss for the treatment of obesity reduces mortality when comorbid conditions such as diabetes, hyperlipidemia, or hypertension are present but is less likely to reduce mortality in the absence of comorbid conditions.[5] The diseases and metabolic disorders that follow have been associated with obesity.

Osteoarthritis

Degenerative joint disease or osteoarthritis of the weight-bearing joints is generally accepted as being more prevalent in obese persons, although not all studies have confirmed a significant correlation. There is also increased likelihood of osteoarthritis in the non–weight-bearing joints, suggesting that the arthritis may not be simply a direct result of mechanical overload. Regardless of whether obesity is the direct cause of the joint disease, it aggravates joint symptoms, exacerbates postural faults, and complicates treatment.

Cancer

In women, obesity has been associated with an increased risk for cancer of the breast, cervix, endometrium, gallbladder, biliary tract, and ovaries; in men it has been associated with cancers of the colon, rectum, and prostate. However, only cancers of the breast and endometrium are associated with obesity after other risk factors are statistically accounted for. In the case of these two cancers, the mechanism may be related to elevated circulating estrogen levels in obese women resulting from increased conversion of androgens (androstenedione and testosterone) to estrogens (estrone and estradiol) in adipose tissue.

Coronary Artery Disease

In general, obese persons are at increased risk for developing coronary artery disease. However, it is still unclear whether uncomplicated obesity is an independent risk factor for coronary artery disease in the absence of co-morbid conditions such as diabetes, hyperlipidemia, and hypertension. Almost 3 decades of observation of the Framingham cohort[6] suggest that body weight is a significant predictor of heart disease independent of other standard risk factors, although not all studies support this conclusion.

Diabetes and Hyperinsulinemia

There is a positive association between the degree and duration of obesity and risk for diabetes mellitus. The prevalence of diabetes is increased about tenfold with moderate obesity and as much as thirtyfold with severe obesity. Elevated plasma insulin levels are uniformly found in obese individuals in both the fasting and glucose-stimulated states, reflecting insulin resistance. Despite this fact, not all obese individuals become diabetic. It is likely that obesity only causes diabetes in individuals who are otherwise predisposed.

Hepatobiliary Disease

Obesity increases the risk of gallstone formation, probably by increasing fasting and residual gallbladder volumes with resultant bile stasis and increasing cholesterol production and bile-cholesterol saturation, which enhances cholesterol crystal nucleation. Women are approximately twice as likely as men to develop gallstones. On average, about 1% to 2% of obese women develop newly symptomatic stones each year. There is no threshold of body weight above which stones occur; (i.e., even a moderate increase in weight can increase risk.) From data collected among women, severe obesity increases the risk of gallstone formation more than sixfold. Individuals who gradually reduce to a normal body weight normalize their risk for gallstones. By contrast, rapid weight loss can increase the chances of stone formation during the period of active dieting by as much as fifteenfold to twenty-fivefold over that of the nondieting obese population. This problem is discussed in the section about weight-loss approaches in this chapter.

Steatosis (fat accumulation within the liver) occurs to some degree in as many as 88% of obese individuals. The hepatic fat content is not directly related to the degree of obesity, and caloric restriction can reduce the fat accumulation even if the obese state persists, suggesting that steatosis is a storage phenomenon rather than a result of a liver function disorder. A liver enlargement noted on a physical exam may be the only sign of the disorder, which is usually asymptomatic with normal liver function tests.

Hyperlipidemia

Most cross-sectional studies have noted a modest positive association between serum triglyceride and cholesterol levels and increasing degrees of obesity; high-density lipoproten (HDL) cholesterol levels tend to be lower in obese persons. Weight reduction generally improves serum lipid levels significantly during the active period of dieting, but the effect is largely a result of energy restriction. After achieving a stable, reduced body weight, lipid levels partially rebound but tend to remain at improved levels as long as the weight loss is maintained.

Hypertension

In population studies there is a small but statistically significant association between body weight and blood pressure. However, the majority of obese persons are not hypertensive. Weight reduction generally improves blood pressure levels, but as with lipid levels the most pronounced effect is from energy restriction (and probably an associated decrease in salt intake) rather than from the weight loss itself. Maximum and permanent improvements in obesity-associated hypertension requires reduction to and maintenance of a normal body weight.

Respiratory Problems

The obesity-hypoventilation or pickwickian syndrome is characterized by marked degrees of obesity, somnolence, periodic apnea (especially during sleep), chronic hypoxemia and hypercapnia (CO_2 retention), and secondary polycythemia. The explanations for the inadequate ventilation and reduced functional lung volume are not clear, although there appears to be decreased efficiency in the functioning of the respiratory muscles, reduced respiratory compliance, a decreased ventilatory response to CO_2, and increased pulmonary dead space and atelectasis. Complications include pulmonary artery constriction resulting in pulmonary hypertension and right heart failure.

Even a moderate weight reduction can reverse the hypoventilation syndrome. Periodic apnea can be caused by intermittent upper airway obstruction distinct from the alveolar hypoventilation syndrome; such obstructions often respond to surgical therapy.

Complications Associated With Increased Intraabdominal Fat

Body fat distribution may be a better predictor of the health hazards associated with obesity than the absolute amount of body fat. Individuals with an upper body fat pattern that reflects an excess of intraabdominal or visceral fat appear to be at greater risk for diabetes, hypertension, hypertriglyceridemia, ischemic heart disease, and death from all causes. The effects of intraabdominal fat appear to be separate from those of total body fat. A practical method for assessing body fat pattern is described in a previous section (see Clinical Assessment of the Obese Patient in this chapter).

TREATMENT
Overview

Not all persons who want to lose weight should do so, and not all treatment programs can be equally endorsed. Table 15-7 offers several criteria to consider when selecting a weight control program. For additional information, see the Suggested Readings for *Weighing the Options,* a report prepared by the National Academy of Sciences Institute of Medicine.

Just as other chronic conditions such as hypertension or diabetes are treated, obesity must be treated. It cannot be corrected by short-term interventions but requires ongoing effort and long-term support to help individuals establish and maintain control of the disorder. The goals of treatment are to establish permanent changes in eating habits and physical activity that become mutually supportive and self-reinforcing.

TABLE 15-7 Criteria for selecting weight control programs

Criteria	Comments
Patient selection	*Special attention:* Patients < 20 or > 65 years old (may have special nutritional needs) BMI > 37 kg/m² History of other eating disorders (anorexia nervosa, bulimia) *Avoid treatment:* Pregnant or lactating patients Patients with a BMI < 20 kg/m² (NOTE: Patients with a BMI < 25, a gynoid pattern of fat distribution, and no comorbidites may not be an appropriate candidate for weight reduction.)
Weight-loss claims	*Look for:* Prescribed rate of weight loss < 1.5% or 1.5 kg/week Direct medical supervision for faster rates of weight loss Outcome data of ≥1 year posttreatment
Therapeutic approach	*Look for:* Team skilled in diet, exercise, behavioral techniques Diet emphasizing self-selection of foods from conventional food supply for long-term weight maintenance Program of physical activity geared to individual needs Behavioral modification, psychosocial support
Medical supervision	*Recommended:* If significant obesity-related comorbidities exist If diet provides < 800 kcal/day

Safe Rate of Weight Loss

A safe rate of weight loss can be recommended on the basis of risk for gallstone formation because it is one of the few objective measures of morbidity associated with various rates of weight loss. Obese persons may transiently compound their risk during the period of active weight loss while attempting to achieve a lower-risk, nonobese state. Active weight loss results in the formation of new gallstones within just 4 weeks, and faster rates of loss appear to enhance stone formation independently of the severity of obesity. Longer *periods* of weight loss increase risk in a linear fashion; however, faster *rates* of weight loss increase risk exponentially. On average, losing less than 1.5 kg per week is associated with gallstone development in less than 10% of dieters, but losing more than 2 kg per week results in stone formation in more than 25% of dieters. These stones do not necessarily produce symptoms. On the basis of this health risk, it is recommended that average weekly weight loss not exceed 1.5 kg or about 1.5% of body weight.

Weight Cycling

Weight cycling or "yo-yo dieting" refers to repeated bouts of weight loss and regain without maintenance of a lower weight. Unquestionably, weight cycling causes frustration on the parts of both the patient and therapist. However, it is less clear whether repeated weight loss/regain cycles are hazardous to health or adversely affect physiologic parameters such as metabolic rate. A recent review by an NIH Obesity Task Force concluded that there is no convincing evidence weight cycling has adverse effects on body composition, energy expenditure, risk factors for heart disease, or the effectiveness of future afforts at weight control.[7] Because the average length of time to regain lost weight is about tenfold longer than the time during which it is lost, it can be argued that the net effect of a weight-loss program, even if not permanent, is likely to be positive in terms of temporarily decreasing health risks. Obese individuals should not allow concerns about weight cycling to deter them from attempting to control their body weight.

Dietary Approach

The dietary approach used to achieve weight loss and long-term weight maintenance must satisfy three criteria: (1) it must be based on a sound scientific rationale, (2) it must be safe and nutritionally adequate, and (3) it must be practical and applicable to the patient's social and ethnic background so that it will be conducive to long-term adherence.

Very Low-Calorie Diets

These diets are designed to provide severe energy restrictions (less than 800 kcal per day) but sufficient protein to minimize loss of lean body mass. Protein losses tend to be less than losses associated with fasting but often continue to occur. The major concern about these diets is they induce rapid weight loss that increases the risk of gallstone formation. They are sometimes useful for patients who are have substantial health risks from severe obesity (e.g., alveolar hypoventilation syndrome) and therefore in whom rapid weight loss is critical. Under these circumstances, direct medical supervision is important.

Moderately Low-Calorie, Balanced Diets

Most persons desiring weight loss may use these diets. Although they can have different characteristics, in general they should meet the three criteria previously outlined, provide at least 800 kcal per day (most often 1000 to 1200 kcal), and emphasize low-fat, high complex-carbohydrate foods. One example of this type of diet is the *EatRight* program used at the University of Alabama at Birmingham that is currently published for public use.[8] Using the concept of time-calorie displacement, this dietary approach is based on the spectrum of calorie densities of the various food groups shown in the box on the following page. The low-calorie, low-fat, high-bulk, slow-eating food groups to the right of the box are emphasized.

Patients are given a list of food in each category from which they can choose items according to their preferences. Most patients who are moderately overweight are

EatRight Approach to Weight Control[8]

| | High-calorie Low-bulk Fast-eating | | [Eat "right"] → | | Low-calorie High-bulk Slow-eating |
	Fat	Meat/dairy	Starch	Fruit	Vegetables
kcal/oz:	225	75	50	15	10
kcal/serving:	45	110	80	60	25
Servings/day:	Maximum 3 to 4	4 to 5	5 to 6	Minimum 4	Minimum 4

instructed to eat the number of servings indicated in each food group in the box. Fats are limited to a *maximum* of 3 to 4 servings per day, whereas the fruit and vegetable prescription is a *minimum* of 4 servings of each per day with no upper limit. By encouraging liberal amounts of complex carbohydrates in the form of vegetables, fruit, and unrefined starch, moderate amounts of low-fat meat and dairy products, and only small amounts of fat, satiety and nutritional adequacy are achieved with a low-calorie intake and without counting calories. Up to 200 kcal/week of sweets and snack foods are permitted as "special-occasion" foods. Studies on the *EatRight* program indicate that it is nutritionally adequate, safe, and effective over the long term. It is also ideal for obesity prevention and with very minor modifications is appropriate for obese children and diabetic patients.

Any dietary approach to weight control must emphasize life-long changes in eating patterns rather than short-term use of diets. The term *diet* implies temporary intervention, whereas the major challenge in treating obesity is not losing weight but maintaining weight loss.

Physical Activity

Physical activity should be included in weight management programs with the objectives of promoting fat loss while maintaining lean body mass and engendering permanent changes in lifestyle without putting individuals at risk.

Increasing physical activity without controlling calorie intake is generally an ineffective means of losing weight. However, repeated studies have demonstrated that a program of routine physical activity is critical for long-term maintenance of weight loss. As a complement to energy restriction, increased physical activity provides the advantages of improving cardiovascular conditioning and insulin sensitivity and according to some studies maintaining muscle mass and bone density while weight is lost. Increased physical activity may best be achieved with a combination of regular exercises several times weekly plus daily "step-losing" activities. When routinely established, step-losing behaviors such as walking or climbing stairs instead of driving or using the elevator may be even more effective than programmed exercise in maintaining weight loss.

For obese persons, aerobic exercises such as walking, swimming, bicycling, and low-impact dance and exercise classes are recommended to minimize damage to weight-bearing joints. The recommendation to "do a little more of what you are doing right now" and keep daily records is a reasonable way to begin increasing physical activity in overweight persons. For the untrained, sedentary person, initially aiming for a pulse rate of 60% to 65% of maximum (220 − person's age) sustained for about 20 minutes several times a week is reasonable. Another rough guide is to be able to maintain a conversation but not be able to sing during the exercise. Table 15-8 lists energy expenditures to expect from selected physical activities.

Behavioral Modification and Psychosocial Support

Behavioral modification and psychosocial support should be included in weight control programs to (1) focus on methods of acquiring new behaviors and not merely on descriptions of desired behaviors, (2) incorporate standard therapeutic modalities including self-monitoring and cognitive restructuring, and (3) provide guidelines for maintaining weight loss, such as resuming record-keeping if weight is regained, practicing controlled intake of "fear" foods, and utilizing family and social support systems.

Patients attempting to modify their diets and physical activity patterns frequently require therapy for psychologic and social problems. Keeping detailed records of dietary intake, exercise, and emotional factors is an important aspect of weight control and appropriately focuses attention on *patterns* and *problems* rather than pounds. An important aspect of behavioral support is to help the patient maintain a positive outlook and emphasize even small, positive behavioral changes rather than setbacks. What patients perceive as major lapses are often no more

Text continued on p. 369.

TABLE 15-8 Energy cost of physical activities (kcal/10 min of activity)[9]

Activity	Level	Body weight (kg/lb)							
		70 155	80 175	90 200	100 220	115 255	125 275	135 300
Inactivity	Sitting, riding in car, watching TV	12	13	15	17	19	21	23
Inactivity	Standing (little movement)	29	33	38	42	48	52	56
Bicycling, stationary	Very light effort (50 W)	35	40	45	50	58	63	68
Bicycling, stationary	Light effort (100 W)	64	73	83	92	105	115	124
Bicycling, stationary	Moderate effort (150 W)	82	93	105	117	134	146	158
Bicycling, stationary	Vigorous effort (200 W)	123	140	158	175	201	219	236
Bicycling	<10 mph, leisured pace	47	53	60	67	77	83	90
Bicycling	10-11.9 mph, slow, light effort	70	80	90	100	115	125	135

Continued

TABLE 15-8 Energy cost of physical activities (kcal/10 min of activity)—cont'd

Activity	Level	Body weight (kg/lb)							
		70 / 155	80 / 175	90 / 200	100 / 220	115 / 255	125 / 275	135 / 300
Bicycling	12-13.9 mph, moderate effort	93	107	120	133	153	167	180
Bicycling	14-15.9 mph, fast, vigorous effort	117	133	150	167	192	208	225
Bicycling	16-19 mph, very fast pace	140	160	180	200	230	250	270
Bicycling	>20 mph; racing, not drafting	187	213	240	267	307	333	360
Conditioning exercise	Calisthenics, •light workout	53	60	68	75	86	94	101
Conditioning exercise	Circuit training, general	93	107	120	133	153	167	180
Conditioning exercise	Weight lifting, light workout	35	40	45	50	58	63	68
Conditioning exercise	Weight lifting, vigorous effort	70	80	90	100	115	125	135
Conditioning exercise	Stair-treadmill ergometer, general	70	80	90	100	115	125	135

Conditioning exercise	Rowing; stationary ergometer, light effort (50 W)	41	47	53	58	67	73	79
Conditioning exercise	Rowing; stationary ergometer, moderate effort (100 W)	82	93	105	117	134	146	158
Conditioning exercise	Rowing; stationary ergometer, vigorous effort (150 W)	99	113	128	142	163	177	191
Conditioning exercise	Rowing; stationary ergometer, very vigorous effort (200 W)	140	160	180	200	230	250	270
Conditioning exercise	Water aerobics, calisthenics	47	53	60	67	77	83	90
Dancing	Aerobic, low-impact	58	67	75	83	96	104	112
Dancing	Aerobic, high-impact	82	93	105	117	134	146	158
Home activities	Sweeping, vacuuming, playing with children	29	33	38	42	48	52	56
Home activities	Cleaning, vigorous effort	53	60	68	75	86	94	101
Home repair	Carpentry, painting, wall papering	53	60	68	75	86	94	101

Continued

TABLE 15-8 Energy cost of physical activities (kcal/10 min of activity)—cont'd

Activity	Level	Body weight (kg/lb)						
		70 155	80 175	90 200	100 220	115 255	125 275	135 300
Walking	<2 mph; very slow strolling	23	27	30	33	38	42	45
Walking	3 mph, moderate pace	41	47	53	58	67	73	79
Walking	4 mph, very brisk pace	47	53	60	67	77	83	90
Running	5 mph (12-min mile)	93	107	120	133	153	167	180
Running	6 mph (10-min mile)	117	133	150	167	192	208	225
Running	8 mph (7.5-min mile)	158	180	203	225	259	281	304
Running	10 mph (6-min mile)	187	213	240	267	307	333	360
Skiing, snow	Downhill, moderate effort	70	80	90	100	115	125	135
Skiing, snow	Downhill; vigorous, racing	117	133	150	167	192	208	225
Swimming	Freestyle, slow	93	107	120	133	153	167	180
Swimming	Freestyle, fast	117	133	150	167	192	208	225
Sports, other	Basketball, nongame	70	80	90	100	115	125	135
Sports, other	Golf	53	60	68	75	86	94	101
Sports, other	Handball	140	160	180	200	230	250	270
Sports, other	Tennis	82	93	105	117	134	146	158
Yard work	Gardening, mowing	58	67	75	83	96	104	112

than exaggerated responses to temporary indiscretions. Reminding patients that they can enjoy a limited amount of "special-occasion" food such as desserts and snack items helps to relieve the feeling of guilt created by eating such food and avoid relapsing into old habits. This is needed to prevent the all-or-none or on/off attitude toward dieting in which patients feel like failures if they eat prohibited food. In addition, it is wise to encourage patients to practice controlled intake of highly desired food that they fear they cannot eat in limited amounts, rather than to suggest total avoidance of the food. This may have to be done in a supervised clinic setting.

Drug Therapy

Thyroid hormones are indicated only for individuals with a clearly established diagnosis of hypothyroidism. Inducing a hyperthyroid state for the sake of weight loss introduces the risk of eroding lean body mass and incurring thyrotoxicosis. Diuretics and digitalis only lower weight by causing fluid loss and are not indicated for the treatment of obesity. Appetite-suppressant drugs include the serotonergic agonists (e.g., fenfluramine), serotonin reuptake inhibitors (e.g., fluoxetine, sertraline), adrenergic agents (e.g., phentermine, diethylpropion, and phenylpropenolamine), and agents with combined adrenergic and serotonergic effects (e.g., sibutramine). These medications have been found to be more effective than placebos in increasing the rate of weight loss during relatively short periods of time (e.g., 3 months), and the FDA has approved many of them for such short-term treatment. However, there are two precautions to consider: (1) whether drugs are used singly or in combination, pharmacotherapy tends to cause only modest amounts of weight loss over that of placebos, and (2) there are currently too few studies available to determine that drugs are safe and sustain weight loss for periods beyond 1 year. Until more data become available, short-term, appetite-suppressant therapy must be considered ineffective in weight management, and data on long-term safety and efficacy are inadequate to justify its use in the general obese population.

Surgical Procedures

Surgery should be limited to individuals who have been severely obese (100 lb or more above or 100% above desirable weight) for at least 3 years, have serious medical conditions related to their obesity, have failed repeatedly at attempts to lose weight, and are judged able to tolerate the operative procedure. The jejuno-ileal bypass procedure developed in the 1970s is no longer an approved procedure because of its high rate of associated complications. By excluding approximately 90% of the absorptive capacity of the bowel, it caused malabsorption and copious diarrhea. Complications included deficiencies of potassium, calcium, magnesium, iron, folate, and vitamins A, B_{12}, and D; nephrolithiasis; arthritis; cholelithiasis; liver disease; and nephropathy. The currently used gastric-reduction procedures are safer but tend to cause less weight loss than the jejuno-ileal bypass procedure, and they depend on changes in eating behavior for sustained weight loss. Complications include vomiting, wound infection, and marginal ulceration. The amount of weight loss can be sizable with both procedures; however, because patients are markedly overweight, most do not achieve their ideal body weight.

References

1. Metropolitan Life Insurance Company, Statistical Bulletin: Build and blood pressure study, 1959.
2. Lee I-M et al: Body weight and mortality: A 27-year follow-up of middle-aged men, *JAMA* 270:2823, 1993.
3. Manson JE et al: Body weight and mortality among women, *N Engl J Med* 333:677, 1995.
4. Durnin JVEA, Womersley J: *Br J Nutr* 32:77, 1974.
5. Williamson DF et al: Prospective study of intentional weight loss and mortality in never-smoking overweight US women aged 40-64 years, *Am J Epidemiol* 141:1128, 1995.
6. Hubert HB et al: Obesity as an independent risk factor for cardiovascular disease: a 26-year follow-up of participants in the Framingham Heart Study, *Circulation* 67:968, 1983.
7. NIH National Task Force on the Prevention and Treatment of Obesity: Weight cycling, *JAMA* 272:1196, 1994.

8. Weinsier R et al: *EatRight— 7 simple steps to lose weight,* Birmingham, AL, Oxmoor House (in press).
9. Ainsworth et al: Compendium of physical activities: classification of energy costs of human physical activities, *Med Sci Sports Exer* 25:71, 1993.

Suggested Readings

Bjorntorp P: Visceral obesity: A "civilization syndrome," *Obesity Res* 1:206, 1993.

Bray GA: Fat distribution and body weight, *Obesity Res* 1:203, 1993.

Kuczmarski RJ et al: Increasing prevalence of overweight among US adults, *JAMA* 272:205, 1994.

NIH National Task Force on the Prevention and Treatment of Obesity: Very low-calorie diets, *JAMA* 270:967, 1993.

NIH Technology Assessment Conference Panel: Methods for voluntary weight loss and control, *Ann Intern Med* 116:942, 1992.

Pi-Sunyer FX: *Obesity.* In Shils ME, Olson JA, Shike M, eds: *Modern nutrition in health and disease,* ed 8, Philadelphia, 1994, Lea & Febiger.

Thomas PR, ed: *Weighing the options: Criteria for evaluating weight-management programs,* Food and Nutrition Board, Institute of Medicine, Washington, DC, 1995, National Academy Press.

16

Diabetes

Diabetes mellitus involves a fundamental alteration in the body's metabolism of glucose that is caused by either a deficiency of insulin, referred to as Type I, juvenile-onset, or insulin-dependent diabetes (IDDM) or a resistance to insulin's actions in peripheral tissues, referred to as Type II, adult-onset, or non–insulin-dependent diabetes (NIDDM). Both types are manifest by elevations in serum glucose levels (hyperglycemia) and glycosuria, and significant long-term complications including nephropathy, retinopathy, neuropathy, and coronary and peripheral artery disease. Cardiovascular disease is the main cause of death. With careful management, persons with diabetes can have virtually normal life expectancies.

PRIMARY GOALS OF DIET THERAPY

Nutrition therapy is essential for successful diabetes management. The overall goal of nutrition therapy is to optimize metabolic control through dietary and exercise habits. Specific goals are listed in the box.

DIETARY GUIDELINES

Successful nutrition therapy begins with a nutritional assessment, requires evaluation of nutrition outcomes, and provides ongoing education. Metabolic parameters such as blood glucose levels, glycosylated hemoglobin, lipids, blood pressure, and body weight in addition to quality of

GOALS OF DIETARY THERAPY IN PATIENTS WITH DIABETES

Types I and II goals

To maintain near-normal glucose levels by balancing diet, insulin (exogenous or endogenous) or oral glucose-lowering medications, and activity

To achieve optimal serum lipid levels to prevent atherosclerosis

To provide adequate energy for attainment or maintenance of reasonable body weight in adults, normal growth in children and adolescents, and increased needs during pregnancy or illness

To prevent and treat short-term complications (hypoglycemia, exercise-related hypoglycemia) and long-term complications (nephropathy, neuropathy, hypertension, cardiovascular disease)

To improve general health through optimal nutrition

Type II goals

To achieve glucose, lipid, and blood pressure goals

To reduce weight to improve glucose control, even if ideal body weight is not achieved

---

life should be monitored for optimum management of diabetes.

Dietary therapy in patients with Type I diabetes must integrate insulin therapy into each patient's lifestyle (eating and exercise) patterns. Consistency in the timing and amount of food consumed is important for diabetic patients receiving conventional insulin therapy (one to two daily insulin injections). However, patients with Type I diabetes do not need to divide meals and snacks into a predetermined pattern. Intensive insulin therapy (multiple daily insulin injections or insulin infusion pumps) allows flexibility in food and exercise regimens. Insulin doses can be adjusted to compensate for changes in meal plans and physical activities.

The primary goal of nutrition therapy in patients with Type II diabetes is to optimize glucose, lipid, and blood pressure levels, which (for most patients) is achieved through a dietary/exercise program aimed at attaining an ideal body weight. Even a modest caloric restriction and small amount of weight loss can greatly improve blood glucose control. Only if metabolic control has not improved after dietary intervention and regular exercise should an oral glucose-lowering medication or insulin be added. General dietary guidelines are listed in the box below.

Protein

There are limited scientific data on which to establish firm recommendations for protein intake in diabetic patients. There is no evidence that diabetic patients have different protein requirements than nondiabetic patients. Protein should supply 10% to 20% of their energy intake. With the onset of nephropathy, a protein intake closer to 0.8 g/kg

---

DIETARY GUIDELINES FOR DIABETIC PATIENTS

10% to 20% of calories from protein
Less than 10% of calories from saturated fats
Up to 10% of calories from polyunsaturated fats
Remainder of calories from monounsaturated fats and carbohydrates
Cholesterol intake of less than 300 mg per day
Carbohydrates individualized for energy needs, eating habits, and glucose and lipid control
Nonnutritive sweeteners used only in moderation (no clear benefits shown from their use in either weight or diabetes control)
Fiber intake of 20 to 35 g per day
Less than 2400 mg sodium per day (perhaps more restrictive in the presence of hypertension)
For insulin-requiring diabetic patients: 2 (or fewer) alcoholic drinks per day (1 drink = 12 oz beer, 5 oz wine, or 1.5 oz distilled spirits)

per day or approximately 10% of total energy is recommended (see Chapter 23).

Fat

Recommendations have changed in the last several years on how to divide the remainder of energy intake between carbohydrate and fat. Abnormalities of lipid metabolism are common in diabetes mellitus, and cardiovascular disease accounts for a majority of deaths (in addition to the fact that diabetes is an independent risk factor for cardiovascular disease). It is therefore desirable to minimize intake of cholesterol-raising fats, particularly saturated fatty acids. The general dietary recommendation of no more than 25% to 30% of calories as fat, 10% of calories as saturated fat, and 300 mg cholesterol daily is appropriate when lipid levels are normal. When the low-density lipoprotein (LDL) cholesterol level is elevated, it is advisable to adhere to the National Cholesterol Education Program Step II guidelines (see Table 11-1 and Chapter 18). Less than 25% of calories should come from total fat, less than 7% from saturated fat, and dietary cholesterol should be less than 200 mg per day. When hypertriglyceridemia from increased very low-density lipoprotein (VLDL) is present, aside from adjusting weight loss and physical activity, attempt to moderate carbohydrate intake and increase monounsaturated fat intake (up to 40% of total calories). In certain susceptible individuals, both fasting and postprandial triglyceride levels may increase after switching to a high carbohydrate intake (regardless of type). This has been found to be a transient phenomenon and may resolve even up to 3 to 6 months later, despite continuation of the high carbohydrate diet. However, if hypertriglyceridemia is persistent the monounsaturated fatty acids (MUFAs) contained in olive, canola, and peanut oils can be used in place of carbohydrate to improve lipid levels (see Chapter 18). Because an increase in fat intake may promote or aggravate obesity, a reduction in all types of dietary fat is generally advisable, especially if serum triglyceride levels are higher than 1000 mg/dl.

Carbohydrates

The percentage of carbohydrate in the diet should be based on the individual's eating habits and glucose and lipid levels. In the past, diabetic patients were taught to avoid "simple sugars" and favor more complex carbohydrates. More recent scientific evidence does not support the idea that simple carbohydrates affect glucose levels unfavorably as compared with starch. Nevertheless, the majority of carbohydrate consumed should come from whole grain, unrefined starch, and fresh or frozen fruit and vegetables in order to guarantee an adequate intake of fiber, vitamins, and minerals. Sucrose-containing food may be added on a "special occasion" basis as long as serum glucose levels are not adversely affected.

Sweeteners

Sorbitol, mannitol, and fructose are commonly used sweeteners with lower glycemic effects than either glucose or sucrose. Mannitol and fructose still provide the same amount of energy as other sugars and should be accounted for in the meal plan. Most low-fat and fat-free food as well as fat substitutes contain carbohydrate or protein and should likewise be accounted for in the meal plan. Sweeteners such as aspartame, saccharin, and acesulfame-K do not contribute significant calories, but if they are included in foods that contain other sources of carbohydrate or fat, the latter need to be taken into account in the meal plan. Because there is no evidence that noncaloric, nonnutritive sweeteners assist in either long-term weight control or diabetes control, it is advisable that they be used only in moderation.

Fiber

Experts' opinions are divided on the effects of fiber on blood glucose levels, but at most the effects are probably modest. Therefore the recommendation for fiber intake mirrors that for the general population because of the potential benefits on serum cholesterol levels, intestinal motility, and colon cancer risk.

Vitamins and Minerals

People with diabetes do not generally require vitamin and mineral supplementation if they consume an adequate diet. The recommendation for sodium intake in diabetic patients is the same as for the general population—less than 2400 mg per day. Potassium supplementation may be needed in patients taking diuretics.

Alcohol

When blood glucose levels are well controlled, diabetic patients may consume alcohol in moderation. For patients who require insulin, up to two alcoholic beverages may be consumed with the usual meal plan. Because it may increase the likelihood for developing hypoglycemia in persons receiving insulin or sulfonylureas, alcohol should be consumed only with meals. When keeping track of energy intake for weight reduction, alcohol is best substituted for fat calories; 1 beverage can be equated to 2 fat servings or exchanges. Alcohol should be avoided by persons with severe hypertriglyceridemia or pancreatitis.

Exercise

Exercise is an important tool for managing diabetes. However, precautions need to be taken by some individuals to ensure maximum benefit. In type II diabetic patients and in well-controlled type I diabetic patients, exercise reduces blood glucose levels and therefore insulin requirements, although self-monitoring is important for adjusting insulin or food with the activity. In general, an hour of exercise requires eating an additional 15 g carbohydrate either before or after exercise. Each additional hour of exercise requires the consumption of another 15 to 30 g carbohydrate. Monitoring blood glucose before and after exer-

| TABLE 16-1 | Diabetic exchange lists[1] | | | |

Groups/ lists	Carbohydrate (g)	Protein (g)	Fat (g)	Calories
Carbohydrate group				
Starch	15	3	1 or less	80
Fruit	15	—	—	60
Milk				
Skim	12	8	0-3	90
Low-fat	12	8	5	120
Whole	12	8	8	150
Other				
carbohydrates	15	Varies	Varies	Varies
Vegetables	5	2	—	25
Meat and meat substitute group				
Very lean	—	7	0-1	35
Lean	—	7	3	55
Medium-fat	—	7	5	75
High-fat	—	7	8	100
Fat group	—	—	5	45

cise allows fine-tuning of insulin and/or carbohydrate intake.

Meal Planning

There are a variety of meal-planning approaches for dietary education, ranging from simple guidelines to complex exchange lists. Selection depends on the educator's assessment of the individual's knowledge base and special needs. In the exchange lists developed by the American Diabetes Association and the American Dietetic Association,[1] foods that are similar in calories, carbohydrate, protein, and fat have been combined into four food groups in which a variety of selections may be made (Table 16-1). These lists may be useful for calculating a meal pattern when metabolic goals have been defined.

References

1. American Diabetes Association and The American Dietetic Association: *Exchange lists for meal planning*, Revised 1995, The Association.

Suggested Readings

American Diabetes Association: *Maximizing the role of nutrition in diabetes,*1994, The Association.

American Diabetes Association: *Medical management of non–insulin-dependent (Type II) diabetes,* ed 3, The Association.

American Dietetic Association: Nutrition recommendations and principles for people with diabetes mellitus: position paper, *Diabetes Care* 18(suppl 1):16,1995.

Franz MJ et al: Nutrition principles for the management of diabetes and related complications, *Diabetes Care* 17:490, 1994.

17

Hypertension

Approximately 30 to 40 million U.S. adults have hypertension, a known risk factor for premature death from cardiovascular disease. In addition, most adults in the United States are at increased risk for heart disease because their blood pressure is above the optimal level (120/80 mm Hg) even if they do not have frank hypertension (higher than 140/90 mm Hg). It has been well established that certain lifestyle factors contribute to hypertension and increases in blood pressure that occur with age in industrialized societies; most notable among these are dietary factors. Although antihypertensive medications are effective, costs, side effects, and potential negative influences on quality of life may limit their usefulness. Therefore lifestyle changes are important in both preventing and treating hypertension.

WEIGHT REDUCTION

As a group, patients with hypertension tend to be overweight, and there is a positive association between blood pressure and body weight that is independent of other factors. The risk of hypertension is increased twofold to sixfold in obese compared to lean individuals. Because obesity is prevalent in the U.S. population, it is estimated that 20% to 30% of hypertension is attributable to this risk factor. Deposition of adipose tissue in the abdomen is particularly detrimental (see Chapter 15).

Weight reduction in obese patients with hypertension

generally reduces systolic and diastolic blood pressure levels and is an important therapeutic maneuver in conjunction with pharmacologic therapy. In fact, blood pressure can usually be improved with as little as 10 lb of weight loss. This is due in part to the acute effects of the energy-restricted and probably sodium-restricted, weight-loss diet. If the hypertension is directly related to the excess adiposity, optimal blood pressure control will require normalization of body weight. In addition to enhancing the effects of antihypertensive medication, weight loss can positively affect other cardiovascular risk factors, including dyslipidemias and glucose intolerance. The mechanism by which blood pressure falls with weight reduction has not been established.

SODIUM RESTRICTION

Sodium is found in almost all food and is a common additive in many prepared and processed foods. Sodium requirements for both children and adults are on the order of less than 200 mg per day, but most societies consume many times that amount, ranging from 6 to 12 g of salt per day (2.5 to 5 g of sodium).

Populations such as the U.S. population that have high sodium intakes tend to have a higher prevalence of hypertension and tendency for blood pressure to rise with age. The effects of salt restriction on blood pressure are likely to increase with age and severity of hypertension and are greater in African-Americans. However, individuals vary in their responses to salt restrictions. Controlled studies of moderate sodium restrictions in patients with hypertension have shown modest reductions of 5 and 3 mm Hg in systolic and diastolic blood pressures, respectively. The mechanism of action is thought to involve a reduction in intravascular volume and vessel wall sodium content and/or a decrease in vascular reactivity.

Because there is no known benefit of consuming more sodium than is needed to meet daily losses, reducing a healthy person's salt intake to less than 6 g (2.4 g of sodium) per day is recommended. This level is achievable and palatable after a brief period of adaptation. This degree of sodium restriction may help control Stage I hypertension in some patients (systolic blood pressure 140 to 159 mm Hg or diastolic pressure 90 to 99 mm Hg). Medication requirements may be decreased by a sodium reduction in patients who still need drug therapy. (See Table 11-5 for guidelines of several levels of sodium restriction.)

ALCOHOL RESTRICTION

Population studies consistently show a higher prevalence of hypertension as alcohol consumption rises. Excessive alcohol intake can cause resistance to antihypertensive therapy, and reduction of intake may prevent hypertension. Possible mechanisms for the relationship include the direct effect of alcohol on the vessel wall, sensitization of resistance vessels to pressor substances, stimulation of the sympathetic nervous system, and increased production of adrenocorticoid hormones. Habitual intake should be limited to no more than two drinks per day (1 oz of ethanol).

OTHER DIETARY CHANGES
Potassium

Animal and human population-based studies have shown an inverse association between blood pressure and potassium intake. The association is apparently even stronger when a low potassium intake is combined with a high sodium intake. It has been suggested that a relatively low potassium intake may account for the high prevalence of hypertension in African-Americans. However, it is unlikely that increasing potassium intake is as important as controlling weight and reducing sodium intake in preventing high blood pressure. Regardless, a liberal intake of potassium-rich foods, particularly fruit and vegetables, is reasonable for most individuals. The usual adult potassium intake ranges from 2 to 6 g per day and is generally from fruit, vegetables, meat, and milk (see Table 11-4).

Calcium

A number of studies have associated low calcium intake with increased levels of blood pressure. However, the relationship is not consistent among subpopulations, and studies have not accounted for the confounding that results from sodium intake. The results of a number of intervention trials have been conflicting or shown no effect of calcium supplementation on blood pressure. The use of calcium supplements to control or prevent hypertension is not established.

Fat

Dietary fat intake or replacement of saturated fat with either monounsaturated or polyunsaturated fat has not been shown to affect blood pressure level. However, reducing total fat intake, particularly saturated fats, is a prudent method for controlling body weight and blood lipid levels. Although large amounts of the omega-3 polyunsaturated fatty acids found in fish oil (such as eicosapentaenoic acid [EPA]) may lower blood pressure, they can also produce adverse effects and are not recommended for preventing or treating hypertension.

Magnesium

Magnesium has a blood-pressure lowering effect under certain circumstances such as preeclampsia. However, trials using magnesium supplementation to lower blood pressure have produced inconsistent results. There are insufficient data to support magnesium supplementation as a modality for decreasing blood pressure or preventing hypertension.

Caffeine

Although caffeine may acutely increase blood pressure, habitual intake has not been associated with blood pressure levels or risk for hypertension.

RECOMMENDATIONS FOR PREVENTING AND TREATING HYPERTENSION

Reduce energy intake and maintain physical activity to achieve a reasonable body weight.

Reduce sodium intake to 2.4 g (6 g salt) or less per day.

Limit alcohol intake to 2 drinks or less per day (1 drink = 12 oz beer, 5 oz wine, or 1.5 oz distilled spirits).

Substitute foods containing complex carbohydrates, especially fruit and vegetables, for foods higher in fat.

RECOMMENDATIONS FOR PREVENTING AND TREATING HYPERTENSION

At least three facts underscore the reason it is so important to initiate populationwide lifestyle changes in the entire population of the United States to minimize the risk for developing hypertension: (1) in most cases hypertension is permanent, (2) many adults in the United States are unaware that they have borderline blood pressure levels (between 120/80 and 140/90 mm Hg), and (3) the increase in blood pressure that occurs in the United States as people age appears to be lifestyle related. Reasonable recommendations for preventing and treating hypertension are listed in the box. Regular aerobic exercise of even low to moderate intensity helps prevent and control high blood pressure, independent of its effect on body weight.

Suggested Readings

Beilin LJ: Non-pharmacologic management of hypertension: Optimal strategies for reducing cardiovascular risk, *J Hyperten* 12:S71, 1994.

Joint National Committee: The fifth report of the Joint National Committee on detection, evaluation and treatment of high blood pressure (JNC V), *Arch Intern Med* 153:154, 1993.

Neaton JD et al: Treatment of mild hypertension study: Final results, *JAMA* 270:713, 1993.

Stamler J, Stamler R, Neaton JD: Blood pressure, systolic and diastolic, and cardiovascular risks: US population data, *Arch Intern Med* 153:598, 1993.

Trials of Hypertension Prevention Collaborative Research Group: The effects of nonpharmacologic interventions on blood pressure of persons with high normal levels: Results of the trials of hypertension prevention, Phase I, *JAMA* 267:1213, 1992.

Cardiovascular Disease

Cardiovascular disease is the leading cause of death in the United States and responsible for 40% of all deaths. The number of cases of coronary heart disease, one form of cardiovascular disease, has declined by 2% per year during the past 2 decades; there has been an even greater decline in the number of cases of strokes. The prevalence of coronary heart disease varies considerably in different population groups, suggesting that environmental factors, especially diet, activity, and cigarette smoking, play prominent roles in its development.

ATHEROGENESIS

The atherosclerotic process begins in childhood with fatty streaks—lesions composed of cholesteryl ester-filled macrophages. Low-density lipoprotein (LDL) particles that are chemically altered by oxidation, acetylation or glycosylation are taken up by activated macrophages. These cells, laden with cholesterol, remain in the arterial wall as the foam-cell components of atherosclerotic plaques and stimulate inflammatory responses. Additionally, oxidized LDL may promote several other steps in the atherogenic process, including endothelial cell damage and synthesis of auto-antibodies. The observation that high-density lipoprotein (HDL) is not a risk factor and even helps decrease the risk of atherosclerosis may relate to its ability to remove cholesterol from macrophages and deliver it back to the liver. Some fatty streaks develop into fibrous plaques (raised lesions with a collagen cap and smooth muscle cell proliferation). The plaques may enlarge and rupture, and if they stimulate thrombosis they can precipitate an acute cardiac event such as a myocardial infarction or sudden death.

CARDIOVASCULAR RISK FACTORS

The relationship between serum total cholesterol and coronary heart disease deaths is curvilinear. The mortality rate from a serum total cholesterol level of 250 mg/dl is twice that of patients with levels of 200 mg/dl, and at 300 mg/dl the risk is fourfold higher. In addition, the risk declines at serum total cholesterol levels less than 200 mg/dl, suggesting that even a serum total cholesterol of 200 mg/dl is not optimal (Figure 18-1).

The relationship between diastolic blood pressure and coronary heart disease death is similar, in that individuals

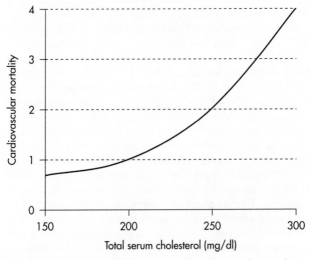

FIGURE 18-1 Relationship of serum cholesterol to cardiovascular risk.

| TABLE 18-1 | Levels of risk associated with lipoprotein levels (mg/dl) | | | |

Lipoprotein	Protective	Desirable	Borderline risk	High risk
Total cholesterol	≤180	<200	200-239	>240
LDL-cholesterol	≤100	<130	130-159	>160
HDL-cholesterol	>60	>45	35-45	<35

in the highest quintile of the population distribution for either serum total cholesterol or blood pressure contribute 50% of the excess risk related to that specific factor. This has led the National Cholesterol Education Program (NCEP) to propose a clinical strategy of diet and medications for individuals in the highest quintile of coronary heart disease risk and a public health approach of lifestyle modifications for the general population. The current mean serum total cholesterol level in U.S. adults is 207 mg/dl, which has decreased during the past 2 to 3 decades. However, the desirable population mean serum total cholesterol level in adults is 175 mg/dl, a level associated with a 30% to 45% lower risk of coronary heart disease. The NCEP has identified levels of risk according to serum lipoprotein levels as shown in Table 18-1. Modifiable and nonmodifiable risk factors for coronary heart disease (factors in addition to abnormal serum total cholesterol and LDL cholesterol levels) are listed in the box.

At any LDL level, the concentration of HDL-cholesterol has an inverse association with coronary heart disease risk. Elevated serum triglyceride levels appear to be an independent coronary heart disease risk factor. High serum triglyceride levels are often associated with a pattern of dyslipoproteinemia characterized by reduced HDL-cholesterol levels and raised levels of chylomicron remnants, very low-density lipoprotein (VLDL) remnants,

RISK FACTORS FOR CORONARY HEART DISEASE

Positive

Age: male 45 years or older; female 55 years or older or premature menopause without estrogen replacement therapy

Family history of premature coronary heart disease

Smoking

Hypertension

HDL-cholesterol level less than 35 mg/dl or 0.9 mmol/L

Diabetes

Negative

HDL-cholesterol 60 mg/dl or higher

---

intermediate-density lipoprotein (IDL), and small, dense, cholesterol-depleted, apolipoprotein (Apo) B-rich LDL. This phenotype is often part of the insulin resistance syndrome, which is accompanied by hypertension, elevated insulin levels, non–insulin-dependent diabetes mellitus, and truncal adiposity.

Both observational studies and controlled clinical trials suggest that each 1 mg/dl increment in the LDL-cholesterol level increases coronary heart disease risk by 1%. Similarly, a 1 mg/dl decrease in the HDL-cholesterol level increases coronary heart disease risk by 2% to 3%. Conversely, lowering serum total cholesterol by 1% is associated with a 2% to 3% reduction in coronary heart disease risk. A number of clinical trials have shown that lowering LDL-cholesterol is effective and safe for primary and secondary prevention of coronary heart disease. In two trials, dietary changes combined with smoking cessation or medication in persons with coronary heart disease resulted in less progression and more regression of coronary artery lesions than did the control regimen. The improvement in artery lumenal diameter correlated with the extent of LDL lowering. In the Lifestyle Heart Trial, a diet with less than 10% of energy from fat and no dietary cholesterol reduced angina in only 1 month, suggesting an immediate impact on vascular relaxation, while later angiograms showed a net regression of coronary heart disease.

DIETARY FACTORS IN CORONARY HEART DISEASE
Fatty Acids and Cholesterol

The recommended diet for dyslipidemia is based on the major nutrients that affect serum total cholesterol. The Keys equation demonstrates that saturated fatty acids raise serum total cholesterol levels twice as much as they are lowered by polyunsaturated fatty acids (PUFAs) and more than the amount they are raised by dietary cholesterol. However, the relationship with dietary cholesterol is curvilinear, so higher dietary intakes have progressively smaller effects on serum total cholesterol levels.

Keys equation: $C = 1.35 (2S - P) + 1.5Z$

where

C = Change in serum total cholesterol (mg/dl)
S = Change in percent energy intake from saturated fat
P = Change in percent energy intake from PUFAs
Z = Difference in square roots of old and new cholesterol
      intakes (mg/1000 kcal)

Saturated fatty acids raise serum total cholesterol levels predominantly by raising LDL-cholesterol levels. However, saturated fatty acids of different chain lengths have variable influences on serum total cholesterol and LDL-cholesterol levels: palmitic (16:0), lauric (12:0), and myristic (14:0) acids raise both serum total cholesterol and LDL-cholesterol levels, whereas stearic acid (18:0) has no effect on them. Reductions in saturated fatty acid intake are generally associated with decreased intake of cholesterol. Because saturated fatty acids and cholesterol interact synergistically to raise LDL, there is the added benefit of decreasing intake of saturated fat.

An important and controversial issue is what should replace the saturated fat in the diet. Four major possibilities are stearic acid, PUFAs, carbohydrate, and monounsaturated fatty acids (MUFAs). The data on stearic acid are too limited to make a population recommendation, and potential promotion of thrombogenesis indicates that caution should be taken. Regarding PUFAs, no population has ever consumed them in high amounts for long periods with proven safety. Because of concerns about suppressing the immune response and promoting tumor development in laboratory animals, it has been suggested that intakes of PUFAs be limited to less than 10% of total energy. On the other hand, high-carbohydrate diets are consumed by many populations that have low rates of coronary heart disease and appear to be safe. Carbohydrates may raise serum triglyceride levels, although the effect is largely transient. If the increased carbohydrate is consumed in the form of fruit and vegetables, the intake of vitamins that function as antioxidants or promote homocysteine metabolism will likely increase, providing additional benefit. If consumed as whole grains and legumes, the increased carbohydrate will increase soluble and in-soluble fiber. In addition, high-carbohydrate diets usually have lower energy densities than high-fat diets, which may lower the prevalence of obesity in the population.

MUFAs, which are rich in the olive-oil based Mediterranean diet, have been suggested as other potential replacements for saturated fat. Although MUFAs were initially thought to be neutral with respect to serum total cholesterol levels, they have now been shown to lower LDL-cholesterol levels without lowering HDL-cholesterol levels as do carbohydrates. The low rates of coronary heart disease in the Mediterranean cohorts in the Seven Countries Study support the efficacy and safety of MUFAs. However, because they are dense in energy, MUFAs could make achievement of ideal body weight more difficult. Overall, both carbohydrates and MUFAs are valid options for replacing saturated fatty acids, with carbohydrate being favored in obesity-prone individuals.

Trans Fatty Acids

Trans fatty acids are isomers of the normal *cis* fatty acids, produced when PUFAs are hydrogenated as they are in the production of margarine and vegetable shortening. The effects of *trans* fatty acids on serum lipids markedly differ from those of the natural *cis* isomer. *Trans* fatty acids uniformly raise LDL-cholesterol levels in humans, whereas the effect of trans fatty acids on HDL-cholesterol levels is small. In addition, *trans* fatty acids raise levels of serum LP(a), an atherogenic lipoprotein.

It remains controversial whether *trans* fatty acids actually increase risk of coronary heart disease, but the effects on lipoproteins are sufficient to indicate that *trans* fatty acids should be avoided. These concerns have stimulated food manufacturers to produce margarine that is lower in *trans* fatty acids.

Fish and Fish Oil

Two types of PUFAs are in the diet: (1) if the terminal double bond is six carbons from the methyl end, the fatty acid is designated n-6; (2) if the terminal double bond is three carbons from the methyl end, it is designated n-3. Linoleic acid (18:2), the major n-6 fatty acid in the diet, is found mainly in plant oils. Fatty acids designated n-3 such as eicosapentaenoic acid and docosahexaenoic acid are found primarily in fatty fish. Observational studies of low coronary heart disease mortality in populations consuming large amounts of fish (200 to 400 g per day) resulted in the hypothesis that n-3 fatty acids may have antiatherogenic and antithrombotic properties. The rarity of coronary heart disease and the low serum triglyceride levels in Greenland Eskimos were linked to their seafood diets. In Japan, platelet aggregability and coronary heart disease mortality were found to be lower in areas where fish intake was higher. In both populations, diets were low in saturated fat and high in n-3 PUFAs.

Several prospective studies found statistically significant inverse trends between fish intake and coronary heart disease mortality. In the Zutphen (the Dutch contribution to the Seven Countries study) and the Chicago Western Electric studies, which involved almost 2800 men free of coronary heart disease at entry, coronary heart disease mortality after 20 to 30 years was inversely related to fish intake. The coronary heart disease mortality was decreased by 35% to 65% with fish intakes of 34 to 44 g per day compared to subjects who had no fish intake. By contrast, in two very large prospective studies (the Physicians Health Study and the Health Professionals Follow-Up Study) with 4- and 6-year follow-ups, there was no evidence for an association between intake of fish and any coronary heart disease endpoint. The explanation for these differences is unclear.

In a controlled clinical trial (the Diet and Reinfarction Trial), men who recovered from an acute myocardial infarction were randomly allocated to two groups, one of which was advised to eat two fatty fish meals per week. Two years later, the fish group had a significant 29% reduction in mortality, although there was no reduction in new myocardial infarctions. In general, patients can be encouraged to consume fish in place of fatty meats to lower their intake of saturated fatty acids and increase n-3 PUFA levels.

Soluble Fiber

The water-soluble fibers include pectin, gums, mucilages, algal polysaccharides, and some hemicelluloses and storage polysaccharides. These fibers are more effective in reducing serum lipid levels than are insoluble fibers. The reduction in serum total cholesterol attributable to soluble fiber may range from 0.5% to 2%/g of dietary fiber intake, and the reduction is greater in patients with initially higher serum total cholesterol levels. Serum total cholesterol levels can be lowered approximately 5% (and almost entirely from LDL) by daily consumption of any of the following: 6 to 40 g pectin, 8 to 36 g gums (e.g., guar gum), 100 to 150 g (0.5 to 0.75 cups) dried beans or leguminous seeds, 25 to 100 g (0.3 to 1.2 cups) dry oat bran, 57 to 140 g (0.7 to 1.7 cups) dry oatmeal, or 10 to 30 g (3 to 9 tbsp) psyllium.

Soluble fiber acts directly by increasing fecal bile acid excretion and slowing absorption of dietary sugars; they act indirectly by displacing fat from the diet. Data from the Health Professionals Follow-Up study suggest that an increase in dietary fiber of 10 g/d decreases the risk of fatal coronary heart disease by 19%. Fiber may have effects on atherosclerosis independent of serum total cholesterol level; supplemental pectin caused atherosclerotic lesions to regress in swine maintained on a high-fat diet without lowering serum total cholesterol concentrations. Average current dietary intake of dietary fiber in adults is 13 g per day, whereas guidelines recommend a total dietary fiber intake of 20 to 25 g per day for adults with about 25% coming from soluble fiber. Adult patients should be encouraged to achieve this with 5 or more servings of fruit and vegetables and 6 or more servings of whole-grain products daily. For children, some authorities have suggested an "age + 5" rule, meaning children more than 2 years old should consume an amount of fiber equal to their age in years plus 5 g per day. Soluble fiber taken in the form of a supplement (e.g., oat bran, gums, or psyllium) may produce additional modest lowering of LDL-cholesterol without affecting HDL-cholesterol and may be useful in treating hypercholesterolemic patients.

Soy Protein

Dietary proteins of plant origin can lower cholesterol levels. In a meta-analysis, replacement of animal protein with soy protein (averaging 47 g per day), without changing dietary saturated fat or cholesterol, resulted in 10% to 12% reductions in serum total cholesterol and LDL-cholesterol without adverse effects on HDL-cholesterol. This model predicted that 25 g per day of soy protein would decrease serum total cholesterol by 9 mg/dl with linear effects through 75 g per day. Two to three servings a day of soy protein equals about 30 g of soy protein.

Alcohol

The relationship of alcohol to coronary heart disease mortality is U-shaped and independent of numerous potential confounders including age, gender, ethnicity, cigarette smoking, education, adiposity, and dietary habits. The overall evidence suggests that alcohol protects persons against coronary heart disease at least in part by raising HDL-cholesterol levels. In addition, some data suggest that alcohol has an antithrombotic effect. However, alcohol consumption at moderate to high levels can raise serum triglyceride levels. Young women who are at low risk for coronary heart disease are more likely to be affected by the adverse effects of alcohol intake than by its benefits. Nondrinkers and established light or moderate drinkers should not be advised to increase their alcohol consumption in order to reduce their coronary heart disease risk.

Homocysteine and Folic Acid

Homocysteine is a sulfhydryl-containing amino acid produced by the demethylation of methionine, an essential amino acid derived primarily from animal protein. To conserve methionine, homocysteine is recycled using a pathway that requires folic acid and vitamins B_6 and B_{12}. In addition to genetic defects in the key enzymes of homocysteine metabolism, marginal deficiencies of these vitamins can elevate homocysteine levels. High levels of homocysteine adversely affect endothelial cells and produce abnormal clotting, so persons with genetic homocystinuria have a high frequency of arterial occlusion and venous thromboembolism in young adulthood. Patients with coronary heart disease and/or peripheral atherosclerosis have significantly higher mean plasma homocysteine levels than do controls. High blood homocysteine levels are prevalent in the U.S. population even in the absence of clear genetic abnormalities. A high homocysteine level combined with other coronary heart disease risk factors appears to be additive or even multiplicative.

The reliable and reproducible association between high homocysteine levels and vascular disease in varied groups employing different study designs suggests that homocysteine is a cause of coronary heart disease independent of other risk factors. In some studies the risk associated with hyperhomocysteinemia was higher than that for hypercholesterolemia, hypertension, and cigarette smoking. The proportion of coronary heart disease attributable to hyperhomocysteinemia was estimated at 4.1%.

Folic acid is the most potent vitamin controlling homocysteine levels. Doses of 0.4 to 1 mg of folic acid reduce fasting homocysteine concentrations. Conclusive evidence of a positive effect of this treatment on coronary heart disease morbidity and mortality will require a randomized, placebo-controlled trial. Dietary changes that can reduce plasma homocysteine concentrations include reducing intake of meat (a rich source of methionine) and increasing intake of vegetables and legumes (increasing folic acid).

Antioxidants

The oxidative modification of LDL and other lipoproteins is important and possibly obligatory in atherogenesis. Thus it has been hypothesized that inhibiting the oxidation of LDL will decrease or prevent atherosclerosis. Vitamin E, β-carotene, and vitamin C (which are all antioxidants) delay and reduce the oxidation of LDL in vitro. It is noteworthy that dietary PUFAs increase the PUFA content in LDL, which increases its susceptibility to oxidation.

Several large observational studies have suggested that vitamin E supplementation reduces coronary heart disease risk, after adjusting for risk factors and for use of multivitamins, β-carotene, or vitamin C. Female nurses who used vitamin E supplements for more than 2 years had a 34% reduction in coronary heart disease risk, and trends toward reduced risk were observed with β-carotene and vitamin C consumption. Similar results (with a 37% reduction in risk) were observed in male health professionals who used vitamin E supplements (100 IU or more per day) for more than 2 years. Randomized prospective trials have thus far confirmed that vitamin E, but not β-carotene, can reduce coronary heart disease risk.

Therefore it is reasonable to recommend antioxidant supplementation (400 IU of vitamin E per day and 1000 mg of vitamin C per day) in high-risk persons such as those with known coronary heart disease and smokers. However, the potential risks of this approach include a false sense of security that may lead to neglect of more certain means of coronary heart disease protection. In addition, a lack of efficacy and possible ill effects of β-carotene have been found in long-term supplementation trials. The most prudent recommendation for the general population is to consume a diet high in dark-green vegetables and deep-yellow fruit and vegetables, which are good sources of antioxidant vitamins.

Iron

Iron is an extremely potent oxidant when it is not bound to protein. It has been suggested that it creates a prooxidant environment in the arterial wall and participates in atherogenic processes such as LDL oxidation, endothelial injury, and myocardial injury during ischemia. Several prospective studies have addressed the relation between iron and risk of coronary heart disease. Although some of these studies support an iron-coronary heart disease link, their results are inconsistent and do not justify changes in nutritional or therapeutic recommendations.

Phytochemicals

Dietary substances from plants can lower serum total cholesterol levels and reduce coronary heart disease risk. Examples of these phytochemicals are phytosterols, tocotrienols, and flavonoids. Phytosterols are plant sterols that inhibit absorption of both endogenous and exogenous cholesterol and lower serum total cholesterol levels. Tocotrienols, which are chemically related to tocopherol, inhibit HMG CoA reductase and lower serum total cholesterol. Garlic that is taken in amounts of one-half to one clove per day decreased serum total cholesterol by 9% in a meta-analysis of five placebo-controlled, randomized studies. The mechanism of action has not been established but may also involve inhibition of HMG CoA reductase. Flavonoids are antioxidant polyphenolic compounds that are ubiquitously present in vegetables, fruit, and beverages of vegetable origin including tea and red wine. Flavonoid intake has been inversely associated with coronary heart disease mortality and explains a significant proportion of the variance in coronary heart disease rates, regardless of its dietary source. This suggests that flavonoids have an impact on coronary heart disease risk that is independent of associated dietary factors. Since the safety and long-term efficacy of phytochemical supplements has not been established, patients should be encouraged to consume a wide variety of vegetables and fruit, which naturally provide these substances and have the added advantage of being low in fat.

OTHER FACTORS IN CORONARY HEART DISEASE
Obesity and Weight Loss

Prospective studies have confirmed a moderate but statistically significant association between obesity and coronary heart disease mortality that is related to the higher prevalence of diabetes, dyslipidemia and hypertension among obese persons. Serum total cholesterol, LDL-cholesterol, and serum triglyceride levels tend to be higher and HDL-cholesterol lower in obese persons. Obesity can contribute to dyslipidemia by increasing secretion of VLDL, which is followed by an increased conversion of VLDL to LDL. Independent of total adiposity, abdominal obesity is associated with disturbances in plasma glucose, insulin, lipid levels, and coronary heart disease mortality. When sustained, weight reduction lowers coronary heart disease risk through its beneficial effects on the lipoprotein profile, insulin resistance, and blood pressure.

Physical Activity

A sedentary person has approximately twice the risk of an acute myocardial infarction and a coronary heart disease death compared to a person who is physically active. Only 22% of adult Americans engage in light to moderate physical activity for at least 30 minutes per day on most days; 54% are only somewhat active, and 24% are inactive. Regular physical activity can increase HDL-cholesterol by 5% to 15%, lower serum triglycerides, enhance insulin sensitivity, and reduce risk for hypertension and obesity. Low or moderate-intensity exercise can lower diastolic blood pressure by 8 mm Hg, which may potentially be associated with a 46% reduction in risk for stroke and 29% reduction in risk for coronary heart disease. The amount of activity is more important than the type or intensity of the activity. The dose-response curve suggests that the greatest health benefits accrue to physically inactive people who introduce some physical activity into their daily lives. The current recommendation is that all individuals should be at least moderately active for 30 minutes per day on most if not all days.

DETECTION AND MANAGEMENT OF DYSLIPIDEMIA
Detection

The NCEP recommends that serum total cholesterol and HDL-cholesterol levels be measured every 5 years in all adults 20 years of age and older. If the fasting serum triglyceride level is also measured, LDL-cholesterol can be estimated using the formula

LDL-cholesterol = Serum total cholesterol −
$$\text{Serum triglycerides}/5 - \text{HDL-cholesterol},$$

where serum triglycerides/5 estimates the VLDL-cholesterol level as long as fasting serum triglyceride levels are less than 400 mg/dl. It is not essential that the patient be fasting for screening, but if an abnormality is detected it should be confirmed after fasting, and the LDL-cholesterol level should be measured directly or lipoprotein fractionation performed. All patients with serum total cholesterol levels of greater than 240 mg/dl and/or HDL levels less than 35 mg/dl and those with serum total cholesterol levels of 200 to 239 mg/dl and two risk factors for coronary heart disease should have lipoprotein levels measured. All patients with evidence of coronary heart disease should have two lipoprotein analyses separated by 1 to 8 weeks and enter into a program of secondary prevention. The levels of risk associated with various lipoprotein levels are shown in Table 18-1.

Persons more than 2 years old who do not have dyslipidemia should be given information on general population dietary recommendations, physical activity, and risk factor reduction. All persons who have high-risk LDL-cholesterol levels and those who have borderline-risk LDL-cholesterol levels plus two additional coronary heart disease risk factors should be evaluated. Secondary causes for high LDL-cholesterol and/or VLDL-cholesterol levels should be ruled out; these include diabetes mellitus, hypothyroidism, nephrotic syndrome, cholestatic liver disease, and medications, particularly progestins, anabolic steroids, and certain antihypertensives, especially thiazide diuretics, and β-blockers. If none of these causes is present, dietary therapy should be instituted. The goal is to lower the LDL-cholesterol level to less than 160 mg/dl when fewer than two other coronary heart disease risk factors are present and less than 130 mg/dl when two or more risk factors are present. Drug therapy is only considered after an adequate trial of dietary therapy has failed to produce adequate results. Levels of LDL-cholesterol to consider for drug therapy in primary prevention are those greater than 190 mg/dl with less than two coronary heart disease risk factors and greater than 160 mg/dl with two or more coronary heart disease risk factors.

For secondary prevention (i.e., in patients with established coronary heart disease) the NCEP has specified a more rigorous LDL-cholesterol goal of less than 100 mg/dl. Patients with coronary heart disease whose LDL-cholesterol level is higher than 100 mg/dl should receive maximal dietary therapy and be considered for drug therapy if the level does not fall below 130 mg/dl. Many physicians consider drug therapy for these patients even if the LDL-cholesterol is between 100 and 130 mg/dl. Supplementation of these patients with vitamin E is also beneficial.

Dietary Management

The NCEP has developed a two-level diet plan for reducing serum cholesterol levels (Table 18-2). The Step I diet is essentially the same as the dietary guidelines for the

TABLE 18-2 Dietary recommendations for lowering serum cholesterol levels

Nutrient*	Step I diet	Step II diet	Average American†
Fat (% energy)	≤30	≤30	34-36
SFA‡ (% energy)	8-10	<7	13-14
MUFA (% energy)	≤15	≤15	14-15
PUFA (% energy)	≤10	≤10	5-6
Cholesterol (mg)	<300	<200	360 (men) 220-260 (women) 200-300 (children)
Total calories	To achieve and maintain desirable body weight		—
Carbohydrate (% energy)	≥55	≥55	~50
Protein (% energy)	~15	~15	14-15

* Calories from alcohol not included.
† Modified from National Health and Nutrition Examination Survey III, 1988-1991.
‡ *SFA*, Saturated fatty acids; *MUFA*, Monounsaturated fatty acids; *PUFA*, Polyunsaturated fatty acids.

general population. The Step II diet is identical to Step I except that it is more restricted in saturated fat and cholesterol. Major sources of saturated fat in the American diet are listed in Table 18-3. The table also shows foods that can be substituted for those high in saturated fat and cholesterol.

Providing adequate nutrition for growth and development is a special dietary consideration in children. Thus the diet should first meet the Recommended Dietary Allowances (RDAs) for all nutrients and especially energy, protein, iron, zinc, and calcium.

Dietary Sources of Saturated Fat and Cholesterol

Approximately 25% to 60% of the fat in animal products is saturated: the proportion of saturated fat increases from fish and poultry at 25% to 30%, to pork at 40%, beef at 50%, and butter fat at 60%. The remainder of their fat content is MUFAs with a small amount of PUFAs. Animal fat generally contains about 1 mg cholesterol/g of fat, whereas butter fat has 3 mg cholesterol/g fat.

Cholesterol is found only in products of animal origin. The cholesterol content of meat is not related to its fat content. Specifically, muscle tissue has 60 to 80 mg cholesterol per 3 oz of meat, but the fat content can vary over a tenfold range. The cholesterol content of most seafood is 50% to 100% of that in meat, except for shrimp, which has 166 mg/3 oz.

Organ meat (i.e., liver, pancreas, kidney, and brains) has a cholesterol content fourfold to fifteenfold higher than muscle. In dairy products, cholesterol and fat content are related. Thus consuming low-fat dairy products significantly reduces their cholesterol contribution to the diet, whereas meat (even lean meat) remains a significant source of dietary cholesterol.

Different fats and oils vary in their fatty acid and cholesterol contents. Tropical oils including palm, palm kernel, and coconut oil are rich in saturated fatty acids (50% to 90%) but like all plant foods do not contain cholesterol. Oleic acid, a MUFA, is the dominant fatty acid in

TABLE 18-3 Major sources of saturated fat in the American diet

Food group (% of saturated fat content of current American diet)	Food to decrease	Food to choose
Meat and mixed dishes (39%)	Hamburgers, beefsteaks, roasts, hot dogs, ham, luncheon meats, pork, bacon, sausage, high saturated-fat dishes* (pizza, soup, casseroles, chili, pot pies)	Fish, shellfish, poultry without skin, lean red meats (if used at all), beans, peas, other meat substitutes
Dairy products (23%)	Whole or 2% milk; whole-milk yogurt, regular cheese, butter, ice cream, and frozen dairy desserts	Skim or 1% milk or buttermilk; low-fat varieties of cheese, cottage cheese, yogurt, and frozen dairy desserts
Sweets and snacks (14%)	High saturated-fat items† (doughnuts, cookies, cakes, chips, milk chocolate)	Angel-food cake, low-fat sweets, fruit, baked goods and chips made with unsaturated oil
Cooking fat/convenience foods (13%)	Hard margarine, animal fat, tropical oil	Unsaturated, unhydrogenated oil (olive, canola, safflower, soybean, peanut, sunflower); margarine, seeds and nuts
Eggs (5%)	Egg yolks	Egg whites, egg substitutes
Invisible fat (3%)	High saturated-fat items† (processed, packaged foods, breads, rolls, and crackers)	Whole-grain breads, low-fat rolls, muffins, crackers and cereals

*Saturated fat content of meal and main dishes defined as >1g/100 g and >10% of calories.
†Saturated fat content of items defined as >1 g/serving and >15% of calories.

avocados and olive, canola, peanut, rice, and hazelnut oils. *Trans* fatty acids, which are formed in the manufacturing of margarine and shortening, are currently considered unsaturated fatty acids on food labels despite the fact that their effects on serum lipids are like those of saturated fatty acids. Major sources of the very long-chain n-3 PUFAs are fatty fish. Recommended vegetable oils include canola, olive, corn, safflower, sunflower, and soybean, which have saturated fat contents ranging from 6% to 25%. Nuts and seeds are rich in oil, containing 4 to 6 g/tbsp of fat and ranging in saturated fatty acid content from 7% in walnuts and pecans to 21% in cashews.

Selection and Preparation of Food Lower in Saturated Fat and Cholesterol

The major food groups needing modification are meat, dairy, and fat and oil. Because the average daily energy intake is 1800 kcal for women and is 2500 kcal for men, the maximum daily saturated fat intake on the Step I and Step II diets is 20 g and 14 g in women, respectively, and 28 g and 19 g in men. Although meat is a concentrated source of protein, iron, zinc, and vitamin B_{12}, there is no requirement for meat in the diet; these nutrients can be obtained from other sources. It is essential that portion size not exceed 6 oz per day, cooked (Step I diet) or 5 oz per day, cooked (Step II diet). (NOTE: A 3-oz serving is about the size of a deck of cards.) All visible fat should be trimmed from meat, and skin should be removed from poultry before cooking. After cooking meat for stew or soup, it should be allowed to cool and the fat skimmed off. The use of soybean protein has the benefit of being low in saturated fat and methionine and inherently cholesterol lowering. Dry beans, lentils, and peas are additional good sources of protein and soluble fiber that may contribute to lowered serum cholesterol levels.

Dairy products are rich sources of protein and supply most of the calcium in the average diet. Preferred choices are skim or 1% milk, nonfat or 1% yogurt, and nonfat or low-fat (less than 2 g/oz) cheese.

Egg yolks provide 213 mg cholesterol and 1.7 g saturated fat per egg. They should be limited to no more than four egg yolks per week on the Step I diet and no more than two per week on the Step II diet. Egg whites contain protein but no cholesterol. Egg substitutes are made primarily of egg white and can replace whole eggs in dishes such as scrambled eggs, omelets, and baked items.

In developing a dietary plan for the prevention or treatment of coronary heart disease, attention must be given to an overall healthy eating pattern and not just fat and cholesterol restriction. Thus the focus is on promoting positive behaviors—the consumption of whole-grain bread and cereal, unrefined starch, fruit, and vegetables—not being fanatic about fat.

Medications for Dyslipoproteinemia

Except in cases of severe dyslipidemia, most patients can be managed with diet and activity modification, and it is essential that the diet and activity programs continue even if medications are required. This approach permits effective control of dyslipidemia with lower dosages of medications and is thus both safer and less costly. Four major classes of lipid-lowering medications will be mentioned briefly.

Bile Acid Sequestrants

Cholestyramine and colestipol lower LDL-cholesterol by 15% to 30%. They are anion-exchange resins that bind bile acids in the intestinal lumen and increase the fecal loss of bile acids. This interruption of enterohepatic circulation of bile acids stimulates increased conversion of cholesterol to bile in the liver, and the depletion of cholesterol stimulates increased LDL receptors and lowers LDL levels. Because this medication can increase serum triglyceride levels, they are indicated for patients with isolated LDL-cholesterol elevations. Their major side effects are gastrointestinal and include reflux, bloating, and constipation. Because of their record of efficacy and long-term safety, they are the only medication recommended for childhood dyslipidemia.

HMG CoA Reductase Inhibitors (Statins)

This widely utilized class of lipid-lowering drugs includes atorvastatin, fluvastatin, lovastatin, pravastatin, and simvastatin. They are competitive inhibitors of the rate-limiting enzyme of cholesterol, synthesis, and by depleting the hepatocellular pool of cholesterol, these drugs stimulate the synthesis of LDL receptors, enhancing the uptake and catabolism of LDL and lowering blood LDL-cholesterol levels. LDL-cholesterol reduction is dose dependent but proportionally less effective at higher dosages. Usual doses (i.e., 50% of the maximum dosage) lower LDL-cholesterol levels by 30% to 35%, lower serum triglyceride levels by 10% to 20%, and increase HDL-cholesterol levels by 8% to 10%. They are generally used to treat patients with significant LDL elevations with or without mild serum triglyceride elevations. Long-term safety data (greater than 5 years) are not available, but these drugs are effective in decreasing coronary heart disease morbidity and mortality in primary and secondary prevention trials. The most common side effects include irritable bowel symptoms like dyspepsia, abdominal cramps, and constipation. Other side effects are increased liver enzyme (transaminase) levels and myopathy.

Nicotinic Acid

Nicotinic acid is the drug of choice for combined hyperlipidemia (i.e., elevated VLDL and LDL levels), which is typically associated with elevated serum triglyceride and total cholesterol levels. The usual dose is 1.5 to 3 g per day of crystalline niacin. Nicotinic acid lowers serum triglyceride levels by 20% to 50%, lowers LDL-cholesterol by 10% to 25%, and increases HDL-cholesterol by 15% to 35%. The major mechanism of action appears to be inhibition of lipolysis, which lowers circulating levels of the free fatty acids that are important substrates for hepatic serum triglyceride synthesis. These effects reduce production of VLDL-containing serum triglycerides and Apo B from the liver. Because VLDL is a precursor of LDL, LDL levels are also reduced. Nicotinic has been shown to be effective in reducing coronary heart disease risk. Adverse effects include flushing symptoms, peptic ulcer disease, diarrhea, hyperglycemia, hyperuricemia, and hepatotoxicity. Combinations of nicotinic acid with statins or resins are very potent in lowering VLDL and LDL levels.

Fibric Acid Derivatives

Gemfibrozil, clofibrate, fenofibrate, benzafibrate, and ciprofibrate are effective in lowering serum triglyceride levels 20% to 50% and raising HDL-cholesterol levels 10% to 15%. Effects on LDL-cholesterol levels are varied in that they decrease high LDL-cholesterol levels and increase low LDL-cholesterol levels. They are most useful for treating severe hypertriglyceridemia or familial dysbetalipoproteinemia. Side effects include an increase in bile lithogenicity, which increases risk of cholesterol gallstone formation. Combination therapy of gemfibrozil with lovastatin has been associated with severe myopathy and rhabdomyolysis.

Suggested Readings

Anderson JW, Johnstone BM, Cook-Newell ME: Meta-analysis of the effects of soy protein intake on serum lipids, *N Engl J Med* 333:276, 1995.

Boushey CJ: A quantitative assessment of plasma homocysteine as a risk factor for vascular disease—probable benefits of increasing folic acid intakes, *JAMA* 274:1049, 1995.

Dattilo AM, Kris-Etherton PM: Effects of weight reduction on blood lipids and lipoproteins: a meta-analysis, *Am J Clin Nutr* 56:320, 1992.

Gould AL et al: Cholesterol reduction yields clinical benefit—a new look at old data, *Circulation* 91(8):2274, 1995.

Hoffman RM, Garewal HS: Antioxidants and the prevention of coronary heart disease, *Arch Intern Med* 155:241, 1995.

Hopkins PN: Effects of dietary cholesterol on serum cholesterol: a meta-analysis and review, *Am J Clin Nutr* 55:1060, 1992.

Katan MB: Fish and heart disease, *N Engl J Med* 332:1024, 1995.

Katan MB, Zock PL, Mensink RP: Dietary oils, serum lipoproteins, and coronary heart disease, *Am J Clin Nutr* 61(suppl):1368, 1995.

Klatsky AL: Epidemiology of coronary heart disease—influence of alcohol, *Alcohol Clin Exp Res* 18:88, 1994.

Kris-Etherton PM et al: *Trans* fatty acids and coronary heart disease risk, *Am J Clin Nutr* 62(suppl):665, 1995.

Wynder EL, Stellman SD, Zang EA: High fiber intake—indicator of a healthy lifestyle, *JAMA* 275:486, 1996.

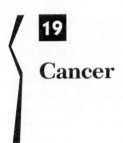

19

Cancer

PREVENTION

The role of nutritional factors in modulating the development of cancer has received a great deal of attention in recent years. Cancer is the second leading cause of death in the United States, and survival figures for the major lethal cancers (those of the lung, breast, and colon) have not substantially increased, so prevention could have a significant effect on the U.S. population.

The risk for cancer is related to nutrients, nonnutritive dietary constituents, and nutritional status in a variety of ways. Part of the complexity stems from the fact that the development of cancer is a multistage process that usually begins with exposure to an environmental substance called a *precarcinogen* that must be activated in vivo. Once active, the carcinogen triggers tumor initiation by producing a mutation that activates an oncogene or inactivates a tumor suppressor gene. This step is necessary but not sufficient for cancer development, as many mutant cells are probably destroyed before they actually form clones. Tumor promotion and progression, which require additional mutations and growth factors and often take many years, must occur before a tumor large enough to produce symptoms develops. It has become clear that nutrition interacts with each of the stages of carcinogenesis, making the relationship complex.

To complicate matters further, the evidence linking nutritional variables to cancer is of many different types and strengths. Evidence for the involvement of particular nutrients in carcinogenesis often begins with epidemiologic observations in human populations. Prospective epidemiologic studies of cohorts, without intervention, have become quite valuable in confirming cross-sectional observations. Yet the diets of individuals are extremely complex, making it difficult to distinguish the effects of single nutrients from those of groups of nutrients and other environmental and lifestyle variables. Animal carcinogenesis studies are often the next step, and perhaps thousands of them have been conducted. Carefully controlled to isolate single variables of interest, these studies allow causal inferences to be drawn, but their correlations with the conditions and metabolism of free-living humans are often uncertain. In vitro investigations such as those conducted on oncogenes provide important insights into the mechanisms of nutrient-cell interactions, but it is often unclear how each observation fits into the overall scheme of cancer development. Randomized, controlled human trials can provide the most definitive causal links in humans but are often quite expensive and lengthy and may use doses of single nutrients or synthetic analogues that are unavailable in the diet.

Nevertheless, taken together the diet-cancer data create a compelling impression. It is conservatively estimated that diet accounts for about 35% of the malignancies experienced in western countries, suggesting that dietary changes would be far from futile. Current evidence can be distilled into the dietary recommendations shown in the

---

DIETARY RECOMMENDATIONS FOR CANCER PREVENTION

Maintain a desirable weight.

Eat a varied diet.

Eat a variety of vegetables and fruit daily.

Eat high fiber food, such as whole-grain cereal, legumes, vegetables, and fruit.

Minimize total fat intake.

Limit intake of alcoholic beverages if consumed at all.

Limit consumption of salt-cured, smoked, and nitrite-preserved foods.

box, which were initially endorsed by the American Cancer Society, the National Cancer Institute, and other groups in 1984 and revised in 1991. These recommendations will be used as an outline for our consideration of the topic.

Maintain a Desirable Body Weight

Obesity was identified more than 30 years ago as a potential risk factor for several cancers. However, after more powerful epidemiologic studies further dissected the relationship, obesity proved to be an independent risk factor for cancers of the endometrium and breast only. The mechanism may be related to alterations in hormone metabolism induced by obesity. Circulating levels of androgens such as androstenedione, which is synthesized in the adrenal glands, are normally quite low in women. However, they are converted in adipocytes to the potential carcinogen, estrone. In obese women the total adipocyte mass is elevated, increasing estrone production and circulating levels, which enhances the risk for endometrial cancer.

As discussed in detail in Chapter 15, all obese persons are not at equal risk for the complications of obesity. Some epidemiologic studies indicate that persons whose excess adiposity is predominantly intraabdominal are at increased risk for endometrial and breast cancer, whereas those with peripheral obesity may have a risk equal to that of lean persons. Although the mechanism for this is not known, it may be caused by differences in hormone metabolism between centrally and peripherally obese persons.

Even when it does not result in obesity, excess energy intake in animals has a profound influence on the appearance of spontaneous or induced cancers. Studies that began in the 1930s demonstrate that allowing rodents to consume food *ad libitum* consistently results in tumor yields of 25% to 300% higher than in animals given energy restrictions of only 10% to 25%. The effect of energy restriction is independent of and more potent than that of dietary fat restriction. There is also evidence that exercising animals to increase energy expenditure may reduce tumor yields, suggesting that absolute energy intake may be less important than the degree to which it matches energy needs.

Although few human studies have specifically addressed energy intake and cancer, those published to date are in general agreement with the animal data. It is probable that total energy intake influences most of the other nutrients correlated with cancer. Mild energy restriction is the most consistent and powerful anticancer "agent" reported.

Eat a Varied Diet

The recommendation to eat a varied diet was added in the 1991 revision of the American Cancer Society guidelines. If one adheres to the other recommendations, it is likely that an adequately varied diet will follow.

Eat a Variety of Vegetables and Fruit Daily

Evidence convincingly indicates that consuming a generous quantity of fruit and vegetables reduces the risk for a number of cancers and the overall cancer death rate. Even without precise knowledge of the relative power of their individual constituents, the evidence that a liberal intake of fruit and vegetables reduces cancer risk is overwhelmingly supported by 128 of 156 studies as of 1992.[1] A large body of literature suggests that a number of nutrients, including β-carotene, folic acid, vitamin C, vitamin E, selenium, and others may be collectively responsible for this effect. It is likely that nonnutritive substances naturally present in fruit and vegetables contribute as well.

The main mechanism through which β-carotene protects against cancer is thought to be the antioxidant properties through which it quenches free radicals produced by metabolism and/or environmental exposure; however, other mechanisms may also be involved. Retinol, as distinguished from β-carotene, comes from animal sources and is a much weaker free-radical scavenger. Nevertheless, it may also have some anticancer activity.

The evidence for the cancer-inhibiting role of the carotenoids and retinoids includes extensive epidemiologic and animal carcinogenesis data plus evidence from in vitro investigations. Most notably, epidemiologic studies show that both smokers and nonsmokers who have lower intakes and/or plasma levels of carotenes are at increased risk for developing lung cancer. It has been known for decades that vitamin A is required for normal epithelial cell differentiation, and deficiency induces potentially premalignant metaplasia in the respiratory, gastrointestinal, and genitourinary tracts of animals. Studies have repeatedly shown that supplementation of animal diets with vitamin A or synthetic retinoids significantly reduces the incidence and number of tumors induced by carcinogen administration. This is true of the mammary gland, lung, skin, and other tissues.

A number of human intervention studies testing β-carotene or synthetic retinoids as cancer chemopreventive agents have been completed. Some of these have confirmed the expected protective effects, but large trials of β-carotene supplementation in smokers showed significant *increases* in lung cancer. This contrary effect may have occurred because carcinogenesis had already progressed in the subjects (who had smoked for many years) beyond the point at which β-carotene could exert a protective effect. When taken by physicians for 12 years, β-carotene supplements produced neither harmful nor beneficial effects. It is quite possible that other constituents of fruit and vegetables are responsible for some of the protective effects attributed to β-carotene.

Because folic acid is required for nucleic acid synthesis and repair and because cells grown in folate-deficient media frequently show chromosomal damage at "fragile sites," folic acid may offer protection against cancer. It is inactivated by certain environmental substances, particularly cigarette smoke, and is marginally sufficient in the diets of many Americans. Therefore localized or systemic folate deficiencies may be relatively common. Cervical dysplasia and bronchial metaplasia, two potentially premalignant conditions, have been associated with lower blood folate levels, and in two trials folic acid supplementation in the diets of smokers with bronchial metaplasia produced improvements in lesions. Women whose cervical cells contained DNA from the human papillomavirus, which is thought to cause cervical cancer, were reported to have an increased risk for cervical dysplasia only if their red blood cell folate levels were in the lowest tertile. This may represent a prototypical interaction between nutritional status and environmental exposure in which the exposure can only produce disease when nutritional status is suboptimal. There is evidence that folate may protect against colon cancer as well.

Vitamin C, another prominent constituent of fruit and vegetables, has been investigated extensively in epidemiologic studies that have shown lower rates of cervical dysplasia and gastric, esophageal, laryngeal, oropharyngeal, and lung cancers in persons with higher intakes of vitamin C. However, many of these observations may be confounded by the association of vitamin C in many foods with carotenoids, folic acid, and other potentially protective compounds. Its most direct role is probably as a water-soluble antioxidant in which it blocks the formation of nitrosamines in the stomach after the ingestion of foods containing nitrates and nitrites. In this way it may reduce the risk of stomach cancer.

The ability of vitamin E to protect lipid membranes against oxidation suggests that it could play a role in inhibiting the actions of carcinogens. Higher cancer rates have been associated with lower plasma levels of vitamin E obtained years earlier; animal studies have been supportive. Another antioxidant, selenium, may provide protection against several cancers, particularly those of the gastrointestinal tract. Because many micronutrients have apparent anticancer properties, a trial of supplementation with various combinations of vitamins and trace elements was undertaken in Linxian, China, which has one of the highest rates of gastric and esophageal cancer in the world. Persons supplemented for 6 years with a combination of β-carotene, vitamin E, and selenium had a 13% decrease in cancer (mainly stomach) mortality and incidence. To date, human trials in western countries have not confirmed these effects.

Nonnutritive substances in fruit and vegetables are probably responsible for some of the benefits of these foods. Many of the substances, including sulforafanes, indoles, protease inhibitors, flavonoids, isoflavones, allylic sulfides, and capsaicin, have demonstrated anticancer actions in vitro. Because they can be obtained only from food, the use of dietary supplements in lieu of dietary change to prevent cancer is foolish. Except in multivitamin/multimineral preparations, Vitamin A and selenium supplements should be particularly discouraged because they can cause significant toxicity. Although it is not clear precisely which nutrients or substances are most responsible, the benefits of consuming fruit and vegetables are beyond dispute.

Eat High-Fiber Food Such as Whole-Grain Cereal, Legumes, Vegetables, and Fruit

Since the inverse association of dietary fiber with colon cancer rates was first described in the 1970s, it has been investigated and discussed extensively. The mechanisms proposed to explain the association include dilution of carcinogens by increased stool bulk, direct binding of carcinogens by fiber, and alterations in colonic bacterial metabolism, which decrease the luminal pH and inhibit the formation of fecal mutagens such as secondary bile acids. The short-chain fatty acid metabolites of fiber also exert a trophic effect on the colonic mucosa, which may help to maintain a better defense against carcinogens.

When subjected to controlled animal studies, fiber has not always proven to be protective against cancer. In some studies only the water-insoluble fibers found in whole grains and wheat bran reduced colon cancer rates in animals. This is reasonable because these fibers tend to exert their effects in the colon rather than in other parts of the intestinal tract. On the other hand, dietary intake of both insoluble and soluble fibers found mainly in legumes, oat or rice bran, fruit, and vegetables has been associated with lower colon cancer risk in human epidemiologic studies.

In human populations, dietary fiber intake varies inversely with dietary fat and directly with the intake of potentially beneficial nutrients, so some of the beneficial effects attributed to dietary fiber may be caused by other factors. Therefore even after more than two decades of investigation a reliable estimate of the independent effect of dietary fiber is impossible to make. Nevertheless, the recommendation to eat more fiber-containing foods is prudent.

Minimize Total Fat Intake

The data supporting this recommendation have generated more controversy than any other aspect of diet and cancer. Epidemiologic studies indicate that countries with high per capita fat consumption have higher age-adjusted death rates from cancers of the breast, colon, prostate, and ovary than do those with lower fat intakes. However, because increased fat consumption tends to be characteristic of more highly developed countries, these studies may be confounded by unmeasured cultural or dietary differences, and studies comparing groups within the same population almost never confirm an association of dietary fat with breast cancer. Almost without exception, animals fed high-fat diets in controlled experiments develop cancers at higher rates than do those on low-fat diets. However, as mentioned previously, this effect may be partly or wholly explained by differences in total energy intake.

The role of dietary fat in colon carcinogenesis is probably the most strongly supported. In the Nurses Health study, which began tracking more than 120,000 nurses in 1976, participants who consumed red meat one or more times per day had a risk for colon cancer that was 2.5 times higher than those who ate virtually no red meat.[2] The effect was not reduced after controlling for intake of energy, fiber, or other known risk factors, and the authors attributed the result to animal fat. No randomized human trials designed to test the dietary fat-cancer hypothesis have been completed, but the Women's Health Initiative that began in 1993 has this as its major objective.

In the midst of all this controversy, it should be emphasized that the recommendation to minimize fat intake makes a great deal of sense. Even if reducing fat to 30% or 20% (or even less) of energy is not guaranteed to reduce the risk for developing breast cancer, it appears likely to do so for colon cancer. Perhaps more important, minimizing fat intake is the most efficient way to reduce total energy intake, and if it is accompanied by higher carbohydrate intake, fat reduction should result in increased intake of vegetables, fruit, and grains.

Limit Intake of Alcoholic Beverages if Consumed at All

Although alcohol is not a carcinogen, it is a promoter of carcinogenesis in several organs. Excessive consumption of alcohol is the major cause of hepatic cirrhosis in the United States, and the incidence of liver cancer is greatly increased in persons with cirrhosis. Excess alcohol acts synergistically with cigarette smoking to dramatically increase the risk of oral, pharyngeal, and esophageal cancer.

Epidemiologic evidence has even linked moderate alcohol intake to increased breast cancer incidence in women. In several studies, including the Nurses Health study, women who consumed as few as three drinks per week had approximately 50% more breast cancer in subsequent years than did nondrinkers. Although they do not indicate that women should abstain from alcohol, it would be prudent to limit consumption to low levels and consider abstaining when other risk factors for breast cancer, such as a family history of the disease, exist.

Limit Consumption of Salt-Cured, Smoked, and Nitrite-Preserved Food

In countries where salt curing and pickling are widely used for food preservation, consumption of such foods is correlated with gastric and esophageal cancers. The ingestion of sodium nitrite, used a food preservative in processed meats, results in the formation of carcinogenic nitrosamines in the stomach and may increase the risk for developing stomach cancer. Because consumption of food preserved by these methods is not high in the United States, their overall contribution to cancer risk is not large. However, individuals who consume them in large amounts would be well advised to moderate their intakes.

Cooking methods that involve intense heat such as charbroiling meat produce or deposit polycyclic aromatic hydrocarbons (from fats) and heterocyclic amines (from proteins) on the meat surfaces. Because many of these compounds are potent carcinogens, it is prudent not to use these cooking methods with great frequency.

There is little evidence that the other food additives commonly used in the United States are responsible for any human cancers. The same is true for caffeine. A number of pesticides are carcinogenic in vitro, but whether they cause cancer in humans is the subject of continuing debate. It has been estimated that human ingestion of naturally occurring carcinogens exceeds that of synthetic carcinogens by a factor of at least 10,000.

TREATMENT

It has been observed for centuries that cancer patients frequently suffer from progressive cachexia. In patients with most tumor types, weight loss heralds a poor prognosis. This is not simply because patients who lose weight have higher tumor burdens; in fact, the correlation between tumor mass and weight loss is poor. The causes of weight loss have been extensively investigated. Reports of energy expenditure in cancer patients are inconsistent, indicating that the contribution of increased resting energy expenditure to weight loss is relatively small. Alterations in the metabolism of carbohydrate, fat, and protein occur in cancer patients, including futile metabolic cycles, glucose intolerance, insulin resistance, increased lipolysis, and increased whole-body protein turnover. Cytokines such as tumor necrosis factor may be activated. However, the major cause of weight loss in cancer patients is poor nutrient intake resulting from anorexia, alterations in sense of taste, and other disease- and treatment-related factors. These are summarized in the box.

The fact that weight loss is associated with poor survival in cancer patients does not necessarily indicate a cause-effect relationship. If weight loss were the cause, reversing it with sufficient nutrients should improve survival. Although this has been attempted in a large number of randomized, prospective trials, the benefits have been

Factors Contributing to Weight Loss in Cancer Patients

Systemic disease-related effects

Anorexia

Changes in perception of taste and smell

Increased sense of fullness, perhaps resulting from decreased digestive secretions, mucosal atrophy, and/or impaired gastric emptying

Changes in metabolism, perhaps induced by cytokines such as tumor necrosis factor

Local disease-related effects

Obstruction of the gastrointestinal tract at any point

Intestinal dysmotility induced by the tumor

Treatment-related effects

Surgery affecting the gastrointestinal tract or head and neck

Chemotherapy, causing mucositis, nausea, vomiting, diarrhea

Radiotherapy, causing decreased saliva, and ability to taste and smell

Psychologic effects

Depression

Conditioned food aversions related to upcoming therapy

minimal and the risks substantial. Some trials tested aggressive nutritional support as adjuncts to chemotherapy and radiation therapy and did not document improvements in survival, tumor response, or tolerance of therapy. Other trials that used aggressive parenteral nutrition for 3 to 10 days before cancer surgery showed that at best, improvements in nutritional status resulted in decreased morbidity and mortality immediately following surgery in patients with preexisting malnutrition, but no long-term benefit was demonstrated. In randomized trials in which total parenteral nutrition (TPN) was administered in conjunction with chemotherapy, higher sepsis rates were consistently seen in TPN-treated patients as compared with controls, prompting some reviewers and the American College of Physicians to suggest that TPN may produce net harm in these patients and should not routinely be used.[3] Very few trials have tested the effects of enteral nutrition.

Concern has been expressed that parenteral feeding may accelerate tumor growth. Some animal feeding studies showed proportional increments in tumor weight and carcass weight, whereas others showed disproportionately greater tumor growth. The few human studies that have addressed the question have not yet answered it positively or negatively.

Therefore it is best to take an individualized approach to nutritional support in cancer patients by monitoring nutritional status carefully and intervening aggressively only when clear indications exist. There is no justification for using enteral or parenteral nutrition to prevent weight loss (except perhaps in bone marrow transplant patients) or treat weight losses of less than 10%. When nutrition support is necessary every effort should be made to use enteral feeding rather than TPN.

Although better outcomes from maintaining adequate nutrition during cancer treatment are uncertain, eating and feeling well nourished contribute to an overall sense of well-being. Paying careful attention to cancer patients' nutritional problems and concerns can help considerably in making them feel stronger and more self-sufficient.

Oral Nutrition

Cancer patients often experience abnormalities in their senses of taste and smell, but because these occur without a predictable pattern, it is best to be aware of individual food preferences and aversions and experiment with various food aromas and seasonings. Cold food tends to be tolerated better than hot food, which may increase nausea and vomiting. Acidic food tends to irritate inflamed mucous membranes. Anorexia and nausea sometimes increase as the day progresses, in which case breakfast meals may be best tolerated. Small meals with between-meal snacks can augment total food intake. Although commercial oral nutritional formulas (see Chapter 12) are helpful, some cancer patients are overwhelmed by the sweetness of the preparations and prefer to drink unflavored "tube-only" formulas.

In the lay press there is much discussion of various "alternative" dietary therapies for cancer, including megadoses of various vitamins. None of these vitamins including vitamin C, which has perhaps received the most attention, improves any outcome variable in cancer patients. However, anorectic cancer patients may rapidly become vitamin deficient without supplemental vitamins, so a daily replacement multivitamin is warranted in these patients; possible preexisting deficiencies in patients undergoing medical and surgical therapy should be considered as well. Zinc and vitamin C supplementation should be taken into account in patients with poor wound healing and sepsis.

Enteral Nutrition

When oral intake is inadequate to maintain nutritional status and the intestinal tract is functional, tube feeding should be used as long as it is consistent with the overall treatment plan. Tube feeding can sometimes provide relief for the anorectic patient who is constantly pressured to eat more while experiencing nausea and food aversions. It can be administered at home to reduce the need for hospitalization. Considerations in choosing a feeding formula are the same as in patients without cancer. Unless there is a contraindication, cachectic patients should be given high-protein formulas.

Parenteral Nutrition

Even with the noted cautions, indications exist for using TPN in cancer patients. Principal among these are intestinal obstruction and major intestinal resection or diversion. Preoperative TPN should be seriously considered for patients who have lost 15% to 20% of their body weight, require major surgery, and cannot be fed enterally by any route. The decision to initiate TPN must be consistent with the prognosis and overall treatment objectives. Thus the ideal candidate is a patient with intestinal obstruction whose prognosis is otherwise reasonably good and for whom additional cancer therapy is planned; however, it is often inappropriate in patients whose malignancies have failed to respond to therapy and are considered terminal. In these cases maintaining hydration with intravenous fluids usually offers comparable benefit and has fewer complications and lower costs.

Home parenteral nutrition, which in the 1970s was considered by many to be inappropriate for cancer patients, is now used more commonly in patients with cancer than in those with any other condition. All of the indications for in-hospital parenteral nutrition now comprise reasons for its use at home. It is particularly effective for prolonging the lives of patients with irremediable intestinal obstruction or massive intestinal resection. In addition, it can reduce the need for hospitalization during chemotherapy and fistula healing, thus decreasing the total cost of care and improving quality of life. However, as with in-hospital TPN, the appropriateness of its use must be carefully considered in terminal care, in which it may provide no more benefit than the maintenance of hydration with intravenous fluids.

References

1. Block G, Patterson B, Subar A: Fruit, vegetables, and cancer prevention: a review of the epidemiological evidence, *Nutr Cancer* 18:1, 1992.
2. Willett WC et al: Relation of meat, fat, and fiber intake to the risk of colon cancer in a prospective study among women, *N Engl J Med* 323:1664, 1990.
3. McGeer AJ, Detsky AS, O'Rourke K: Parenteral nutrition in cancer patients undergoing chemotherapy: a meta-analysis, *Nutrition* 6:233, 1990.

Suggested Readings

Work Study Group on Diet, Nutrition, and Cancer: American Cancer Society guidelines on diet, nutrition, and cancer, *CA* 41:334, 1991.

Gastrointestinal and Liver Diseases

GASTROINTESTINAL DISEASES

Because the primary function of the gut is to absorb nutrients (Figures 20-1, 20-2, and 20-3, and Table 20-1), it is not surprising that gastrointestinal diseases have an impact on nutrition or that nutritional manipulations are integral to the management of gastrointestinal diseases.

Malabsorption

Many gastrointestinal diseases result in malabsorption, which is a failure of the gastrointestinal tract to absorb ingested nutrients. Malabsorption results from surgical resections and many types of gastrointestinal diseases, such as pancreatic or biliary insufficiency and primary bowel conditions (such as infiltrative, inflammatory, or neoplastic diseases). However, it is best to classify malabsorption on the basis of its physiologic effects. Processes that cause malabsorption affect either the intraluminal or the mucosal phase of digestion and absorption.

Intraluminal

The intraluminal phase is the phase in which ingested food is mixed with pancreatic enzymes and bile salts to decrease the size of carbohydrates and proteins so that they can be absorbed by the mucosa. Fats are also converted to simpler forms, but bile salts are needed to help them migrate to the intestinal mucosa. This process is disturbed in

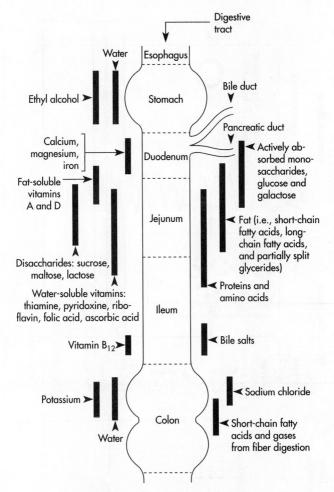

FIGURE 20-1   Sites of nutrient absorption.

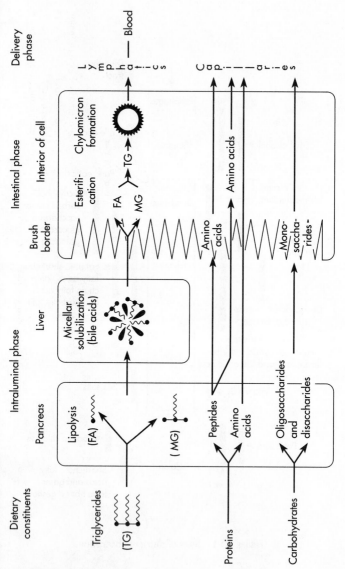

FIGURE 20-2 Digestion and absorption of triglycerides, proteins, and carbohydrates.[1]

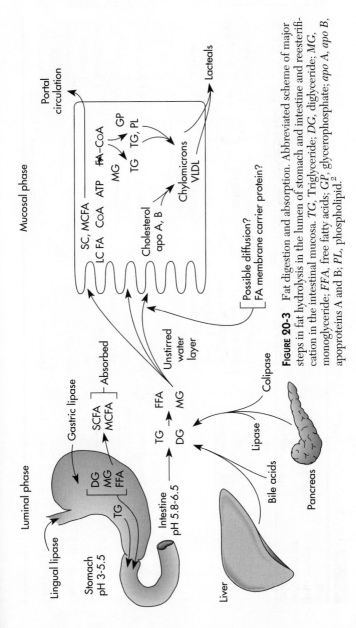

FIGURE 20-3 Fat digestion and absorption. Abbreviated scheme of major steps in fat hydrolysis in the lumen of stomach and intestine and reesterification in the intestinal mucosa. *TG,* Triglyceride; *DG,* diglyceride; *MG,* monoglyceride; *FFA,* free fatty acids; *GP,* glycerophosphate; *apo A, apo B,* apoproteins A and B; *PL,* phospholipid.[2]

TABLE 20-1 Intraluminal and mucosal digestion of carbohydrates[3]

Diet (percentage of carbohydrate intake)	Luminal enzymes	Oligosaccharides and disaccharides presented to mucosa	Mucosal enzymes	End products
Starch (60%) Amylopectin	Salivary and pancreatic alpha-amylases →	Maltose, maltotriose, and other oligosaccharides (α-1,4 linkage)	Glucoamylase (maltase) →	Glucose
		Alpha-dextrins (α-1,6 linkage)	Alpha-dextrinase (isomaltase) →	Glucose
Amylose	Salivary and pancreatic alpha-amylases →	Maltose, maltotriose, and other oligosaccharides	Glucoamylase (maltase) →	Glucose
Sucrose (30%)	→	Sucrose	Sucrase →	Glucose and fructose
Lactose (10%)	→	Lactose	Lactase →	Glucose and galactose
Trehalose	→	Trehalose	Trehalase →	Glucose

patients with chronic pancreatitis (in which insufficient pancreatic enzymes are produced) and biliary cirrhosis (in which insufficient amounts of bile salts are excreted). In pancreatic insufficiency, oral replacement of the enzymes can improve absorption.

Mucosal

All nutrients must cross the intestinal mucosa to enter circulation, and most do so by specific mechanisms. Anything affecting the length or mass of the intestinal mucosa, such as inflammatory conditions (e.g., Crohn's disease [regional enteritis]), giardiasis, gluten enteropathy, infiltrative processes, lymphoma, and intestinal resection, will decrease absorption. Problems can also occur when a specific mucosal digestive or transport mechanism is missing or damaged, such as in lactose intolerance. Some types of malabsorption are corrected when the underlying disease such as giardiasis, gluten enteropathy, or lactose intolerance, is treated. However, many other diseases require considerable manipulation. Intestinal resections have become one of the more significant causes of malabsorption, because surgical resections may be necessary for treating an intestinal infarction, congenital malformations, inflammatory diseases, cancer, and trauma.

Resection

Gastrointestinal resections can alter the physiology of digestion and absorption in a variety of ways depending on the portion removed. There may be a change in transit time, reduction in overall surface area, inability to absorb nutrients requiring specialized portions of the intestine, and altered bacterial colonization. Long-term parenteral nutrition is usually required when less than 2 feet of jejunum or ileum are intact; when there is 1 foot or less, parenteral nutrition is necessary for survival.

Resection of the Stomach

The gastric pylorus normally functions as a gate, retaining the gastric contents until they are isotonic and then releasing them into the duodenum. Most gastric operations alter the pylorus, increasing the rate of gastric emptying. Premature passage of hyperosmolar contents into the upper small intestine can result in rapid shifts in the amount of fluid entering the small intestine (referred to as *dumping syndrome*) and maldigestion caused by inadequate mixing of ingested food with bile and pancreatic secretions.

A total gastrectomy removes the sources of intrinsic factor that are required for ileal absorption of dietary and enterohepatically recirculated vitamin B_{12}, placing the patient at risk for B_{12} deficiency. With decreased gastric acid and pepsin secretion after gastric removal, absorption of heme-iron is impaired because its reduction to the ferrous form is hampered. Iron is normally absorbed in the duodenum, but the jejunum can adapt to perform this function if the duodenum is removed.

Resection of the Small Intestine

The symptoms and signs of small intestinal disease depend on the extent of the resection that was performed. For inflammatory and other diseases the severity of the disease is equally important. For most patients with a small bowel resection or disease, steatorrhea (fat loss in the stool) and its consequences are the most significant resulting problems. Although fluids and electrolytes are also absorbed in the jejunum and ileum, the colon has a tremendous capacity for absorbing the increased output from the small bowel. Therefore fluid loss or liquid diarrhea is generally not a problem unless the colon is also damaged or missing.

The most consistent and often earliest manifestation of steatorrhea is increased stool bulk. Patients may have one to three very large bowel movements a day rather than small watery stools and may not complain of diarrhea. Because of their high fatty acid and air contents, the stools may be frothy and float, are often foul smelling, and may be associated with flatulence. Weight loss is a common but inconsistent finding in patients with malabsorption, because many patients compensate for poor absorption by increasing their energy intake.

Fat malabsorption can lead to secondary problems. Cramping and paresthesias (numbness and tingling) of the hands and feet are a manifestation of hypocalcemia and/or hypomagnesemia. These conditions develop when unabsorbed free fatty acids form insoluble precipitates (soaps) with calcium and magnesium ions, rendering them unabsorbable. Patients with steatorrhea are at risk for developing calcium oxalate kidney stones, which result from high urinary oxalate excretion (hyperoxaluria). The latter is caused by enhanced absorption of dietary oxalate resulting from increased free oxalate in the adapted remnant bowel lumen when calcium, which normally binds oxalate and impedes its absorption, is trapped by free fatty acids.

Patients with steatorrhea also malabsorb the fat-soluble vitamins A, D, E, and K. Bleeding into the skin, especially without trauma, suggests a vitamin K deficiency. However, because colonic bacteria produce vitamin K, a deficiency does not generally develop unless the colonic flora are destroyed by antibiotics. Decreased dark adaptation because of a vitamin A deficiency tends to present initially as reduced visual acuity on entering a dark room such as a theater or when driving at night and looking into the lights of an oncoming car. Bone loss and increased risk of fractures may result from chronic malabsorption of both calcium and vitamin D. Vitamin E has significant antioxidant effects and is needed in young children for proper nerve growth. Dietary carotene is poorly absorbed and serum levels are frequently low, providing a useful diagnostic test to support the impression of fat malabsorption—as long as the patient consumes several servings of carotene per day from yellow and green vegetables and fruit (which many Americans do not).

Digestion and absorption of most nutrients occurs primarily in the jejunum; however, the ileum can perform these functions if the jejunum is resected. By contrast, the jejunum cannot replace specific terminal ileal functions such as the active absorption of bile salts and vitamin B_{12}. Diarrhea can develop from the increased amount of bile salt entering the colon. Both unabsorbed fatty acids and bile acid interfere with colonic sodium and water absorption and may cause fluid secretion and severe diarrhea. Bile salt malabsorption also predisposes patients to cholesterol gallstone formation. Resection or disease of the most distal portion of the ileum prevents the absorption of intrinsic factor-bound vitamin B_{12}. Macrocytic anemia in the setting of malabsorption is strongly suggestive of vitamin B_{12} deficiency or in some situations folate deficiency. This may require several years to manifest. Although the clinical manifestations of zinc deficiencies are less commonly seen in patients with malabsorption, the frequently low blood zinc levels should be addressed because of the potential for the development of poor wound healing and immune compromise.

The presence or absence of the ileocecal valve is a critical determinant of bowel function in individuals with significant intestinal resection or disease. This structure regulates the entrance of small bowel contents into the colon and protects the small intestine from colonization by colonic organisms. If these bacteria enter the small intestine after resection of the ileocecal valve, bacterial overgrowth of the small intestine can occur, possibly producing diarrhea. Regardless of the extent of the small bowel resection, a patient with an intact ileocecal valve is generally much less symptomatic than a patient without the valve.

Resection of the Colon

The major role of the colon in the digestive process is to absorb electrolytes and water. Unabsorbed carbohydrates are fermented by colonic bacteria, producing hydrogen, carbon dioxide, and short-chain fatty acids; the colon can absorb these, providing 5.7 kcal/g. However, a large production of short-chain fatty acids decreases the colonic pH to less than 5.5, disturbing sodium absorption by the colon mucosa and tending to cause diarrhea (as does the presence of the osmotically active fatty acids in the lumen of the colon). Patients who have had extensive resections of both the colon and small bowel usually have profuse, watery diarrhea. Patients with externally-draining jejunostomies sometimes have fluid losses large enough to require long-term parenteral nutrition. Although removing the colon protects patients who have had terminal ileum resections against bile acid colitis, the colitis can usually be managed with cholestyramine.

Nutritional Management Following Intestinal Resection

Though certain aspects of malabsorption are predictable, no two patients with malabsorption are identical. Survival and rehabilitation after intestinal resection depend on the length, location, and condition of the remaining intestine; capacity of the intestinal remnant to adapt by increasing its absorptive capacity; and adequacy of nutritional support. Even after massive intestinal resections, patients with short bowel syndrome often find that they are able to readapt to using enteral feeding as their sole nutritional support. However, this result requires judicious use of both parenteral nutrition and a carefully designed oral refeeding regimen to facilitate intestinal adaptation.

Nutrition and Bowel Adaptation

Although the mechanisms of intestinal adaptation after partial resections are not well understood, the anatomic and physiologic changes are well documented. The remaining bowel dilates, mucosal hyperplasia occurs, crypt length increases, and absorption per unit length of bowel increases. However, this adaptation only takes place when enteral feeding is being used to stimulate the bowel and pancreatic and biliary secretions. Parenteral nutrition without enteral feeding is not sufficient.

After extensive small bowel resections, optimal intestinal function and nutritional status are achieved through a combination of graduated oral feeding and parenteral nutrition. In this way, nutritional needs can be met and weight maintained or gained while the intestines are challenged incrementally and adaptation is taking place. To accomplish this goal, the refeeding regimen described in Chapter 11 is recommended for all patients undergoing drastic intestinal resectioning and for those who have suffered significant weight loss and malnutrition because of malabsorption.

General Nutrition Guidelines

Once the patient has progressed through the refeeding regimen for 1 to 3 weeks, the diet should consist of small frequent meals, avoidance of milk (because of expected lactose intolerance), and restriction of fat (less than 30 g per day). As intestinal adaptation takes place in 3 to 4 months, intake of fat may be gradually increased to about 40 g per day and then to 50 or 60 g per day. Medium-chain triglyceride (MCT) oil may be supplemented if increased calories are needed. Supplemental enteral formulas can be useful as long as they are lactose free and low in fat. Although it may be useful to run a therapeutic trial in difficult cases, special formulas containing prehydrolyzed proteins (peptides and/or crystalline amino acids) have no proven advantage in terms of intestinal function or nitrogen balance and are generally higher in osmolarity and cost.

Minerals and Vitamins

When deficiencies of the divalent cations calcium and magnesium exist (as evidenced by hypocalcemia and/or hypomagnesemia), restriction of dietary fat to less than 30 g per day is an even more essential part of patient management. Calcium and vitamin D supplementation are often needed to maintain the serum calcium level but are often inadequate without fat restriction. Hypomagnesemia also dictates a need for fat restriction, because oral magnesium supplements cause diarrhea and are tolerated only in small doses.

Treatment to avoid deficiencies of the fat-soluble vitamins A, D, E, and K should be guided by appropriate blood tests. Large oral doses of vitamins A, D, and E are often needed to sustain normal blood vitamin levels and (in the case of vitamin D) maintain a normal serum calcium. Vitamin K supplements are not required unless the prothrombin time is prolonged.

Patients with malabsorption usually do not develop deficiencies of most of the water-soluble vitamins because they are efficiently absorbed in even short segments of the small intestine. However, patients with ileal disease or resections usually require periodic injections of vitamin B_{12}. Alternative methods of vitamin B_{12} supplementation that are sometimes effective include large oral doses (1000 μg/day) and nasal gel. Folate deficiencies sometimes develop in patients with small intestinal disorders and usually respond to supplementation with 1 mg per day. Iron deficiencies are infrequent in these patients because maximal iron absorption occurs in the duodenum, which is left intact after most bowel resections. However, serum levels of vitamin B_{12}, folate, and iron should be tracked and appropriate supplements used if they drop to unacceptably low levels.

Treat patients with hyperoxaluria or a history of oxalate-containing renal stones by increasing fluid intake and administering oral calcium supplements to increase binding of oxalate in the intestine.

Therapeutic multivitamin-multimineral supplements are often helpful in patients with significant malabsorption, especially in those with short bowel syndrome. Suggested dose ranges are shown in Appendix C. A few commercial multivitamin preparations are designed to provide these doses, but they often contain insufficient amounts of one or two vitamins such as A and D. Individual nutrient supplements are outlined in more detail in Table 20-2.

Medications

Several medications commonly used in patients with malabsorption are also listed in Table 20-2. Pancreatic enzyme supplements containing high lipase activities may

TABLE 20-2   Supplements and agents that may be used in maldigestiion or malabsorption

Agent	Dosage	Route	Comment/precautions
Minerals			
Calcium gluconate or	5-10 mg t.i.d.	p.o.	Should monitor serum Ca^{++}
Calcium carbonate (500 mg Ca^{++} tab)	500mg b.i.d. to q.i.d.	p.o.	Should monitor serum Ca^{++}
Magnesium gluconate (500 mg-tab)	1-4 g q.i.d.	p.o.	—
Ferrous sulfate (325 mg-tab)	325 mg t.i.d.	p.o.	One tablet taken at bedtime
Vitamins			
Vitamin A (25,000 U-cap)	100,000-200,000 U b.i.d.	p.o.	Maintenance dose: 25,000 to 50,000 U
Vitamin D (10,000-50,000 U-cap)	30,000-50,000 U/day	p.o.	Can increase dose to make serum Ca^{++} normal
Vitamin K (menadione)	4-12 mg/day	p.o.	—
Vitamin K_1 (Mephyton)	5-10 mg/day	p.o.	—

Folic acid (1 mg-tab)	5 mg/day for 1 wk, then 1 mg/day	p.o.	—
Vitamin B_{12}	1000 μg loading dose; then 100 μg q 1-2 mo	IM	—
Vitamin B complex	1-2 tabs daily	p.o.	—
Pancreatic enzymes			
Pancrease, Viokase (0.3 g), or Cotazyme	3 tabs with meals	p.o.	Effect may be improved by taking 300 mg cimetidine q.i.d. to decrease lipase inactivation
Antibiotics/antibacterials			
Metronidazole	250 mg t.i.d.	p.o.	—
Antidiarrheal agents			
Loperamide (2 mg tab)	2-4 mg p.r.n.	p.o.	—
Bile acid-binding resin			
Cholestyramine	4 g t.i.d.	p.o.	—

improve fat digestion and steatorrhea in some patients after intestinal resections. Usually, large and frequent doses are required, and responses are variable in patients with bowel disease or resections, whereas they are usually effective (and diagnostic) in patients with maldigestion caused by pancreatic insufficiencies. In patients who have had 100 cm or less of ileum resected, bile acid-induced diarrhea may respond to 8 to 12 g of cholestyramine per day. This binding resin reduces the irritating effects of the bile acids in the colon. In patients with more extensive resections, cholestyramine is of little help and may aggravate the steatorrhea by further depleting the bile acid pool.

Bacterial colonization of the small bowel can contribute to diarrhea and malabsorption, especially when the ileocecal valve is removed. When colonization is suspected, a trial of oral antibiotics such as metronidazole may bring symptomatic improvement.

Gastric hypersecretion commonly develops during the first several weeks after intestinal resections and is thought to be a result of increased gastrin secretion. Antacids and ranitidine are sometimes used in this setting, but hypersecretion is not a constant finding and tends to disappear with time.

Gastrointestinal Problems Without Malabsorption

Many of the common gastrointestinal diseases and conditions do not have malnutrition components, although nutritional management is an important component of their treatment. Following are the most common of these conditions.

Irritable Bowel Syndrome

A poorly understood condition, irritable bowel syndrome can cause abdominal pain, constipation, diarrhea, and abdominal distention. It is most likely a motility disorder and can be triggered by stress and certain food. While the offending food varies from patient to patient, caffeine should always be eliminated from the diet. Supplementing the diet with up to 30 g per day of fiber has very beneficial effects in most patients.

Constipation

Although constipation can be treated with laxatives and stool softeners, a high-fiber diet can be equally effective, cheaper, and provide added benefits. Whether used for constipation or irritable bowel syndrome, a high-fiber diet must be consistently consumed and accompanied by sufficient fluid intake to be effective.

Gastroesophageal Reflux

Defined as the movement of gastric acid and other gastric contents into the esophagus, gastroesophageal reflux can produce pain, heartburn, and esophageal strictures. Certain dietary changes can decrease the severity of the reflux. It is important to eliminate caffeine from the diet because it relaxes the lower esophageal sphincter. In addition, even decaffeinated coffee may need to be eliminated because the oils in coffee seem to potentiate reflux.

LIVER DISEASES

The liver orchestrates a wide variety of major metabolic processes in the body including carbohydrate, fat, and protein metabolism, protein synthesis, and detoxification and excretion of both endogenous and exogenous waste products. The liver has an enormous functional reserve (which performs satisfactorily when only 20% of its cells are functioning) and an excellent ability to repair itself after injury. However, severe impairment of any of its functions regardless of the cause can create widespread and diverse metabolic derangements that often affect nutritional status through anorexia, fat malabsorption, depressed protein synthesis, and other mechanisms. Conversely, impairment of nutritional status may further exacerbate abnormal liver function by hampering the liver's ability to regenerate itself. The goal of nutritional therapy in liver disease is to support liver function and optimize the liver's ability to regenerate if the injury is repaired or resolved.

Carbohydrate and Fat Metabolism

The liver plays a central role in blood glucose homeostasis. When exogenous calories fail to meet the body's requirements, the liver initially maintains blood glucose levels by metabolizing glycogen (glycogenolysis). As starvation continues, there is a gradual transition toward synthesis of glucose from amino acids (gluconeogenesis). In patients with severe hepatic insufficiency, these processes are impaired and hypoglycemia may occur.

The liver also plays an important role in fat metabolism. Fatty acids from both endogenous and exogenous sources are converted to energy via the Krebs cycle. When adapting to starvation, the liver forms ketone bodies that can be utilized by parts of the body including the brain as an alternative to glucose. By sparing gluconeogenesis and its amino acid substrates, muscle protein is conserved. The liver also synthesizes, packages, and interconverts cholesterol, bile acid, and lipoprotein.

In patients with hepatic injuries, all of these functions may be impaired. Malabsorption of fat and fat-soluble vitamins may occur because of diminished bile salt production and/or excretion by the liver into the bile, where they are needed to facilitate fat absorption.

Protein Metabolism

As with carbohydrate and fat, the liver processes endogenous and exogenous amino acids. Endogenous proteins are continuously hydrolyzed to amino acids and resynthesized into proteins. Through hepatic transamination, amination and deamination reactions, there is a constant interchange between the amino acids and the energy-producing substrates of carbohydrate and fat metabolism. Ammonia, a byproduct of amino acid catabolism, is converted to urea by the liver for excretion in the urine.

Altered protein metabolism is probably the most significant metabolic disturbance that develops in patients with liver disease (Figure 20-4). It is characterized by altered plasma amino acid profiles and manifests clinically by muscle wasting and encephalopathy. As hepatic insuffi-

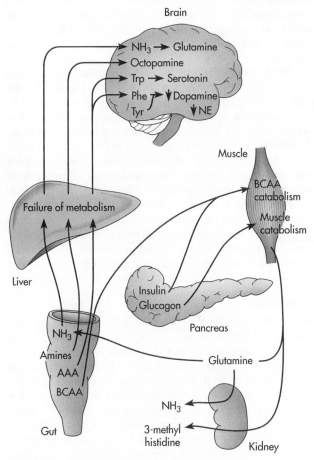

FIGURE 20-4 Pathogenesis of amino acid imbalances leading to hepatic encephalopathy. *BCAA*, Branched-chain amino acids; *AAA*, aromatic amino acids.[4]

ciency develops, the liver provides the body with glucose less efficiently. As a consequence the branched-chain amino acids—leucine, isoleucine, and valine—are utilized locally by several tissues to produce energy and their blood levels decrease. In contrast, the aromatic amino acids—phenylalanine, tyrosine, and tryptophan—and methionine are not metabolized normally by the liver and their levels rise, resulting in a low branched-chain amino acid to aromatic amino acid ratio. The ratio of free tryptophan to protein-bound tryptophan in the blood also increases.

Encephalopathy (neuromuscular irritability, stupor, and coma) sometimes develops when a patient with chronic liver disease becomes infected or dehydrated, consumes alcohol, or ingests more protein than the liver can handle. The mechanism is multifactorial but appears to relate at least in part to the alterations in amino acid metabolism. Manipulation of the plasma amino acids to resolve this sometimes improves encephalopathy. Chronic liver disease with superimposed encephalopathy differs metabolically from acute fulminant hepatic failure, in which plasma branched chain amino acid levels are often normal but those of all other amino acids are increased. This difference may explain the apparent ineffectiveness of manipulation of the plasma amino acids in this condition.

Treatment

Severe hepatic insufficiency places the patient in a difficult position nutritionally. Encephalopathy may develop even with normal amounts of protein intake, and inadequate protein synthesis threatens the functioning of all organ systems as well as immune mechanisms. Therefore the overall approach in treating liver disease is to meet the estimated energy needs and give enough protein to maintain nitrogen balance without precipitating encephalopathy. Keeping these principles in mind, the guidelines in the box on the following page may be used to formulate nutritional support goals.

NUTRITIONAL SUPPORT IN HEPATIC INSUFFICIENCY

A nutritional assessment (see Chapter 8), including a 24-hour urinary urea nitrogen assessment, should be used to estimate energy and protein needs and the level of catabolism. Major effort is sometimes required to prevent weight loss.

Fluid and sodium restrictions are indicated when ascites and/or edema is present.

Standard oral sources of protein and standard enteral and parenteral formulas can usually be used. If there is no history or high likelihood of encephalopathy, a normal protein balance should be maintained. If the patient has a history of protein intolerance or encephalopathy, protein intake should be restricted to about 0.5 to 0.7 g per kg of "dry" body weight per day. This can be increased judiciously by about 10 to 15 g per day to determine protein tolerance.

If encephalopathy develops, particularly if it does not respond to other therapies, or mild encephalopathy prevents the intake of adequate protein to maintain nitrogen balance, branched-chain amino acid-enriched formulas should be considered. The formulas designed for enteral use are listed in Table 12-1; Hepatamine 8% (McGaw) is used parenterally. Though their usefulness is not universally accepted, adequate doses (1.2 to 1.5 g/kg per day) frequently appear to result in improvement of encephalopathy.

Dietary fat restriction is unnecessary unless fat malabsorption is symptomatic.

Vitamin and mineral replacement therapy should be initiated and monitored periodically, because deficiencies are common.

Electrolyte and fluid balance disturbances should be treated as they are encountered.

Periodic nutritional reassessments should be done to evaluate the effectiveness of the nutritional support regimen.

References

1. Silverman A, Roy CC, eds: *Pediatric clinical gastroenterology*, St Louis, 1983, Mosby.
2. Tsang RC, Nichols BL, eds: *Nutrition during infancy*, St Louis, 1988, Mosby.
3. Silverman A, Roy CC, eds: *Pediatric clinical gastroenterology*, St Louis, 1983, Mosby.
4. Munro HN: Metabolic integration of organs in health and disease, *J Parenter Enteral Nutr* 6:271, 1982.

Suggested Readings

Maddrey WC: Branched chain amino acid therapy in liver disease, *J Am Coll Nutr* 4:639, 1985.

Roy CC, Silverman A, Alagille D, eds: *Pediatric clinical gastroenterology,* St Louis, 1995, Mosby.

Schiff L, Schiff E, eds: *Diseases of the liver,* ed 7, Philadelphia, 1993, Lippincott.

Sleisenger M, Fordtran J, eds: *Gastrointestinal disease,* ed 5, Philadelphia, 1993, WB Saunders.

21

Critical Illness

Various critical illnesses, especially those resulting from trauma or severe sepsis, share many metabolic and nutritional features. Regardless of whether they are septic, many critically ill patients exhibit a constellation of systemic inflammatory responses that impair immune function and tissue healing and can lead to lung, kidney, and liver dysfunction (multiple organ failure syndrome), prolonged hospitalization, and high mortality.

METABOLIC RESPONSE TO INJURY AND INFECTION

Since the 1930s, scientists and clinicians have been aware of the marked catabolic response involving breakdown of body tissues that occurs in injured patients even when they are receiving what appears to be adequate nutritional support. In fact, injury and infection induce the most accelerated breakdown of body tissue observed in the practice of medicine, with burns and head injuries heading the list of causes of the most severe degrees of catabolism. However, only in recent years has there been documentation that the rapid mobilization of the body's fuel and tissue reserves can be offset by aggressive and appropriate nutritional intervention.

The major components of the metabolic response are hypermetabolism, proteolysis and nitrogen loss, and accelerated gluconeogenesis and glucose utilization. The most evident metabolic change is a shift from storage to utilization of protein, fat, and glycogen reserves. The degree of substrate mobilization is closely related to the extent and severity of the insult and mediated largely through the release of cytokines and counterregulatory hormones—tumor necrosis factor, interleukins 1 and 6, catecholamines (epinephrine and norepinephrine), glucagon, and cortisol (see Table 7-3). These hormones are "counterregulatory" to the effects of insulin, the primary hormone of anabolism. Although circulating levels of insulin tend to be high in patients in a stressed state, tissue responsiveness is severely blunted (especially in skeletal muscle) as a result of insulin resistance caused by the other hormones. Regardless of the nutritional support being used, only when the critical illness has subsided do the hormone levels return to normal.

Hypermetabolism

Hypermetabolism (increased energy expenditure) occurs in proportion to the severity and duration of the critical illness (Figure 21-1). Because it is a systemic response, even when an injury is localized to one area of the body, increased oxygen consumption occurs throughout the body, including in the skeletal muscle, splanchnic bed, and kidneys. The increase in metabolic rate is partly a result of the inefficiency with which glucose is utilized in the area of injury or infection. Glucose becomes the sole source of energy and is converted to lactate via anaerobic glycolysis under hypoxic conditions in the unstructured "front-line" of repair where blood perfusion is limited. Lactate is then returned to the liver where it is converted back to glucose and returned to the injured area (Cori cycle). Two moles of ATP are generated per mole of glucose degraded to lactic acid, whereas 4 moles of ATP are consumed per mole of lactic acid cycled back to regenerate glucose, resulting in a net loss of 2 moles of ATP per rotation of the Cori cycle. In effect, the localized area of injury or infection represents an energy drain on the rest of the body and hence contributes to the hypermetabolic state.

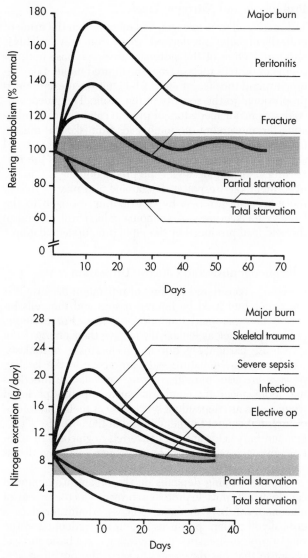

FIGURE 21-1 Changes in metabolic rate and nitrogen excretion with various types of physiologic stress. Normal ranges are indicated by shaded areas.[1]

Proteolysis and Nitrogen Loss

The increased urea nitrogen loss measured in the urine of critically ill patients is derived largely from muscle. This is also a reflection of the systemic stress response and not simply of protein release from the injured tissue. Like energy expenditure (see Figure 21-1), nitrogen excretion is proportional to the severity of the insult. The glucocorticoids are major mediators of protein catabolism, accelerating the movement of amino acids from skeletal muscle to the liver where they serve as sources of glucose and acute-phase proteins for host defense. Alanine is the major precursor of glucose for the production of ATP in the hypermetabolic response. Glutamine also plays a role in the glucogenic process by contributing nitrogen to the kidneys for synthesis of ammonia, which will neutralize the acid load produced by the rapid protein degradation.

Gluconeogenesis and Glucose Utilization

Glucose is considered the fuel of reparation because it is the major fuel used by injured tissues and the cells involved in repair and immune processes. For example, polymorphonuclear leukocytes receive their energy from glycolysis, particularly during phagocytosis; fibroblasts, which in their immature stage are active in the healing process, are also "pure glycolyzers;" and all cells functioning under anaerobic conditions such as poorly perfused wound sites are dependent on glucose as their sole source of fuel. Fat cannot be metabolized in the absence of oxygen and fatty acids are not converted to glucose. In addition, glycogen reserves are too small to provide significant amounts of glucose for tissue repair.

Hence, healing depends on the organism's ability to cannibalize its muscle protein to provide glucose by way of gluconeogenesis. Exogenous glucose administered to a critically ill patient produces little if any reduction in the rate of protein breakdown, suggesting it is a basic survival response that has developed to serve the organism at a time when food intake is not possible. By contrast, even small amounts of exogenous glucose markedly reduce protein catabolism in nonstressed, fasting individuals.

For example, under the influence of the counterregulatory hormones, hepatic glucose production increases from normal rates of about 200 g per day to approximately 400 g per day in patients with bacteremia. Hyperglycemia often results, and the high circulating concentrations of glucose can be preferentially provided to the reparative tissues. Because of insulin resistance, little glucose is utilized by resting skeletal muscle. Instead, fatty acids become the main fuel used by skeletal muscle and the liver and is therefore a major energy source, justifying its use in nutritional support of these patients.

NUTRITIONAL CONSEQUENCES OF INJURY AND INFECTION
Circulating Proteins

Physiologic stress results in both catabolism and decreased synthesis of proteins. Thus reduced circulating levels of proteins such as albumin and transferrin (or total iron binding capacity) are expected consequences of critical illnesses. Hypoproteinemia may complicate an illness and its treatment and has been associated with reduced wound healing, wound dehiscence, decubitus ulcer formation, reduced immune responsiveness, delayed gastric emptying, and reduced small intestinal mobility and absorption. Hypoproteinemia is not necessarily an indication of malnutrition but a reflection of the severity of the stress. As the stress subsides, it is only with adequate nutritional support that protein synthesis can return circulating levels to normal.

Body Composition

Without adequate nutritional support, profound weight loss and erosion of essential body compartments accompany critical illness. Loss of more than 10% to 20% of body weight that occurs rapidly in the setting of acute illness can seriously compromise physical performance and increase operative morbidity and mortality.

Weight loss in patients with physiologic stress cannot be justified by the assumption that it primarily reflects loss of body fat reserves. In fact, in the presence of stress, lean body mass is more likely to be the largest component lost. For example, without nutritional support a septic individual with a resting energy expenditure (REE) of 1.5 times normal and total nitrogen losses of 16 g per day is catabolizing about 0.4 kg of muscle tissue vs. only 0.3 kg of adipose tissue per day (see Chapter 7). Accompanying the loss of muscle are proportional losses of potassium, phosphorus, magnesium, and zinc.

NUTRITIONAL SUPPORT OF CRITICALLY ILL PATIENTS

The traditional belief that an injury is accompanied by about 6 weeks of catabolism, only after which nutritional repletion may take place, is no longer valid. With improved understanding and modern techniques of nutritional support, it is now possible to achieve energy and nitrogen balance throughout critical illness and by doing so improve survival and reduce the length and cost of hospital stay.[2,3]

Enteral vs. Parenteral Nutrition

The advantages of enteral over parenteral nutrition discussed in Chapter 9 are particularly relevant to the critically ill patient. Although not conclusively proven in humans, enteral feeding may maintain a healthier intestinal mucosa and thus prevent the translocation of intestinal bacteria and toxins and reduce the risk of multiple organ failure syndrome. Given its other proven benefits, every effort should be made to feed critically ill patients enterally.

Energy and Protein Requirements

Although the metabolic response to stress is essentially unaltered by nutritional support, nutrient supply can be increased to match losses. Thus weight loss in patients with trauma or sepsis is not obligatory. The energy requirements of most injured or septic patients are in the range of 1.2 to 1.5 times their calculated basal energy expenditure (BEE; see Chapter 9). Only in cases of extensive injury such as burns covering more than 40% of the body surface area do energy requirements rise above this range. Energy needs for burned patients can be estimated as shown in the box below.

ESTIMATING 24-HOUR ENERGY EXPENDITURE IN BURN PATIENTS (KCAL/DAY)

Toronto formula[4] (probably most accurate)

$$= -4343 + (10.5 \times \% \text{ TBSA}) + (0.23 \times \text{CI}) + (0.84 \times \text{BEE}) + (114 \times \text{Temp}) - (4.5 \times \text{PBD})$$

Modified Curreri formula (for TBSA ($\leq$ 40%; may overestimate requirements)

$$= (20 \text{ kcal} \times \text{Wt}) + (40 \times \% \text{ TBSA})$$

Traditional method (for TBSA > 40%; may overestimate requirements)

$$= \text{BEE} \times 2$$

where

TBSA = Percent total body surface area burned (*whole number*, not decimal), estimated on admission and corrected where needed for amputation

CI = Number of calories received in the previous 24 hours, including all dextrose, total parenteral nutrition (TPN), and tube feeding

Temp = Average of hourly rectal temperature (°C) in the previous 24 hours

PBD = Number of days postburn on the *previous* day

BEE = Basal energy expenditure estimated by the Harris-Benedict equations

Wt = Body weight in kilograms

Critically ill patients should not be given energy loads that exceed their needs. In fact, excess calories especially in the form of glucose may increase catecholamine production and metabolic rates even further. Humans cannot sustain energy expenditures above about 2.1 times the BEE. Therefore feeding patients above this level cannot be justified except to produce weight gain, and this should only be attempted after the acute stress has resolved.

Protein requirements are calculated using the 24-hour urinary urea nitrogen (UUN) excretion (see Chapter 8). Calorie intake must be adequate for protein needs to be met. Although carbohydrate calories do not effectively suppress nitrogen mobilization in the stress state, sufficient energy is necessary for ingested protein to be used to replace nitrogen losses rather than to meet energy needs.

For patients with burn injuries the UUN calculation can be modified as shown in the box below to account for protein lost directly through the skin.

ESTIMATING PROTEIN CATABOLIC RATE IN BURN PATIENTS (G/DAY)

$$= (UUN + 4 + [0.2 \text{ g} \times \% \ 3°] + [0.1 \text{ g} \times \% \ 2°]) \times 6.25$$

where

UUN = Measured urinary urea nitrogen in grams

% 3° = Percent body surface area with 3° (full-thickness) burns (*whole number*, not decimal)

% 2° = Percent body surface area with 2° (partial-thickness) burns (*whole number*, not decimal)

Example: for a patient with the following—
24-hr UUN of 13 g, 35% 3° burns, 15% 2° burns
$$= (13 + 4 + [0.2 \times 35] + [0.1 \times 15]) \times 6.25$$
$$= 159 \text{ protein catabolized}$$

As with other patients, to ensure positive nitrogen balance, the goal for protein intake should be about 10 g per day higher than protein loss. (In the previous example about 170 g per day would be provided.)

Micronutrient Requirements

Early in the course of stressful illnesses, serum levels of many micronutrients decrease significantly because they are either consumed, excreted, or sequestered in the liver and reticuloendothelial system.[5] Zinc is sequestered in the liver, zinc and vitamin A are excreted in the urine, and vitamin C is consumed at an accelerated rate. Because zinc and vitamins C and A figure importantly in immune competence and the healing of wounds, it is prudent to supplement them. A suggested empirical approach to micronutrient supplementation of critically ill patients is shown in the box below. Doses in the upper ends of the ranges are appropriate for patients with extensive injury such as burns, and lower doses may suffice for patients who are less stressed.

In general, avoid using iron supplementation in acutely ill patients. Their serum iron levels are often low,

---

MICRONUTRIENT SUPPLEMENTATION OF CRITICALLY ILL PATIENTS

Enteral approach

One multivitamin tablet containing vitamin A, 1 to 4 times daily

Ascorbic acid 500 to 2000 mg daily in divided doses

Zinc sulfate 220 mg 1 to 3 times daily

Parenteral approach

MVI-12 or the equivalent, 1 to 4 doses daily

Ascorbic acid 500 to 2000 mg daily in divided doses

Zinc as sulfate 5 to 10 mg daily

because the body sequesters iron in the reticuloendothelial system in response to stress (not because it is lost from the body). Therefore the serum iron level is an unreliable indicator of iron status in this setting (see Table 24-3). Because the iron binding capacity is frequently low in the stress state as well, treatment with iron can result in the circulation of unbound iron, making it more available for bacterial uptake and thus infection. Patients with anemia should be treated with transfusions during acute illness, and investigation of iron deficiencies should be postponed until after the stress resolves.

Specialized Nutritional Support

Much research has gone into developing nutritional formulas specially designed for critically ill patients. A number of intriguing findings from basic and clinical research have been explored to determine whether alterations in the intake of specific nutrients will provide benefits beyond those of basic macronutrient and micronutrient support. However, before specialized formulas are put into practice, clinical trials must demonstrate superior outcomes that justify their inevitably higher costs.

Because branched-chain amino acids are particularly catabolized by stressed patients and can be used as a fuel by muscle tissue, enteral and parenteral formulas enriched in these amino acids (different from those developed for hepatic encephalopathy; see Chapter 20) were marketed for these clinical situations. These formulas allowed earlier attainment of a positive nitrogen balance but did not lead to improved outcomes.

Glutamine is a conditionally essential amino acid that is mobilized in large quantities from skeletal muscle and lung when a patient has a critical illness. It is used directly as an energy source by enterocytes; contributes to ammoniagenesis (which counteracts acidosis); and supports lymphocyte and macrophage proliferation, hepatic gluconeogenesis and ureagenesis, and fibroblast function in healing wounds. A trial using glutamine-enriched parenteral nutrition showed improved nitrogen balance, a lower incidence of clinical infection, and shorter hospital stay in bone marrow transplant patients.[3] Additional trials are needed to confirm these effects. Although glutamine-enriched enteral formulas are commercially available, their efficacy is not yet clear.

Because small peptides are more rapidly absorbed by the gastrointestinal tract than whole proteins, and critically ill patients often have intestinal dysfunction including mucosal atrophy, a number of enteral formulas containing small peptides from hydrolyzed proteins have been promoted. Although efficient absorption has been well documented, clinical trials have not demonstrated improved outcomes such as faster nutritional recovery, shorter intensive care unit or hospital stays, or lower mortality rates.

Several nutrients and dietary substances have been reported to improve immune function and reduce infection rates in injured animals by stimulating lymphocyte proliferation, enhancing macrophage and killer-cell function, and other mechanisms, which almost directly led to the marketing of enteral formulas containing these nutrients. A clinical trial of one of these formulas, which contains arginine, nucleotides, and fish oil, demonstrated a reduction in length of hospital stay and frequency of acquired infections in critically ill patients as compared to patients using a standard formula.[2] However, because of their cost and lack of proven superiority in other patients, their use should be restricted to critically ill patients. It seems likely that other formulas with varying modifications will be developed in coming years; however, before committing to use these formulas, clinicians should require evidence of safety and efficacy from randomized, controlled clinical trials.

Monitoring the Patient

As with other patients, the main parameters to be tracked during the course of nutritional support are body weight, adequate nutrient delivery, nitrogen balance, and serum albumin level. Common sense dictates the frequency of measurement and interpretation of changes in body weight, but it is helpful to measure it at least 2 to 3 times weekly. Dietary records of energy and protein intake should be reviewed daily. The 24-hour UUN should be measured 1 to 2 times weekly to monitor nitrogen balance. Serum albumin and/or other circulating proteins should be monitored once or twice weekly. Although in stressed patients the albumin level falls acutely, roughly in proportion to the severity of the injury, its nadir is generally within 7 to 10 days of the initial insult. A gradual upward trend thereafter usually reflects adequate nutritional support. Failure to rise and/or periodic declines in the albumin level suggest persistent or intercurrent stress or inadequate nutritional support. Additional information is obtained from serial measurements of electrolytes, BUN, creatinine, phosphorus, magnesium, and anthropometrics.

References

1. Long CL et al: Metabolic response to injury and illness: Estimation of energy and protein needs from indirect calorimetry and nitrogen balance, *JPEN* 3:452, 1979.
2. Bower RH et al: Early enteral administration of a formula (Impact) supplemented with arginine, nucleotides, and fish oil in intensive care unit patients: results of a multicenter, prospective, randomized, clinical trial, *Crit Care Med* 23:436, 1995.
3. Ziegler TR et al: Clinical and metabolic efficacy of glutamine-supplemented parenteral nutrition after bone-marrow transplantation: a randomized, double-blind, controlled study, *Ann Intern Med* 116:821, 1992.
4. Allard JP et al: Validation of a new formula for calculating the energy requirements of burn patients, *JPEN* 14:115, 1990.
5. Louw JA et al: Blood vitamin concentrations during the acute-phase response, *Crit Care Med* 20:934, 1992.

Suggested Readings

Souba WW, Wilmore DW: Diet and nutrition in the care of the patient with surgery, trauma, and sepsis. In Shils ME, Olson JA, Shike M, eds: *Modern nutrition in health and disease,* ed 8, Philadelphia, 1994, Lea & Febiger.

Torosian MH, ed: *Nutrition for the hospitalized patient,* New York, 1995, Marcel Dekker.

22

Pulmonary Disease

Patients with acute and chronic respiratory failure are at high risk for developing malnutrition. Malnutrition is common among patients with chronic obstructive pulmonary disease (COPD), especially those with emphysema, who frequently have reduced weight-for-height and triceps skinfold measurements, midarm muscle circumferences, and creatinine/height indexes. Patients with COPD have increased work of breathing, which can increase caloric needs. The degree of weight loss generally correlates with the reduction in air flow as measured by spirometry. Thus, COPD can create a cycle in which respiratory dysfunction promotes weight loss, and weight loss further hinders respiratory function.

When patients with COPD are hospitalized for ventilatory failure, the clinical outcome is affected by nutritional support. Among a number of ways discussed below, it is notable that studies have demonstrated patients who receive adequate nutritional support are more readily weaned from mechanical ventilators than those whose diets are deficient in protein and energy.

NUTRITIONAL EFFECTS ON THE RESPIRATORY SYSTEM

Nutrition impacts patients with pulmonary disease at several levels. Nutritional status affects all components of the respiratory system, including central hypoxic and hypercapnic drives, respiratory muscles, and lung tissues (parenchyma) themselves. The amount and composition of energy intake affect the metabolic rate, O_2 consumption, and CO_2 production. Hypophosphatemia can have a profound effect on ventilation. Nutritional status is also important to the integrity of the immune system.

Ventilatory Drive

Ventilatory drive (the body's increase in minute ventilation in response to hypoxia or hypercapnia) is closely associated with metabolic rate. When the metabolic rate increases, as it does during exercise, tissue oxygen levels drop (hypoxia), producing a compensatory increase in ventilation. However, in patients that are underfed (e.g., receiving only 5% dextrose infusions), the ventilatory response to hypoxia is depressed, impairing their ability to maintain adequate ventilation. Fortunately, these changes tend to normalize with refeeding and are prevented if semistarvation is initially avoided. Therefore underfeeding a patient with pulmonary disease is detrimental to the respiratory drive.

Respiratory Function

As body weight is lost, there is a proportional reduction in the weight and strength of the diaphragm and function of respiratory muscles. In patients with emphysema, the hyperinflated lungs alter the fiber length of the respiratory muscles and impair their efficiency. Decreased respiratory muscle strength is evidenced by reduced maximal inspiratory and expiratory pressures, vital capacity, and maximal voluntary ventilation. Respiratory muscle fatigue can occur when the demand for energy surpasses its supply (e.g., during semistarvation). Undernutrition also affects the pulmonary parenchyma by diminishing collagen synthesis and increasing proteolysis. This may be manifest as decreased surfactant production and alveolar collapse.

Metabolism, O_2 Consumption, and CO_2 Production

One of the hallmarks of respiratory insufficiency is abnormal gas exchange, with resultant hypoxemia and/or hypercapnia. Patients with pulmonary failure often have limited abilities to expire CO_2, and therefore it is retained. Because the total energy intake and composition of the feedings affect the body's CO_2 production and O_2 consumption, nutrient intake can be altered to influence metabolism and gas exchange favorably.

Energy Intake

Giving excess energy, particularly as carbohydrate, to acutely ill patients with respiratory insufficiency can increase the metabolic rate, and thus O_2 consumption and CO_2 production. The synthesis of fat from excessive carbohydrate calories is also associated with production of a large amount CO_2. In patients with limited pulmonary reserves, this may precipitate respiratory failure from CO_2 retention. It is important to remember that hypermetabolic, stressed patients respond differently to excessive calories than semistarved patients or normal persons (see Chapter 9).

Carbohydrate/Fat Mix

The oxidation of carbohydrate, fat, and protein to yield energy requires O_2 and produces CO_2 and H_2O, in proportions unique to each substrate. The ratio of moles of CO_2 produced to moles of O_2 consumed—the respiratory quotient (RQ)—is 1 for carbohydrates, 0.7 for fat, and approximately 0.8 for protein. The synthesis of fat from carbohydrate yields an RQ of greater than 1. Thus the oxidation of carbohydrate generates more CO_2 per unit of energy produced than does fat or protein, and overfeeding can dramatically increase CO_2 production through a combination of increased conversion of carbohydrate to fat and increased metabolic rate (and in turn, CO_2 production). Therefore if the predominant nonprotein energy source in the diet is carbohydrate, the amount of CO_2 that must be expired is greater than if the source is fat. Reducing CO_2 production by substituting fat for carbohydrate may prevent the need for mechanical ventilation and facilitate weaning from the ventilator. Conversely, relying on carbohydrate can worsen respiratory failure or make ventilator weaning more difficult. Of the two effects, overfeeding has a greater impact on CO_2 production than does the carbohydrate and fat mix, and therefore it is important not to exceed a patient's estimated energy requirements during the weaning process.

Reports in the 1970s indicated that rapid infusions of intravenous lipid emulsions could impair pulmonary O_2 diffusion, which created some concern over the use of lipid emulsions in patients with hypoxemic lung disease. However, this has not proved to be of clinical significance as long as the lipid is infused in 12 to 24 hours and not more rapidly.

Some lipids should be provided in all cases, because the prostaglandins and leukotrienes formed from essential fatty acid metabolism affect the bronchial and vascular smooth muscle tissues and immune response. For example, prostaglandins E_2 and E_3 and prostacyclin are antiinflammatory and bronchodilatory agents. Thus, provision of lipids as a source of essential fatty acids—enterally or parenterally—is a fundamental part of nutritional support of all patients, and especially those with respiratory compromise.

Hypophosphatemia

Hypophosphatemia has a particularly deleterious effect on respiratory muscle function, by impairing its diaphragmatic contractility. Hypophosphatemia with decreased 2,3-diphosphoglycerate in red blood cells and diminished levels of ATP may complicate acute respiratory failure by impairing tissue oxygen delivery and respiratory muscle function, respectively. Therefore hypophosphatemia should be prevented and when present treated vigorously (see Chapter 9).

Immune Function

Because respiratory failure is often complicated by pneumonia and sepsis, impairment of the immune system from malnutrition adversely affects recovery. Epidemiologic studies have found a strong link between malnutrition and pneumonia. Malnutrition is associated with decreased cell-mediated immunity, altered immunoglobulin production, and impaired resistance of the tracheobronchial mucosa to bacterial infections (see Chapter 27).

NUTRITIONAL SUPPORT IN PULMONARY DISEASE

Guidelines for nutritional support in patients with pulmonary disease are summarized in the box. An initial nutritional evaluation of the patient with respiratory failure is important. Malnutrition should be diagnosed and appropriate plans made for refeeding.

Optimization of total energy intake is the cardinal principle in therapy; both overfeeding and underfeeding should be avoided. Generally, giving 1.2 to 1.5 times resting energy expenditure (REE) is adequate; cachectic patients with pulmonary disease should be refed with particular care. When there is a question about energy requirements or the effect of nutritional support on gas exchange, indirect calorimetry is indicated (see Chapter 9). The data

---

NUTRITIONAL SUPPORT OF PATIENTS WITH PULMONARY DISEASE

Perform a complete nutritional assessment.

Evaluate energy needs and provide an appropriate amount. (Do not overfeed or underfeed).

Ensure protein balance.

Monitor fluids and electrolytes, especially phosphorus.

Evaluate vitamin and mineral status as indicated.

Consider high-fat, low-carbohydrate feedings in patients with hypercapnia.

generated from indirect calorimetry indicate the REE as well as the RQ, and can be used to tailor nutritional support. Reduction of energy intake to a level equal to or below the REE may facilitate weaning but should be avoided in catabolic patients and never prolonged. If weight gain is desired and the patient is stable and ambulatory, intake may be increased to 2 times the REE, as long as it does not impair respiratory function.

In patients who are not hypercapnic, calories may be distributed conventionally; 50% to 60% as carbohydrate, 20% to 30% as fat, and 15% to 20% as protein. For patients with hypercapnia (whether ambulatory or ventilator-dependent), giving 25% to 30% of calories as carbohydrate and 50% to 55% of calories as fat may be beneficial. This should be individualized to determine the lowest percentage of fat that maintains an acceptable pCO_2 level. However, it is noteworthy that providing an appropriate amount of energy is generally more important than fine-tuning the ratio of dietary fat and carbohydrate.

Suggested Readings

DeMeo MT et al: Nutrition in acute pulmonary disease, *Nutr Rev* 50:320, 1992.

McMahon MM, Farnell MB, Murrary MJ: Nutritional support of critically ill patients, *Mayo Clin Proc* 68:911, 1993.

Pingleton SK, Harmon GS: Nutritional management in acute respiratory failure, *JAMA* 257:3094, 1987.

Rothkopf MM et al: Nutritional support in respiratory failure, *Nutr Clin Pract* 4:166, 1989.

Talpers SS et al: Nutritionally associated increased carbon dioxide production. Excess total calories vs high proportion of carbohydrate calories, *Chest* 102:551, 1992.

23

Renal Failure

The kidneys play a crucial role in maintaining the body's physiologic milieu by excreting, secreting, synthesizing, regulating, and degrading metabolic substances and participating in erythropoiesis (formation of blood) and the metabolism of hormones. When these functions deteriorate as a result of renal failure, various metabolic abnormalities occur that impinge on nutritional status, including the following:

- Impaired clearance of urea and other nitrogenous products of protein metabolism
- Impaired regulation of sodium, potassium, phosphorus, calcium, magnesium, water, and hydrogen ions
- Impaired vitamin D metabolism
- Anorexia and loss of body mass

The severity of these changes reflects the type and duration of renal failure (acute or chronic) and the degree of catabolic stress the patient experiences. The role of nutritional support in renal failure is to prevent or reverse associated malnourished states, minimize the adverse effects of substances that are inadequately excreted, and favorably affect the progression and outcome of renal failure.

CHRONIC RENAL FAILURE

Chronic renal failure is caused by a variety of prolonged renal insults such as diabetes mellitus, hypertension, and primary renal diseases such as glomerulonephritis. The broad spectrum of abnormalities in chronic renal failure correlates with the number of functioning nephrons. More than 50% of normal renal function must be lost before the serum creatinine level begins to rise and nutritional interventions are needed. However, because cardiovascular events are the primary cause of mortality in end-stage renal disease patients, efforts to maintain optimal serum lipid levels are indicated as early as possible.

Patients with 20% to 50% of normal renal function (pre–end-stage renal disease) usually have serum creatinine levels between 2 and 5 mg/dl, mild anemia, and mild retention of sodium, potassium, magnesium, phosphorus, and water. For these patients, nutritional regulation is paramount. Progressive chronic renal failure produces anorexia and increased protein catabolism, resulting in wasting of lean body mass, reduced growth rates in children, and diminished synthesis of proteins including albumin. By careful dietary management it may be possible to stabilize the progression of chronic renal failure and avoid or postpone dialysis.

In patients with end-stage renal disease who have less than 10% of normal renal function (serum creatinine greater than about 7 mg/dl), nutritional regulation is not usually sufficient to control uremic symptoms, and dialysis is often required. Nutritional management is still important after dialysis has begun, but the restrictions are less rigorous. With an incidence of 18 per 100,000 Americans and an estimated total annual cost of more than $40,000 per patient, end-stage renal disease is a major consumer of U.S. health care dollars.

ACUTE RENAL FAILURE

Patients with acute renal failure have an abrupt and marked decrease in renal glomerular filtration rate caused by a variety of insults to the kidney such as infection, trauma, dehydration, shock, and exposure to exogenous nephrotoxins such as drugs. Urine output may be normal (nonoliguric), reduced (oliguric), or absent (anuric). The fluid and electrolyte balances become rapidly deranged through defective renal regulation. A patient with acute renal failure is often highly catabolic because of the underlying disease process.

Using dialysis, the fluid and electrolyte abnormalities of acute renal failure can be regulated and uremic symptoms reduced. However, the ravages of catabolism including poor wound healing, the risk of infections, and increased mortality cannot be prevented by dialysis alone. Nutritional support must be used to maintain nutritional status until the acute renal failure improves. In a sense, dialysis relieves renal excretory insufficiency so that nutritional support can be administered.

NUTRITIONAL ASSESSMENT IN RENAL DISEASE

In chronic renal failure it is particularly important to monitor nutritional status. In pre–end-stage renal disease, simple assessments such as weight and triceps skinfold on a regular basis are sufficient to detect significant changes in body composition. Assessment of the nutritional status in patients with end-stage renal disease as well as those on dialysis is commonly biased by deteriorated social conditions (unreliable sources of diet history) and variability in hydration status, which demands special caution in interpreting anthropometric and biochemical parameters. Therefore a combination of different methods must be used to monitor nutritional status. The box lists criteria for detecting risk for malnutrition and need for aggressive nutritional support in patients with renal failure.

In end-stage renal disease it has been well established that serum albumin levels below 3.5 g/dl are associated with increased mortality.[1] Therefore it is reasonable to give greater weight to albumin when using the previously mentioned criteria. Dietary records or recall are the only practical techniques for estimating energy intake in outpatients. However, it should be noted that these methods may underestimate or overestimate by considerable amounts.

CRITERIA FOR PRESENCE OF MALNUTRITION IN PATIENTS WITH CHRONIC RENAL FAILURE

10% or greater decrease in dry body weight° in less than 1 year or a weight of 85% or less of ideal (see Table 15-2)

15% or greater decrease in anthropometry (e.g., triceps skinfold thickness or midarm muscle circumference) in less than 1 year

Serum albumin level less than 3.5 g/dl

Total lymphocyte count of less than 1500/mm^3

Plasma transferrin level of less than 150 mg/dl

Energy intake of less than 35 kcal/kg ideal body weight

°The weight at which a patient is neither hypertensive nor hypotensive compared to usual blood pressure.

NUTRITIONAL SUPPORT IN RENAL FAILURE

For concise information on therapeutic diets for renal disease, see the tables in Chapter 11.

Energy Requirements

The general principles of nutritional support discussed in Chapter 9 apply to patients with renal failure. Although most patients with renal insufficiency require about 25 to 40 kcal/kg of their ideal body weight or 1.2 to 1.5 times the calculated basal energy expenditure, these guidelines must be applied with caution, because physical activity varies substantially among individuals. Maintaining sufficient energy intake to avoid weight loss can be difficult when other nutrients are restricted. For this reason and because vigilance is required to sustain good dietary habits, the help of a dietitian is invaluable in the management of patients with renal failure. Because environmental factors such as poverty and disability commonly interfere with food availability, an interdisciplinary approach is highly recommended.

Protein Requirements

Under normal conditions the renal glomeruli filter amino acids and up to 30 g of intact protein each day, virtually all of which is reabsorbed in the proximal tubules. Renal disease often increases the glomerular permeability to proteins and/or decreases tubular reabsorption, resulting in proteinuria. Urea is also filtered and only about half is reabsorbed; the excretion of the remaining urea is one of the most important functions of the kidneys. As the glomerular filtration rate (GFR) decreases, urea is not adequately filtered and the blood urea nitrogen (BUN) level rises. The term *uremia* refers to the constellation of signs and symptoms associated with chronic renal failure, regardless of cause or of BUN level.

The common practice of restricting protein intake in patients with chronic renal failure to about 0.6 g/kg per day to control uremic symptoms or delay the onset of end-stage renal disease was shown in a multicenter trial to provide only small benefit,[2] so slightly more generous guidelines can be recommended (Table 23-1). However, because the American's average protein intake is around 100 g per day or 1.5 g/kg per day, which is much higher than recommended, some dietary adjustments are almost always needed; changes in diet are also required for treating the most common underlying causes of chronic renal failure, diabetes and hypertension (see Chapters 16 and 17).

In chronic renal failure patients who are not on dialysis, very low-protein diets (0.28 g/kg per day) in combination with essential amino acid or ketoacid supplementation have been shown to reduce uremic symptoms and stabilize BUN levels while maintaining nitrogen balance. The limited protein intake may enhance nitrogen recycling from ammonia by urea-splitting bacteria in the gut. However, no delay in the development of end-stage renal disease or death has been demonstrated with this approach.[2] In patients with acute renal failure, limitation of nonessential amino acids cannot be assumed to be beneficial either, because they are required for the synthesis of acute-phase proteins and the repair of the kidneys themselves. Many patients with acute renal failure are treated

TABLE 23-1 Recommended intake of protein and phosphorus according to severity of chronic renal failure[1,3]

Stage		Glomerular filtration rate (ml/min)	Recommended protein intake (g/kg IBW/day)*	Recommended phosphorus (mg/kg IBW/day)
Pre-ESRD	—	>60	No restriction	No restriction
	—	25-60	0.6-0.8	8-12
	—	10-25	0.6	5-10
	Diabetes	10-60	≥ 0.8	8-12
	Nephrotic syndrome	10-60	0.8-1	8-12
ESRD	Hemodialysis	—	1.1-1.4	<17
	Peritoneal dialysis	No peritonitis	1.2-1.5	<17
		Peritonitis	1.5-2	No restriction
Post-transplant	First month	—	1.3-2	Varies†
	Subsequent months	—	1	17-20

*IBW, Ideal body weight; ERSD, end-stage renal disease.
† Urinary calcium and phosphorus may be high in the first weeks after transplantation.

with antibiotics that destroy the colonic urea-splitting bacteria necessary for hypothetical nitrogen recycling. In addition, randomized trials using these formulas have not shown that they can improve the resolution of acute renal failure or survival rates in patients with acute renal failure.

Therefore a balanced mixture of essential and nonessential amino acids is recommended for treatment of both chronic renal failure and acute renal failure. When enteral or parenteral feeding is used, a formula that will meet the patient's energy and protein needs should be chosen. The objective is for the patient to take only as much protein as necessary to meet protein requirements. Because a patient with a larger-than-average body mass or physiologic stress or who is receiving steroid treatment (e.g., after renal transplantation) may require more protein than other patients, each patient's needs should be documented and tracked using measurements of 24-hour urine urea nitrogen (UUN) to determine the actual protein requirement (see Chapter 8). In patients whose urine output is minimal or absent and/or whose BUN levels are changing, the 24-hour UUN is unreliable. Calculation of urea nitrogen appearance (UNA), including measurement of UUN in any urine produced, provides a suitable estimate of individual protein needs (see Chapter 8 or Appendix B). UNA is best calculated using the changes in BUN and body water during one- to three-day periods between dialyses. If the patient is dialyzed during the collection period, the dialysate urea nitrogen must be measured, adjusted to grams per day, and added to the UUN.

It is often assumed that in stressed patients with renal disease dietary protein intake should not be increased to meet protein requirements calculated by UUN or UNA; there is a fear that doing so will increase ureagenesis, tax the kidneys further by increasing the renal urea load, and raise the BUN level. However, if protein intake only matches and does not exceed protein requirements, it does not increase ureagenesis. On the contrary, a negative nitrogen balance is as deleterious to patients with renal impairment as it is to others and should be avoided.

Replacement of protein lost in the urine of a patient with a nephrotic syndrome does not correct disordered plasma or tissue protein pools; protein supplementation increases glomerular permeability, exacerbating urinary albumin losses. Therefore protein requirements in these patients should be estimated as they are in other patients with renal disease—without adjusting for their protein-uria.

Lipids

Hypertriglyceridemia is quite common in patients with chronic renal failure primarily because of defective catab-olism of lipoproteins. In the nephrotic syndrome other factors contribute to increased triglyceride-rich, very low-density lipoprotein (VLDL) levels. Aggressively lowering triglycerides has not been shown to lower morbidity or mortality, but a Step I lipid-lowering diet (see Table 11-1 and Chapter 18) is recommended for use with nonuremic patients to prevent coronary artery disease, the leading cause of death in patients with end-stage renal disease.

Because hypertriglyceridemia may impair a patient's tolerance of intravenous lipid emulsions, triglyceride lev-els should be monitored in chronic renal failure patients treated with parenteral nutrition. Fat emulsions do not need to be restricted unless serum triglyceride levels con-sistently exceed 350 mg/dl.

Fluids and Electrolytes
Sodium and Water

Normally, sodium and water are filtered by the renal glomerulus and reabsorbed by the tubules and/or col-lecting ducts (sodium actively and water passively). When the GFR is reduced in patients with either chronic or acute renal failure, filtration is impaired and reabsorption is fixed and therefore unable to adapt to changes in sodium intake. The resulting retention of sodium and wa-ter may produce edema, hypertension, and congestive heart failure. In this instance, restriction of sodium and water intake is appropriate depending on the level of renal failure and urine volume. A suitable starting point is 1 to 3 g per day of sodium and a fluid intake 500 ml greater than the urine output to account for insensible water losses. Adjustments can be made according to body weight and serum sodium levels to eliminate edema and normalize blood pressure and serum sodium levels. In patients with the nephrotic syndrome, sodium restriction is always indicated.

In contrast, when the primary defect is in the renal tubule, ineffective reabsorption of sodium and water sometimes results in dehydration, hypotension, and further reduction in the GFR. Restriction of sodium and water is inappropriate in this circumstance, and their judicious addition may be required.

Potassium

Like sodium, potassium is filtered by the renal glomeruli and reabsorbed mainly in the proximal tubules. It is then actively secreted into the late distal tubules and collecting ducts for excretion. Renal tubular damage from acute renal failure or chronic renal failure often impairs potassium filtration. This can lead to hyperkalemia, which can result in fatal arrhythmias. Potassium should be restricted to about 60 mEq per day when this occurs. Hyperkalemia is especially likely if acidosis, oliguria, or catabolism is present.

Phosphorus and Calcium

When renal glomerular filtration of phosphorus is hampered in chronic renal failure, the serum level rises, leading to depression of serum calcium. This stimulates parathyroid hormone, which restores homeostasis by obtaining more calcium from bone, intestines, and kidneys and increasing renal phosphorus clearance. This can lead eventually to hyperparathyroidism and progressive loss of bone (renal osteodystrophy). Hyperphosphatemia and hyperparathyroidism may not only cause morbidity, they may themselves inflict further renal damage.

Therefore patients should be instructed as soon as possible about dietary phosphate restriction (see Table 23-1) and use of phosphate-binding antacids to keep the serum phosphorus level as low as possible, even prior to its first elevation. Calcium carbonate is the preferred antacid because although aluminum hydroxide antacids bind phosphorus more strongly, aluminum accumulation in the brain and bone can lead to dementia and osteomalacia. In addition, calcium carbonate (which is best given between meals) provides needed supplemental calcium and corrects mild acidosis.

Magnesium

Magnesium is also normally excreted by the kidney, but it is often retained in patients with both acute and chronic renal failure. Dietary restriction of the other nutrients discussed usually reduces magnesium intake sufficiently. Magnesium-containing antacids, enemas, or laxatives should be avoided because they can result in dangerously high magnesium levels.

pH

Metabolic acidosis is often present in patients who are not on dialysis with acute and chronic renal failure because of retention of metabolic acids and/or renal loss of bicarbonate. It can produce profound malaise, promote muscle proteolysis, and increase bone dissolution and should therefore be rigorously treated. Calcium carbonate is useful for treating mild acidosis, but sodium bicarbonate is necessary when acidosis is severe. Dialysis is indicated if these measures are ineffective in controlling acidosis. When total parenteral nutrition (TPN) is used, using acetate as the anion to accompany sodium and/or potassium helps to ameliorate acidosis.

Vitamins

Water-soluble vitamin deficiencies are common in patients with chronic renal failure because of poor oral intake, decreased renal reabsorption (e.g., of vitamin B_6), and losses from dialysis. Patients with chronic renal failure, whether or not they are treated with dialysis, should receive supplements that at least provide the Recommended Daily Allowance (RDA) of all water-soluble vitamins and folic acid (0.8 to 1 mg) and vitamin B_6 (5 mg in patients not receiving dialysis treatments and 10 mg in those receiving dialysis treatments).

Because a diseased kidney cannot adequately remove retinol binding protein from circulation, hypervitaminosis A may occur in patients with chronic renal failure; therefore, vitamin A supplements should be avoided. Functional vitamin D deficiency can occur in chronic renal failure patients because the renal hydroxylation of 25-hydroxycholecalciferol (calcifediol) to the metabolically active 1,25-dihydroxycholecalciferol (calcitriol) is impaired. This results in reduced intestinal calcium absorption and exacerbates the derangement in bone metabolism and the hypocalcemia caused by phosphorus retention. Vitamin D deficiency can be prevented by supplementing the patient with calcitriol (Rocaltrol), starting with a dose of 0.25 to 0.50 µg/day. It is uncertain just when vitamin D supplementation should begin, but a slight excess of vitamin D probably does not affect renal function or bone turnover. However, calcitriol can cause hypercalcemia and hyperphosphatemia, so serum calcium and phosphorus levels must be closely monitored.

Trace Elements

Iron deficiency is common in chronic renal failure patients because of both poor oral intake and intestinal absorption of iron and increased blood loss from occult gastrointestinal bleeding, phlebotomy for laboratory tests, and hemodialysis. The hematologic and iron statuses of chronic renal failure patients should be monitored, and supplementation with 325 mg of ferrous sulfate up to 3 times daily used if needed. Although some studies indicate that the use of zinc sulfate in doses of about 220 mg daily may improve taste acuity, appetite, and sexual dysfunction, it has not been firmly established that patients with renal failure should be routinely supplemented with zinc.

References

1. Owen WF et al: The urea reduction ratio and serum albumin concentration as predictors of mortality in patients undergoing hemodialysis, *N Engl J Med* 329:1001, 1993.
2. Klahr S et al: The effects of dietary protein restriction and blood-pressure control on the progression of chronic renal disease, *N Engl J Med* 330:877, 1994.
3. American Dietetic Association—renal Dietitians Dietetic Practice Group: *National renal guide: professional guide,* 1993, The Association.

Suggested Readings

Kopple JD: *Nutrition, diet, and the kidney.* In Shils ME, Olson JA, Shike M, eds: *Modern nutrition in health and disease,* ed 8, Philadelphia, 1994, Lea & Febiger.

Mitch WE, Klahr S: *Nutrition and the kidney,* ed 2, Little, Brown, 1993.

Shuler CL, Wolfson M: *Nutrition in acute renal failure.* In Rombeau JL, Caldwell MD, eds: *Clinical nutrition: enteral and tube feeding,* ed 2, Philadelphia, 1990, WB Saunders.

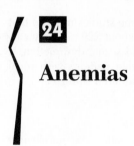

24

Anemias

DEFINITION

Anemia is a deficit of circulating red blood cells (RBCs) associated with diminished oxygen-carrying capacity of the blood. Anemia is diagnosed when the hemoglobin concentration is less than 12 g/dl in adult females or 14 g/dl in adult males or the hematocrit is less than 36% in females or 42% in males.

Signs and Symptoms

Anemia is a multisystem disorder with symptoms that often depend less on the severity of the anemia than on the pace of its development. Thus symptoms are more likely to occur when anemia is caused by acute gastrointestinal bleeding than by long-term occult blood loss from aspirin use. Symptoms of severe anemia include being easily fatigued and poor exercise tolerance. In patients with iron deficiencies, exercise tolerance is further impaired by lack of iron for myoglobin synthesis and the functioning of energy-releasing, heme-containing enzymes in mitochondria. Resting tachycardia with a pulse rate of greater than 100 beats/min reflects the body's attempt to compensate for the diminished oxygen-carrying capacity in the blood. Other symptoms may include palpitations, dizziness, syncope (loss of consciousness), or amenorrhea. Pallor of the mucous membranes (conjunctiva, buccal cavity, tongue) and skin may provide a clue to the presence of anemia but unfortunately does not correlate closely with the hematocrit. Other signs of anemia include a wide pulse pressure, systolic ejection murmurs, and a cardiac venous hum.

Nutritional anemias are often accompanied by deficiencies of other vitamins and minerals. Because vitamin C and folic acid coexist in many foods, patients with folate-deficiency anemia may also have scurvy. In addition, anemia is not usually an isolated finding; a nutritional deficiency that limits RBC production usually affects other cells with high turnover rates, such as leukocytes, platelets, and enterocytes. Most cases of megaloblastic anemia are accompanied by reddening and soreness of the tongue, loss of lingual papillae (slick tongue), and megaloblastic changes in the intestinal tract.

Etiologies

The major hematopoietic nutrients are iron, vitamin B_{12}, and folic acid. Because of the particular hematopoiesis steps in which these nutrients function, the causes of nutritional anemias are suggested by the morphologic appearance of cells in peripheral blood or bone marrow smears. The mean corpuscular volume (MCV) provides the first clue to the etiology of anemias (Table 24-1). Anemias are classified as microcytic (small-cell) when the MCV is less than 80 μ^3, in which case the major nutritional cause is iron deficiency. Normocytic anemias (with an MCV of 80 to 100 μ^3) are common in patients with protein-energy malnutrition (PEM), and macrocytic anemias (with an MCV of greater than 100 μ^3) can be caused by vitamin B_{12} or folic acid deficiencies. Microcytic and macrocytic cells can coexist; for example, a patient can have both iron and folate deficiencies. In these cases, the MCV may be deceptively normal and suggest a normocytic anemia, but the blood smear shows a dimorphic population of RBCs. The diagnosis of a nutritional anemia is confirmed by measuring the blood level of the suspected nutrient and sometimes by examination of the bone marrow. Final proof of the diagnosis is provided by a therapeutic response to replacement of the deficient nutrient. Table 24-

TABLE 24-1	Differential diagnosis of nutritional anemias by RBC MCV	
Category (MCV)	Nutritional causes	Other causes
Microcytic ($<80\ \mu^3$)°	Iron deficiency (common), pyridoxine deficiency (uncommon), copper deficiency (uncommon)	Chronic disease, thalassemias, hemoglobin E disorders, sideroblastic anemia (lead toxicity)
Normocytic ($80\text{-}100\ \mu^3$)°	Protein-energy malnutrition	Chronic diseases
Macrocytic ($>100\ \mu^3$)°	Folic acid deficiency (common), Vitamin B_{12} deficiency (common)	Alcoholism, liver disease, hemolysis

° Normal values for MCV vary among hospitals; these values are representative.

1 also lists nonnutritional conditions that can cause anemias of each morphologic type.

Anemias are caused by three basic mechanisms: (1) diminished erythropoiesis (RBC production), usually caused by nutritional deficiencies or bone marrow failure, (2) blood loss, and (3) increased hemolysis (RBC destruction), either hereditary or acquired. Thus anemia is a manifestation of not only nutritional deficiencies, but many different conditions. An anemia is considered nutritional in origin when one or more nutrients essential to RBC formation is deficient. Such deficiencies may occur with normal dietary intake if there are increased requirements (e.g., as a result of hemolytic disease or alcoholism) or external losses (e.g., chronic gastrointestinal blood loss or pregnancy). The major mechanisms by which an individual becomes nutrient deficient include inadequate ingestion, malabsorption, impaired utilization, elevated requirements, increased excretion, or increased destruction.

Diagnostic Steps

The investigation of anemia involves obtaining a thorough patient history and physical examination. It is important to discover whether the patient has a history of drug exposure, because many medications interfere with nutrient metabolism (see Chapter 14 and the related discussion at the end of this chapter). Laboratory data including complete and differential blood cell counts and examination of the blood smear are mandatory. In addition, a count of reticulocytes (immature cells recently released from the bone marrow) is also helpful information. A variety of other tests (see following discussion) such as those providing vitamin and mineral levels can provide important evidence about etiology. A bone marrow aspirate and/or biopsy is often necessary to make a definitive diagnosis.

MICROCYTIC ANEMIAS

Microcytic anemias are characterized by small cells and an MCV of less than 80 μ^3. Although the major nutritional cause is iron deficiency, other conditions including pyridoxine and copper deficiencies may also cause microcytic anemias (see Table 24-1).

Iron Deficiency

Iron deficiency anemia can result from inadequate intake, inadequate absorption, or excessive losses (bleeding); the latter are most often the cause in the United States. Iron deficiency anemia is the most common nutritional anemia and perhaps the most common nutritional deficiency in the world.

Pathophysiology

Iron is present in the body in functional and storage forms. In its functional form, iron is incorporated into heme and myoglobin and is part of enzymes such as cytochrome oxidase, peroxidase, and catalase. Its storage form is ferritin and hemosiderin.

Dietary iron is composed of heme iron, which is mainly from meat, and nonheme iron, which is principally from vegetables and cooking vessels. It is largely absorbed in the upper small intestine, especially the duodenum. Heme iron is about 20% bioavailable, whereas nonheme iron is only 3% bioavailable. Net absorption of the two forms combined is about 10%. The absorption of *nonheme* iron can be enhanced up to threefold by the simultaneous ingestion of high-quality protein and 25 to 75 mg of vitamin C. The vitamin C aids in the conversion of ferric (Fe^{3+}) iron to the more readily absorbed ferrous (Fe^{2+}) form. Absorption of *heme* iron is unchanged by these factors. When necessary, (e.g., in pregnancy, after blood loss, or in anemic states), mucosal cells of the upper small intestine can respond to the body's need for more iron by increasing absorption. However, it is not always possible to meet these requirements through diet alone. Therefore daily supplementation with 30 to 60 mg of iron during pregnancy is recommended (see Chapter 3).

Each day in normal adults, about 1% of the red blood cell mass is destroyed, releasing approximately 30 mg of iron into the reticuloendothelial system and circulation. Of the 30 mg released, about 29 mg is salvaged and utilized for the synthesis of new hemoglobin and only 1 mg must be replaced. In adult males, nutritional equilibrium is maintained by the absorption of about 1 mg per day from a diet containing the Recommended Dietary Allowance (RDA) of 10 mg iron. Premenopausal women need an additional 0.5 mg per day to compensate for menstrual losses or a total of 1.5 mg per day to maintain equilibrium; therefore the RDA for adult women is 15 mg per day. The RDA of iron is 30 mg during pregnancy and returns to 15 mg during lactation.

The greatest risk for iron deficiency occurs during the following four stages of the life cycle: (1) between 6 months and 4 years of age, (2) in early adolescence, (3) during menstruating years, (4) and during pregnancy.

When an iron deficiency occurs during growth and development, it usually results from inadequate iron intake rather than increased losses. In adults who are not pregnant, blood loss is most often the cause of iron deficiencies, so it is crucial to find the source of and stop the blood loss as well as to replace the iron deficit. In addition to alcohol abuse, large doses of aspirin or other nonsteroidal antiinflammatory drugs frequently cause gastrointestinal blood loss. Blood loss in premenopausal women is usually from menstruation, so if the patient's history and physical examination provide no other information about the source of the loss, it is justifiable to recommend a 30-day therapeutic trial of oral iron supplementation without searching for additional sources. However, this method of treatment is almost never justified in males, in whom iron deficiency is most often caused by chronic, occult blood loss from the gastrointestinal tract. Multiple stool specimens should be tested for occult blood, and complete examination of the gastrointestinal tract with x-rays and/or endoscopy is often indicated. In hospitalized patients, repeated blood sampling for laboratory tests may lead to significant iron losses. One unit of donated blood (450 ml) contains about 225 mg of iron that may require 2 to 4 months to replace. There are increased numbers of cases of iron deficiencies among populations in which pica is practiced (ingestion of clay, laundry starch, ice, etc.).

Diagnosis

In addition to physical findings generally associated with anemia, other physical manifestations that may occur in patients with iron deficiencies include glossitis and (infrequently) koilonychia (spooning of the nails). Esophageal webs may form (Plummer-Vinson syndrome) in patients with severe, prolonged deficiencies.

Table 24-2 presents the characteristic laboratory findings in patients with nutritional anemias. Iron deficiencies occur in stages: first, the bone marrow iron is depleted; next, the serum iron level drops and the total iron-binding capacity increases; finally, there are low MCV and hemo-

TABLE 24-2 Morphologic findings and laboratory values in nutritional anemias[1]

Deficiency	None	Iron	Folic acid	Vitamin B_{12}
RBC morphology	Normocytic	Hypochromic, microcytic	Macrocytic	Macrocytic
MCV (μ^3)	80–100	<80	>100	>100
MCHC* (%)	32–36	<32	>32	>32
Hypersegmented neutrophils	Absent	Absent	Present	Present
Bone marrow morphology	Normal	Normoblastic	Megaloblastic	Megaloblastic
Bone marrow iron	Normal	Absent	Normal/high	Normal/high
Serum iron (μg/dl)	42–135	<42	Normal/high	Normal/high

Serum TIBC (μg/dl)	270-400	>400	Normal/high	Normal/high
Serum ferritin (ng/ml)	10-300	<10	Normal/high	Normal/high
Plasma folate (ng/ml)	3-10	3-10	Usually <3	Normal/high
RBC folate (ng/ml)	140-360	140-360	<140	Normal
Plasma vitamin B_{12} (pg/ml)	200-700	200-700	Normal/high	<200
Serum homocysteine (μmol/L†)	5.4-16.2	5.4-16.2	High	High
Serum methylmalonic acid (nmol/L†)	73-271	73-271	Normal	High

* MCHC, Mean corpuscular hemoglobin concentration; TIBC, total iron-binding capacity.
† Normal range, mean ± two standard deviations.

globin levels. The diagnosis of iron deficiency should be considered when the red cells are small (microcytic) and pale (hypochromic). An MCV of less than 80 μ^3 and a mean corpuscular hemoglobin concentration (MCHC) of less than 32% usually indicate iron deficiencies, but they can also be caused by thalassemias, which are particularly common among African Americans and Asian Americans. The diagnosis of iron deficiency can be more certain when there is a low serum iron value (usually less than 42 µg/dl) and high total iron-binding capacity (greater than 400 µg/dl). The serum iron level is normally 15% or more of the total iron-binding capacity; lower values indicate that the available binding sites on transferrin are not saturated and suggest the patient may have an iron deficiency. A high total iron-binding capacity is important for distinguishing an iron deficiency from other causes of low serum iron, such as PEM, injury, infection, or chronic inflammatory disease (Table 24-3), which can lower both iron and total iron-binding capacity levels. Severe physiologic stress, such as stress resulting from burns and sepsis, can result in serum iron levels as low as zero, even when iron stores are normal. The low serum iron levels are a result of the body sequestering iron in the reticuloendothe-

TABLE 24-3   Conditions affecting iron parameters[2]

Lab findings	Injury, infection, chronic inflammation	Iron deficiency	PEM†
Serum iron	Low	Low	Generally low
Serum TIBC°	Normal or low	High	Low
Serum ferritin	Normal or slightly high	Low	Generally low
Marrow and liver iron stores	Present	Absent	Low to absent

° *TIBC,* Total iron-binding capacity.
†*PEM,* Protein-energy malnutrition.

lial system, apparently reducing the risk of infections by inhibiting infectious organisms from using free iron for growth.

Another laboratory finding that can make the diagnosis of an iron deficiency more certain is a serum ferritin value of less than 40 ng/ml; a level of less than 10 ng/ml is virtually diagnostic. Caution must be used in interpreting ferritin levels when the patient also has liver disease or acute stress, because these conditions can raise the ferritin level even when an iron deficiency is present. A ferritin level of up to 70 ng/ml in patients with these conditions does not rule out iron deficiencies. The gold standard for diagnosing an iron deficiency is a bone marrow with greatly diminished or absent iron stores. When both iron and total iron-binding capacities are low and the ferritin level is equivocal, examination of the bone marrow is often the only method that can be used to establish the diagnosis; in addition it helps identify rare cases of iron-loading (e.g., sideroblastic) anemia and thalassemia in which the patients has hypochromic and/or microcytic anemia but adequate or excessive stores of iron.

Dietary Sources

The iron density of the American diet is 5 to 6 mg/1000 kcal. About 10% to 15% of the iron comes from heme sources such as meat and seafood, and 85% to 90% comes from nonheme sources including dried beans and peas, greens, enriched bread and cereal, dried fruit, and egg yolks. Phytates, oxalates, and tannins decrease nonheme iron absorption, whereas it is increased by reducing sugars, ascorbic acid, amino acids, and animal protein.

Treatment

Iron deficiencies can usually be treated effectively with iron preparations such as ferrous sulfate given orally in doses of 325 mg (60 mg elemental iron) 1 to 3 times daily with meals. Therapy should be continued for 4 to 6 months to restore normal hemoglobin levels and iron stores. Depending on the cause of deficiency, long-term, low-dose therapy may be required.

Parenteral iron is seldom needed but is available as iron dextran (Imferon), which provides 50 mg/ml of elemental iron. This should be used only when oral therapy is ineffective and is best given intravenously, because intramuscular injections are poorly tolerated. A small test dose should be given initially to detect hypersensitivity. When necessary, it can be admixed with total parenteral nutrition, preferably in doses no larger than 50 mg per day.

MACROCYTIC ANEMIAS

Macrocytic or large-cell anemias are characterized by an MCV of greater than $100 \, \mu^3$. When caused by a deficiency of folic acid or vitamin B_{12}, they are also called *megaloblastic anemias* because large, immature red cell precursors (megaloblasts) accumulate in the bone marrow. Not all macrocytic anemias are megaloblastic; in those associated with alcoholism, liver disease, and hemolysis, the red cells are large for other reasons, and megaloblasts are not present in the bone marrow. In addition, artifactual macrocytosis without anemia can be caused by cold agglutinins, hyperglycemia, and marked leukocytosis.

Vitamin B_{12} Deficiency

Vitamin B_{12} deficiency anemia is most often caused by impaired absorption. Although not rare, it is much less common than iron deficiency.

Pathophysiology

Vitamin B_{12} (cobalamin) is a cobalt-containing molecule with a porphyrin-like structure that facilitates the metabolism of fatty acids and the conversion of methylmalonyl CoA to succinyl CoA. Most vitamin B_{12} originates from bacterial synthesis, which occurs particularly in the rumen of ruminants. The vitamin B_{12} ingested by humans in food is bound to proteins called *R-binders* that are secreted by the salivary glands and stomach. After passing into the small intestine, pancreatic enzymes remove vitamin B_{12} from the R-binders, and it is then bound to intrinsic factor (IF), a glycoprotein secreted by the acid-producing parietal cells of the stomach. Vitamin B_{12} must be bound to IF to be absorbed at specific receptor sites in the distal ileum. Because it is excreted in the bile but very efficiently reabsorbed in the distal ileum (enterohepatic recirculation), it takes many years for an individual to deplete vitamin B_{12} stores on a vitamin B_{12}-free diet, as long as the intestinal and hepatobiliary systems are intact. The total body pool of vitamin B_{12} in normal adults is about 2500 μg; the largest storage site is the liver.

Because of the small amounts required and the efficiency with which the body regulates its vitamin B_{12} stores, anemia resulting from inadequate vitamin B_{12} intake is rare. Strict vegetarians (vegans) who consume no dairy products, eggs, or meat are at increased risk for deficiencies, but even bacterial contamination of food provides some deficiency protection. Drinking water contaminated by feces of ruminant animals may actually serve as a source of dietary vitamin B_{12} for vegetarians living in poor areas of the world.

The main cause of vitamin B_{12} deficiencies is pernicious anemia (PA), a condition affecting primarily elderly white persons of North European ancestry in which gastric secretion of IF becomes markedly reduced, leading to vitamin B_{12} malabsorption. Intestinal disorders can also cause vitamin B_{12} deficiencies even when dietary intake is adequate. Absorption is disrupted by a total gastrectomy because the site of IF secretion is eliminated. Regional enteritis (Crohn's disease), bacterial overgrowth of the small bowel (which occurs in a variety of intestinal disorders), and ileal resection interfere with vitamin B_{12} utilization by impairing or eliminating the site of absorption. Severe pancreatic disease and a total pancreatectomy also hinder vitamin B_{12} absorption by altering the normal transfer of cobalamins from R-binders to IF. The length of time required to deplete stores of and induce a vitamin B_{12} deficiency is usually at least several years. For example, if vitamin B_{12} is not replaced after a total gastrectomy, megaloblastic anemia does not typically occur until 4 to 5 years later.

The RDA for vitamin B_{12} is 2 µg per day for both men and women. During pregnancy the RDA is 2.2 µg and during lactation is 2.6 µg. Drugs that can induce B_{12} malabsorption are listed in Chapter 14. Long-term use of omeprazole may also impair B_{12} status.

Diagnosis

In addition to the general physical findings associated with anemia, prolonged vitamin B_{12} deficiencies affect the central and peripheral nervous systems, causing loss of vibratory and position sense, numbness and tingling in the hands and feet, unsteadiness, and even delusions and psychosis.

In patients with vitamin B_{12} and folic acid deficiencies, the morphologic appearance of cells in peripheral blood and bone marrow are indistinguishable. Macrocytes and hypersegmentation of neutrophils are found on the peripheral smear; there is hypersegmentation if 5% of the neutrophils have more than 5 lobes or the average number of lobes per cell exceeds 3.5. Hypersegmentation may also be congenital or caused by chronic renal failure or pyruvate kinase deficiency. Macrocytes are also present in patients with hypothyroidism, reticulocytosis, and liver failure.

A vitamin B_{12} deficiency should be considered when the plasma vitamin B_{12} concentration is less than about 150 to 200 pg/ml. If there is a deficiency of vitamin B_{12}, the plasma folate level may be elevated to 15 or 20 ng/ml because of impaired tissue folate uptake and turnover (methyl-folate trap). However, not all patients with low cobalamin levels have vitamin B_{12} deficiencies, and conversely, serum cobalamin levels are normal in a significant minority of patients with vitamin B_{12} deficiencies. The causes for these inconsistencies are not clear. Some individuals with low plasma vitamin B_{12} levels who do not have deficiencies may have plasma IF inhibitors that interfere with the vitamin B_{12} assay, giving falsely low results.

Useful tests for distinguishing true vitamin B_{12} deficiencies include elevated serum homocysteine and methylmalonic acid levels.[1]

When a vitamin B_{12} deficiency is found, it is important to establish or exclude the diagnosis of PA because it requires lifelong vitamin B_{12} replacement. If PA is mistakenly treated with folic acid, the anemia may disappear, but degeneration of the posterolateral spinal cord will progress. It is because of the risk of masking pernicious anemia with large doses of folate that the folate content of over-the-counter multivitamins is limited to 400 µg.

The diagnosis can be confirmed by the Schilling test, which compares the intestinal absorption of vitamin B_{12} bound to IF with that of unbound vitamin B_{12} after a vitamin B_{12} injection of 1000 µg is given to saturate plasma binding sites. PA patients absorb the IF-bound vitamin B_{12} normally (as demonstrated by urinary excretion of more than 10% of the isotope in 24 hours) but do not absorb the unbound B_{12} well. If both isotopes are not absorbed well, intestinal dysfunctioning (not PA) is the likely cause, so it is very important to perform both stages of the test to make this distinction. PA is also suggested by the presence of antiparietal cell antibodies in the serum. Not all patients with PA have abnormal Schilling tests, because some patients can absorb crystalline vitamin B_{12} well but not vitamin B_{12} associated with food proteins. This has led to the use of a "food" Schilling test. In these cases, antiparietal cell antibodies and elevated serum gastrin levels may also be present.

The development of a vitamin B_{12} deficiency occurs in stages. The first stage is characterized by a negative vitamin B_{12} balance, during which the plasma vitamin B_{12} level is marginal, and only vitamin B carriers in the plasma (transcobalamins) may be abnormally low. Subsequently, the plasma vitamin B_{12} level falls. When the level reaches 100 to 150 pg/ml, neutrophils begin to appear hypersegmented. Finally, macroovalocytes appear, the MCV is elevated, and the hemoglobin level drops. Anemia develops in the later stages of vitamin B_{12} deficiencies as it does in iron deficiencies.

Dietary Sources

Vitamin B_{12} is found only in food of animal origin. Most meat and dairy products contain B_{12}; beef liver is an especially rich source.

Treatment

Remission of the signs and symptoms of vitamin B_{12} deficiency begins with a single intramuscular injection of 100 to 1000 μg of cyanocobalamin or hydroxocobalamin. Daily administration of 100 μg for several days is advisable. Reticulocytosis, indicating hematologic response, begins after 5 to 7 days. For PA patients and others who need continued parenteral therapy, injections of 100 μg every month are generally adequate. Large oral doses of 1 mg daily or nasal gel supplying 400 μg monthly may suffice in some cases, but therapy should be individualized according to the patient's hematologic response and plasma B_{12} levels.

Folic Acid Deficiency

In contrast to vitamin B_{12} deficiencies, folic acid deficiencies from insufficient intake are common. Aside from anemia, suboptimal folate intake during early pregnancy, even without other manifestations of folate deficiency, is a major risk factor for neural tube birth defects.

Pathophysiology

Folate is the generic term for the folic acid coenzyme in the body. It consists of a pteridine ring, a para-aminobenzoic acid moiety, and a glutamate side chain. Folate acts as a coenzyme in numerous one-carbon transfer reactions in the body, including the methylation of homocysteine to form methionine, formation of purines, and methylation of deoxyuridylate to form deoxythymidylate.

Folic acid is present in food in the form of polyglutamates with numerous glutamate side chains in an amide linkage. Absorption occurs in the upper small intestine after the glutamate side chains are hydrolyzed by conjugase to form the monoglutamate. Folate stores in the liver are estimated to be 5 to 10 mg. The RDA for folate was reduced in 1989 to 3 µg/kg per day or about 180 µg/day for females and 200 µg/day for males. During pregnancy the RDA is 400 µg per day and during lactation it is 260 to 280 µg/day. For a number of reasons including prevention of neural tube defects, a higher average daily intake is appropriate and can be achieved with reasonable dietary practices.

By any standard the dietary folate intake of many individuals in the United States is inadequate. Persons who rarely consume green leafy vegetables or other sources of folate can exhibit low plasma folate levels in a few weeks and signs of deficiency after several months. Folate malabsorption is associated with a variety of intestinal disorders such as Crohn's disease, celiac disease, and tropical sprue. Alcoholics are also commonly deficient in folate. The average plasma folate levels of cigarette smokers are lower than those of nonsmokers, partly from poor diets but probably also from smoke-induced destruction.

Folate-deficiency anemia can also result from drug-nutrient interactions (see Chapter 14). Abnormal utilization of folate has been observed with certain anticonvulsants (phenytoin, phenobarbital), diuretics (triamterene), antibiotics (trimethoprim, sulfasalazine), and antimalarials (pyrimethamine) as well as conventional folic acid antagonists (methotrexate).

Diagnosis

The hematologic characteristics of folate-deficient anemia in both the peripheral blood and bone marrow are indistinguishable from those of vitamin B_{12}-deficient anemia. A folic acid deficiency is indicated by a plasma folate level of less than 3 ng/ml. However, because plasma folate levels fluctuate with recent dietary intake, the RBC folate level is a more reliable indicator of tissue stores; levels less than

140 ng/ml indicate deficiencies. The serum homocysteine level is also elevated in patients with folic acid deficiencies, indicating an inability to remethylate homocysteine to form methionine.

Like iron and vitamin B_{12} deficiencies, folate deficiencies develop in stages. The first stage is characterized by a negative folate balance, manifest by a low serum folate level. Next, the RBC folate level decreases and neutrophils appear hypersegmented. Finally, macroovalocytes appear, the MCV is elevated, and the hemoglobin level drops.

Dietary Sources

Folic acid is widely distributed in yeast, liver and other organ meat, legumes, leafy vegetables, fresh fruit, and enriched bread and cereal products. Orange juice is the highest contributor of folic acid to the American diet. Between 50% and 90% of the folate in foods can be destroyed by prolonged cooking and processing.

Treatment

Folic acid deficiencies are readily resolved in most patients with a 1 mg daily oral supplement. In patients with malabsorption, initial treatment with parenteral folate is advised, but thereafter maintenance with oral therapy usually suffices. Plasma levels should be used to guide therapy.

OTHER NUTRITIONAL ANEMIAS

Although less common, anemia can be caused by deficits of other trace elements and vitamins, some of which are involved with the normal utilization of iron, folate, and vitamin B_{12}. For example, copper is essential for the normal production of hemoglobin; a copper deficiency leads to hypochromic anemia and low serum iron levels. The mechanism leading to these conditions is believed to be an impaired iron transport system resulting from lack of a copper-containing enzyme necessary for iron oxidation. Vitamin A deficiencies may also produce anemia and low serum iron levels. Riboflavin deficiencies are reported to cause reversible aplasia of RBC precursors in the bone marrow. An atypical sideroblastic anemia responsive to vitamin B_6 (pyridoxine) has also been found. Vitamin E deficiencies in low birth weight infants can lead to mild hemolytic anemia, particularly if the infant is exposed to the oxidant effects of an iron salt.

References

1. Allen RH et al: Diagnosis of cobalamin deficiency I: usefulness of serum methylmalonic acid and total homocysteine concentrations, *Am J Hematol* 34:90, 1990.

2. Beisel WR: Iron nutrition: immunity and infection, *Res Staff Phys*, 27:37, 1981.

Suggested Readings

Beck WS: Diagnosis of megaloblastic anemia, *Annu Rev Med* 42:311, 1991.

Colon-Otero G, Menke D, Hood CC: A practical approach to the differential diagnosis and evaluation of the adult patient with macrocytic anemia, *Med Clin N Am* 76:581, 1992.

Guyatt GH et al: Laboratory diagnosis of iron-deficiency anemia: an overview, *J Gen Intern Med* 7:145, 1992.

Massey AC: Microcytic anemia: differential diagnosis and management of iron deficiency anemia, *Med Clin N Am* 76:549, 1992.

25

Eating Disorders

Anorexia nervosa is self-imposed starvation that is associated with an excessive concern with weight and an irrational fear of becoming fat. Individuals with the disorder are characterized by extremely low body weights and an obsessive, narrowed focus on body fat. Patients with anorexia nervosa deny they have problems and have distorted perspectives of their body shapes. There are two subtypes of anorexia nervosa: (1) the restricting type in which patients severely limit energy intake (often consuming less than 600 kcal per day) and/or engage in excessive exercise, and (2) the binge-eating/purging type in which patients engage in compensatory behaviors, such as self-induced vomiting or abuse of laxatives or diuretics, after they believe they have eaten excessive amounts of food (although the amounts may not be objectively large).

Bulimia nervosa is also accompanied by a preoccupation with weight and fear of becoming fat. Bulimic patients overemphasize the importance of their body weight or shape in evaluating their self-worth. Individuals with bulimia alternate between periods of rigid control over energy intake and episodes of excessive consumption, or binges. An intense fear of weight gain prompts compensatory behaviors to counteract the effects of the binge episodes. Individuals with the purging subtype of bulimia nervosa engage in self-induced vomiting or laxative or diuretic abuse, and those with the nonpurging subtype engage in methods such as fasting or excessive exercise to compensate for binge eating.

Preoccupation with food, changes in eating habits, irritability, depression, social withdrawal, and poor sleep patterns are all associated with eating disorders. In addition, patients often tend to be perfectionists and set rigid standards for themselves.

DIAGNOSIS

Anorexia nervosa and bulimia nervosa are identified as mental disorders by the American Psychiatric Association; their diagnostic criteria are listed in the box on the following two pages. The two disorders share several common features, including an irrational fear of being fat or gaining weight. The box on p. 498 contains signs that may indicate a patient has an eating disorder.

Another diagnostic category, *eating disorder not otherwise specified* (ED-NOS), has recently been added to accommodate pathologically disordered eating that does not meet the full criteria for anorexia or bulimia nervosa. Examples of patients included in this category include females who meet the criteria for anorexia nervosa but have regular menses or females who meet the criteria for bulimia nervosa but only engage in binge eating and inappropriate compensatory behaviors less than twice weekly or have engaged in them for less than 3 months. A specific case of an ED-NOS is a *binge eating disorder* (BED), a recently described eating disorder that is characterized by patients engaging in binge-eating episodes at least twice weekly on average over the previous 6-month period. These binges often extend throughout the day, more similar to "grazing" rather than the discrete periods of rapid eating that are common in bulimia nervosa. Individuals with BED do not engage in regular compensatory behaviors such as self-induced vomiting, fasting, or exercise and are therefore likely to be overweight.

A patient suspected of having an eating disorder should have a psychologic and psychiatric evaluation to establish a diagnosis. In addition, the patient should be asked to keep an eating and activity log for one week that includes a record of inappropriate compensatory behaviors. Such

Diagnostic Criteria for the Eating Disorders[1]

307.10 Anorexia nervosa

A. Refusal to maintain body weight at or above a minimally normal weight for age and height (e.g., weight loss leading to maintenance of body weight less than 85% of that expected or failure to make expected weight gain during period of growth, leading to body weight less than 85% of that expected)

B. Intense fear of gaining weight or becoming fat, even though underweight

C. Disturbance in the way in which body weight or shape is perceived, undue influence of body weight or shape on self-evaluation, or denial of the seriousness of the current low body weight

D. In postmenarcheal females, amenorrhea (i.e., the absence of at least three consecutive menstrual cycles; periods occur only following hormone—e.g., estrogen—administration)

Specify type

Restricting type
During the current episode, no regular participation in binge-eating or purging behavior
Binge-eating/purging type
During the current episode, regular participation in binge-eating or purging behavior (i.e., self-induced vomiting or the misuse of laxatives, diuretics, or enemas)

307.51 Bulimia Nervosa

A. Recurrent episodes of binge eating characterized by both of the following:
   1. Eating, in a discrete period of time (e.g., within any 2-hour period), an amount of food that is definitely

DIAGNOSTIC CRITERIA FOR THE EATING DISORDERS[1] — CONT'D

      larger than most people would eat during a similar period of time and under similar circumstances

  2. A sense of lack of control of eating during the episode (e.g., a feeling that eating cannot be stopped or controlled)

B. Recurrent inappropriate compensatory behavior to prevent weight gain, such as self-induced vomiting; misuse of laxatives, diuretics, enemas, or other medications; fasting; or excessive exercise

C. Participation in binge eating and inappropriate compensatory behaviors, on average, at least twice a week for 3 months

D. Excessive influence of body shape and weight on self-evaluation

E. Disturbance not exclusively during episodes of anorexia nervosa

Specify type

Purging type

During the current episode, regular participation in self-induced vomiting or the misuse of laxative, diuretics, or enemas

Nonpurging type

During the current episode, use of other inappropriate compensatory behaviors, such as fasting or excessive exercise, but no regular participation in self-induced vomiting or the misuse of laxatives, diuretics, or enemas

CLUES TO POSSIBLE EATING DISORDERS

Amenorrhea for several consecutive months

Because menstrual irregularity is one of the earliest manifestations of anorexia nervosa, an anorexic patient often initially seeks help from her general practitioner or gynecologist. Patients in their early teens are often brought to the physician by their parents because of this problem. Unless there has been dramatic weight loss, the diagnosis of anorexia nervosa may be missed. Women with bulimia nervosa also commonly experience menstrual irregularities.

Complaints of fatigue, dizziness, diarrhea, headaches, or muscle cramps

These symptoms may result from abuse of laxatives or diuretics or from long periods of fasting in either bulimic or anorexic patients.

Rigid, arbitrary definitions of fattening food or avoidance of certain food groups (e.g., starch, fat, or sugar) or types (desserts)

Compulsive, intense aerobic exercise

requests must be made with great sensitivity, because patients with bulimia or a BED are likely to be embarrassed by their behavior patterns; those with anorexia nervosa may resist acknowledging their patterns all together. Treatment should be carried out by a multi-disciplinary team of physicians, psychologists or psychiatrists, and nutritionists experienced in treating patients with eating disorders.

PREVALENCE

The majority of anorexia and bulimia patients are adolescent women. By contrast, a BED generally affects women who seek treatment in their 30s. The onset of anorexia nervosa generally occurs at two critical times—around the ages of 14 and 18—and it affects between 0.5% and 1% of adolescent females. Bulimia nervosa most commonly develops between 18 and 22 years of age and affects approximately 1% to 2% of women. Substantially more women report experimenting with binge/purge behavior without developing the full bulimic syndrome. The BED appears to be the most common eating disorder, affecting 2% to 3% of individuals in the general population and as many as 30% of patients who seek treatment for obesity. Unlike anorexia and bulimia, a BED is about as prevalent among men as among women. However, women with BEDs are more likely to seek treatment.

PREDISPOSING FACTORS

Currently, no known physical disorders have been identified that contribute to the development of any of the eating disorders. Though some researchers believe that a hypothalamic dysfunction may be an etiologic factor, evidence does not support this. However, there is high comorbidity between eating disorders and affective disorders. Otherwise, the features most frequently associated with the disorders are social and psychologic.

The subgroups of women who are most prone to develop eating disorders include those from higher socioeconomic groups and adolescents who are dieting, as well as women in certain professions like dancing, gymnastics, and modeling. A family history of eating disorders and/or affective illness (e.g., depression) is common. A history of sexual victimization does not appear to be a specific risk factor for eating disorders, but as in patients with other psychiatric disorders high rates have been noted in this patient group. Similarly, high lifetime rates of substance abuse (alcohol and/or other drugs) are common.

The significance of societal pressures in the development of eating disorders is underscored by the fact that the preponderance of reported cases of anorexia and bulimia nervosa are found in industrialized western countries. The mass media consistently support the notion that "you can't be too rich or too thin." Whether in a fashion magazine, movie, or television program, the successful, happy young woman is thin. The number of women dieting to reach this ideal has been steadily increasing over the past few decades, as has the prevalence of eating disorders, suggesting that these two events are directly related.

PHYSICAL FEATURES AND COMPLICATIONS

A summary of the physical features of patients with eating disorders is given in Table 25-1. The characteristics associated with patients who have anorexia nervosa are related to reductions in metabolic rate and protein synthesis and other physiologic adaptations observed in starvation. Most of the conditions are reversed when energy intake in-

TABLE 25-1 Physical manifestations of anorexia nervosa and bulimia nervosa[2]

Manifestation	Anorexia nervosia	Bulimia nervosa
Endocrine/ metabolic	Amenorrhea	Menstrual irregularities
	Euthyroid sick syndrome	
	Decreased norepineph- rine secretion	
	Decreased levels of somatomedian C	
	Elevated levels of growth hormone	
	Decreased or erratic vasopressin secretion	
	Abnormal temperature regulation	
Cardio- vascular	Bradycardia, arrhythmias	
	Hypotension	
Renal	Blood urea nitrogen (BUN) increased by dehydration or decreased by low protein intake	Hypokalemia (induced by diuretics or laxatives)
	Decreased glomerular filtration rate	

creases. However, osteopenia and osteoporosis can be a source of lifelong morbidity.

The complications of bulimia are largely related to binge/purge behaviors rather than metabolic alterations. The most serious complication is a gastric rupture after a binge, which carries an 80% mortality rate. A variety of oral and dental abnormalities also develop, especially dental enamel erosion probably resulting from exposure to gastric acid.

Although a number of laboratory abnormalities can be found in patients with eating disorders, including endocrine changes in patients with anorexia nervosa and electrolyte abnormalities in patients with bulimia, they do

TABLE 25-1 Physical manifestations of anorexia nervosa and bulimia nervosa[2]—cont'd

Manifestation	Anorexia nervosia	Bulimia nervosa
Renal—cont'd		
	Renal calculi	
	Edema	
Gastro-intestinal	Decreased gastric emptying	Parotid enlargement
	Constipation	Dental enamel erosion
	Elevated levels of liver enzymes	Esophagitis
		Mallory-Weiss tears, esophageal rupture
		Acute gastric dilatation, rupture
Skeletal	Decreased bone mass, osteoporosis	—
Hematologic	Anemia, leukopenia, thrombocytopenia	—
Integu-mentary	Lanugo hair, hair loss	—
	Hypercarotenemia	

not help establish the diagnosis and should be used primarily to monitor complications.

TREATMENT

Individuals with eating disorders can generally be treated on an outpatient basis, depending on the severity of the problem, physical status of the patient, social support available, and presence of any associated psychopathology. A key factor in successful treatment is the establishment of a therapeutic alliance between the clinician and the patient, which is accomplished by involving the patient in decision-making and acceding to the patient's requests when possible. If granting a particular request is not wise, a clear, direct explanation should be given. Frequently a compromise can be reached that will satisfy both parties (e.g., controlled exercise in exchange for increased calorie intake and weight maintenance for an anorexic patient). In addition, informing the patient in advance of potential adverse side effects of therapy (e.g., transient edema as weight gain begins or purging ceases) will help the patient develop trust in the clinician. Finally, setting limited, achievable goals allows the patient to improve slowly and minimizes the anxiety that occurs with normalization of eating habits or with weight gain.

Anorexia Nervosa

The treatment of anorexia nervosa is a long, tedious process with limited success in many cases. Exhorting the patient to eat more food does little more than contribute to the struggle. Unless the patient has a coexisting depression, medication is of little value to the treatment process. A host of psychologic approaches have been reported, ranging from long-term psychodynamic treatment to briefer behavior modification. Regardless of the psychologic orientation, the initial concern is the stabilization of body weight with adequate nutritional intake.

Adequate nutritional status in an anorexic patient may be reestablished in several ways, depending on the patient's physical state and current attitudes. In severe cases, tube or intravenous feedings may be necessary; however, these should be employed only as a last resort and should be used cautiously, as rapid refeeding of cachectic patients is risky and occasionally fatal. Often the patient can slowly increase calorie intake to an acceptable level with the aid of nutritional counseling. Some patients will increase their overall nutrient intake if they can be taught how to do so without gaining what they consider excessive weight. Even 1000 calories per day may be enough to stabilize the patient's body weight and if well planned will increase protein and micronutrient intake to safer levels. Such strategies require attention to a patient's beliefs about massive weight gain following caloric increase. Setting up "empirical experiments," assuring the patient that it is not your goal to make her obese, and "testing out" the rate of weight gain associated with increments in energy intake are often effective in establishing a collaborative treatment relationship.

Once an anorectic patient is stabilized, a course of dietary monitoring and psychotherapy is critical to further improvement. Therapy must deal with a number of issues including body image, self worth, and independence. Individuals with anorexia nervosa harbor irrational beliefs about themselves and their weight that must be corrected for long-term success. The demand for perfection must also be addressed and attitudes toward achievement modified.

Bulimia Nervosa

Hospitalization of bulimic patients is rarely justified unless the binge/purge cycle is nearly continuous or physical complications require careful monitoring. As with anorectic patients, treatment involves psychotherapy emphasizing behavioral and cognitive techniques. Antidepressant medication may be helpful for patients who have a primary affective disorder, but medication alone is insufficient.

Success is determined by the ability of the patient to modify rigidly-held attitudes about the importance of maintaining a slender body weight for personal worth and to adopt more realistic standards for self-evaluation. Developing methods to interrupt the binge/purge cycle and establish new coping strategies for situations that trigger the cycle is also critical. Bulimic patients typically respond to negative feelings such as anger, frustration, and anxiety by binge eating and purging and must be helped to find more appropriate responses. Erratic eating patterns perpetuate feelings of loss of control, so more regular dietary habits must be developed as well as a tolerance to a greater variety of food. Therefore nutrition education and behavior modification are often incorporated into effective treatment programs.

Binge Eating Disorder

Because patients with this disorder are commonly overweight, treatment must address the concerns of both binge-eating behavior and weight loss. Cognitive-behavioral interventions that address the obsessive concern about weight and body shape and establish coping strategies to prevent or stop binges are currently considered the treatment of choice. After patients regain some control of their eating habits, a sensible approach to weight loss that features moderate restriction and emphasizes flexibility can be introduced.

References

1. American Psychiatric Association: *Diagnostic and statistical manual of mental disorders*, ed 4, Washington DC, 1994, The Association.
2. Herzog DB, Copeland PM: Eating disorders, *N Engl J Med* 313:295, 1985.

Suggested Readings

Fairburn CG, Wilson GT, eds: *Binge eating: nature, assessment, and treatment*, New York, 1993, Guilford Press.

Halmi KA: *Behavioral management for anorexia nervosa*. In Gardner DM, Garfinkel PE, eds: *Handbook of psychother-*

apy for anorexia nervosa and bulimia, New York, 1985, Guilford Press.

Mitchell JE et al: Medical complications and medical management of bulimia, *Ann Intern Med* 107:71, 1987.

Smith DE, Marcus MD, Eldredge KL: Binge eating syndromes: a review of assessment and treatment with an emphasis on clinical application, *Behavior Therapy* 25:635, 1994.

26

Metabolic Bone Disease

OSTEOPOROSIS
Definition and Classification

Osteoporosis is a metabolic bone disease involving an imbalance between bone formation and bone resorption, causing a reduction in bone mass that greatly increases the risk of traumatic or atraumatic bone fractures. The definition of osteoporosis as defined by the measurements of dual-energy x-ray absorptiometry (DEXA) is a bone mineral density 2.5 or more standard deviations below that of a "young normal" standard. Bone densities between 1 and 2.5 standard deviations below this standard are termed *osteopenia*. It was estimated that 26 million Americans suffered from osteoporosis in 1995; of these, 20 million were women. The annual cost to our health care system is approximately $10 billion.

Osteoporosis can be classified as primary (no clear cause) or secondary (related to a specific cause, such as hypogonadism), and has both high- and low-turnover forms, reflecting the level of activity of osteoblasts and osteoclasts. Type I osteoporosis affects trabecular bone in early postmenopausal women and produces vertebral crush fractures and distal radial (Colles') fractures. Type II osteoporosis involves loss of both cortical and trabecular bone in men and women and is related to aging. Fracture sites are mainly in the hip and vertebrae, but fractures of the humerus, tibia, and pelvis also occur. Type III osteoporosis is mainly induced by drugs such as corticosteroids and affects both trabecular and cortical bone in men and women.

Risk Factors

A number of factors related to lifestyle, genetics, hormones, and medical conditions and therapies affect the risk for developing osteoporosis (Table 26-1).

Age and Gender

Bone mass increases until to approximately age 30. After a period of stabilization, age-related bone loss begins in both females and males. Bone loss is associated with aging itself, partly because of a decline in intestinal calcium absorption. Females are more affected than males because bone loss accelerates when estrogen levels decline at menopause. However, osteoporosis is not a certain consequence of aging.

Peak Bone Mass

Peak bone mass, which occurs in the third decade of life, is one of the most important modifiers of risk for osteoporosis. A greater absolute bone mass means there is a greater bone reserve, and therefore more bone can be lost during the aging process or as a result of other factors before symptoms of osteoporosis occur (i.e., fractures). Therefore a person with a low peak bone mass at age 30 is at greater risk for osteoporotic fractures.

Heredity

The quantity and quality of bone mass attained by maturity is associated with numerous inherited factors. Reduced bone mass is associated with being female, white or Asiatic, of small stature, lean, having long-term lactose intolerance, or a family history of osteoporosis. Conversely, being male, black, of large stature, or obese are correlated with higher bone mass.

Nutrition

Among other dietary factors, bone mass is related to calcium intake throughout life, but especially during the first

TABLE 26-1 Risk factors for low bone mineral density

Risk factor category	Associated risks
Nutrition and lifestyle	Low dietary calcium and/or vitamin D intake
	High protein or salt intake
	Excessive alcohol or caffeine intake
	Lack of weight-bearing exercise
	Excessive exercise producing amenorrhea
	Smoking
Genetics	Lactose intolerance
	Asthenic (small, lean) body habitus
	Family history of osteoporosis
	White or Asian heritage
Hormones and life cycles	Advanced age
	Early menopause (surgical or natural)
	Postmenopausal estrogen deficiency (lack of replacement)
	Late menarche, nulliparity
	Hypogonadism (low testosterone levels in males)

30 years, when peak bone mass is developing. The dietary calcium intake recommended by the NIH Consensus Development Panel on Optimal Calcium Intake is shown in Table 26-2.[1] Unfortunately, calcium intake in many age categories for both males and females in the United States is substantially below these levels.

Excessive protein intake enhances calcium excretion in the urine and therefore places a burden on calcium balance. The Western cultural emphasis on meat consump-

TABLE 26-1	Risk factors for low bone mineral density—cont'd
Risk factor category	**Associated risks**
Medical comorbidities	Gastric or intestinal resection, malabsorption, long-term parenteral nutrition
	Eating disorders
	Renal failure, dialysis
	Cardiopulmonary or renal transplantation
	Cushing's syndrome
	Diabetes mellitus
	Prolactinoma
	Hyperparathyroidism
	Hyperthyroidism
	Rheumatoid arthritis
Medications	Corticosteroids, cyclosporin A
	Anticonvulsants
	Phosphate-binding antacids
	Excessive thyroid replacement therapy
	Gonadotropin-releasing hormone agonists or antagonists
	Heparin
	Methotrexate
	Extended tetracycline use

tion often results in a protein intake more than twice that needed for good health and may contribute to the development of osteoporosis. Moderation of protein intake is advisable.

Excessive sodium intake, which is typical among Americans, can lead to negative calcium balance by increasing urinary calcium excretion and has been associated with increased bone loss. It has been suggested that lowering sodium intake can reduce the need for a high-calcium diet, which may be difficult for persons who are lactose intolerant.[2] Data also suggest that caffeine may have an adverse effect on calcium balance.

Other Lifestyle Habits

Alcohol intake and tobacco use have adverse effects on bone mass, as does a sedentary lifestyle. Exercise throughout life, especially weight-bearing exercise, helps to maintain the health of the skeleton. However, exercising so much that amenorrhea results is detrimental to skeletal health. For persons who already have osteoporosis, avoid-

TABLE 26-2 Optimal calcium intakes[1]

Age group	Optimal calcium intake (mg)
Infants	
Birth-6 months	400
6 months-1 year	600
Children	
1-5 years	800
6-10 years	800-1200
Adolescents/young adults	
11-24 years	1200-1500
Men	
25-65 years	1000
>65 years	1500
Women	
25-50 years	1000
>50 years (postmenopausal)	
Taking estrogen replacement	1000
Not taking estrogen replacement	1500
>65 years	1500
Pregnant or nursing	1200-1500

ing falls (e.g., by properly arranging the home and environment) has a significant influence on decreasing fracture risk.

Hormonal Factors

Normal sex hormone status is one of the most important factors in maintaining bone mineral density. Hypogonadism in males can cause osteoporosis. The decline in estrogen at menopause greatly accelerates the rate of bone loss in the early postmenopausal period. Nulliparity also increases the risk of osteoporosis.

Medical Conditions and Medications

Many medical and/or surgical conditions and drug therapies have adverse effects on bone mineral density, including resection of the stomach, malabsorption, renal failure, hyperparathyroidism, hyperthyroidism, long-term use of corticosteroids or anticonvulsants, or excessive thyroid hormone replacement.

Pathophysiology

Osteoporosis is the end result of defects in the bone remodeling cycle. Bone remodeling is a dynamic process in which older bone is resorbed by osteoclasts, osteoblasts are recruited, and osteoid bone matrix is deposited and ultimately calcified. When bone resorption outpaces formation, bone mineral density declines. Osteoporosis involves either a high- or low-bone turnover state. In high-turnover disease there is accelerated bone resorption. In low-turnover disease, resorption exceeds formation without a net increase in bone turnover.

Diagnosis

The diagnosis of osteoporosis is made by combining historical data, clinical examinations, laboratory tests, plain radiographs, and specialized radiographic procedures.

History and Physical Examination

When completing a patient's history, emphasis should be placed on obtaining information about genetic and lifestyle factors, medical conditions, and medications that can affect bone mineral density. Current height may be compared to the patient's height at age 18 or the height on the driver's license. Because clinical manifestations of osteoporosis can be silent, posture, skeletal deformities, and gait are important factors to note. A characteristic change in posture results from vertebral fractures; changes include loss of height (best measured with a stadiometer), a humped back (the dowager's hump), loss of waistline contour, and a protuberant abdomen. Vertebral fractures may be painful just after they occur, but subsequent pain is generally from paraspinous muscle tenderness.

Laboratory Tests

Laboratory tests are used to rule out secondary causes of osteoporosis such as thyrotoxicosis, metastatic bone cancer, and hyperparathyroidism, as well as to quantify the rate of bone turnover. A reasonable battery of laboratory tests includes a complete blood count with differential, erythrocyte sedimentation rate, chemistry panel, and serum and urine protein electrophoresis if malignancy is suspected. Free thyroxine and thyroid-stimulating hormone levels can rule out thyrotoxicosis or excessive thyroid replacement. Luteinizing hormone, follicle-stimulating hormone, estradiol, and testosterone levels can help detect hypogonadism. Parathyroid hormone levels are measured to diagnose hyperparathyroidism. A variety of vitamin D metabolites, such as 25-hydroxyvitamin D and 1,25-dihydroxyvitamin D can also be measured. A variety of specialized markers for bone formation is available. Serum osteocalcin serves as a marker; normally, bone formation and bone resorption are balanced, and when they are unbalanced or uncoupled then osteocalcin is said to be a reasonable marker of bone formation.

A measurement of 24-hour urine calcium and creatinine helps detect impaired calcium absorption and hypercalciuria. Urinary hydroxyproline or pyridinoline and deoxypyridinoline can serve as markers of bone resorption. However, urinary hydroxyproline is also affected by dietary collagen intake.

Radiographs

Plain radiographs are useful in evaluating underlying disorders such as rheumatoid arthritis, the morphology of bones, and the presence of fractures. Because standard radiographs can only detect losses of greater than 30%, they are relatively insensitive indicators of bone mass. A lateral radiograph of the spine is useful to check for vertebral compression fractures. Plain radiographs can also be useful for ruling out other causes of back pain such as lumbar spinal stenosis.

A number of more sophisticated tests can be used to assess bone mineral density, such as single-energy x-ray absorptiometry (SXA), DEXA, quantitative computed tomography (QCT), and radiographic absorptiometry (RA). DEXA is currently the most accurate method. It generates a T-score that relates the bone density to that of a "young normal," and a Z-score that compares it to that of an "age-matched" control. Indications for DEXA include the following: parathyroid disease, chronic prednisone therapy, malabsorption, incidental osteopenia noted on plain films, and hypogonadism. It is also useful in the perimenopausal period, when a relatively low bone mineral density makes postmenopausal hormone replacement advisable.

Bone Histomorphometry and Biopsy

A bone biopsy is another useful test for establishing the diagnosis of metabolic bone disease. If the patient takes tetracycline before the biopsy, the rate of bone formation can be assessed.

Prevention and Treatment

Most cases of osteoporosis can be prevented by eliminating modifiable risk factors (see Table 26-1). Guidelines are summarized in the box. Like prevention of osteoporosis, treatment of established osteoporosis is focused on slowing bone loss but also includes attempts to reverse some bone loss, the prevention of falls, and possibly drug therapy.

Lifestyle

All possible lifestyle factors should be modified. Smoking, excessive alcohol intake, and inactivity should be addressed. Weight-bearing exercise and weight training are especially useful in increasing and/or maintaining bone mass. In women who have amenorrhea from excessive exercise, the intensity of exercise should be decreased to establish regular menstrual cycles.

Diet

A rational approach to achieving adequate calcium intake (see Table 26-2) is to maximize dietary sources and if necessary take supplements. Because bone health is influenced by other nutrients such as protein and sodium (see Table 26-1), a good diet is the cornerstone of both prevention and therapy. Dairy products, canned salmon with

---

GUIDELINES FOR PREVENTING OSTEOPOROSIS

Consume adequate amounts of dietary calcium and avoid excessive protein and sodium intake; if necessary, take a calcium supplement.

Consume adequate dietary vitamin D and get a reasonable amount of sun exposure.

Participate in regular weight-bearing exercises.

Do not smoke.

Consume alcohol in moderation, if at all.

Consider estrogen replacement after menopause.

bones, collard and turnip greens, spinach, broccoli, and cooked, dried beans (e.g., kidney, lima, and navy) all contribute calcium to the diet. If dairy products are consumed, use low-fat varieties to minimize the intake of saturated fat. Lactose-reduced (e.g., cultured or lactase-treated) products can be used by individuals who have lactose-intolerance. Calcium-fortified products such as calcium-fortified orange juice and cereal can also add calcium to the diet.

Nutritional Supplements

The amount of calcium contained in commonly used supplements are listed in Table 26-3. Calcium carbonate is the most commonly used supplement and is available in numerous commercial preparations that contain a variety of doses; some of the other forms have only one manufacturer. Preparations that contain bone meal or dolomite can be contaminated with heavy metals and should not be

TABLE 26-3 Elemental calcium content of commonly prescribed supplements

Preparation	Percent elemental calcium	Amount (mg) providing 500 mg elemental calcium
Calcium carbonate (various)	40	1250
Calcium phosphate tribasic (Posture)	39	1280
Calcium acetate (Phos-Ex, PhosLo)	25	2000
Calcium citrate (Citracal)	21	2380
Calcium lactate (various)	13	3850
Calcium gluconate (various)	9	5550
Calcium glubionate (Neo-Calglucon)	6.5	7700

used. To optimize absorption, it is recommended that no more than 500 mg of elemental calcium be consumed at one time. It is best to take calcium supplements between meals, unless patients have achlorhydria, in which case the calcium carbonate is better absorbed with food. Calcium citrate is a useful preparation for patients with achlorhydria.

There are theoretical concerns about the adverse effects of calcium supplements on the absorption of other nutrients such as iron, although calcium citrate and calcium supplements containing ascorbic acid do not interfere with iron absorption.

Vitamin D (as cholecalciferol) intakes in the range of 400 to 800 IU per day are also helpful in maintaining bone mineral density. The lower dose is contained in virtually all replacement multivitamins (see Appendix C). Combined calcium-vitamin D supplements are also available.

Drug Therapy

Several drug therapies are now available for treating established osteoporosis, and many of them lower the rate of bone resorption. Calcitonin can be injected subcutaneously or inhaled nasally. Because of its analgesic effect, calcitonin is especially useful in treating recent compression fractures. Another class of drugs, bisphosphonates, become integrated into the hydroxyapatite crystal and down-regulate osteoclast activity. A variety of estrogen-progesterone combinations, which can be given orally or topically, is available to treat postmenopausal osteoporosis. The decision to use hormone replacement therapy must be balanced with a concern for its associated risks, including a possible increased risk for breast cancer. Although fluoride therapy has been found to increase bone mineral density, the bones are more prone to fracture. There have been recent promising results using slow-release sodium fluoride with continuous calcium citrate supplementation.

OSTEOMALACIA
Definition

Osteomalacia and rickets are disorders of mineralization of bone osteoid. Rickets occurs in growing bones and involves the epiphyses as well as trabecular and cortical bone. Osteomalacia occurs after growth has ceased.

Pathophysiology

In patients with vitamin D deficiencies there is inadequate calcium and phosphorus absorption from the intestine, which causes secondary hypocalcemia. Hypocalcemia increases the secretion of parathyroid hormone, which in turn increases bone resorption by osteoclasts to normalize serum calcium and phosphorus concentrations. Increased parathyroid hormone levels also increase the reabsorption of calcium and excretion of phosphorus in the kidney. The major causes of rickets and osteomalacia are vitamin D, calcium, and phosphorus deficiencies. Vitamin D deficiencies occur (1) when there is lack of adequate sunshine to produce calciferol in the skin, (2) when dietary vitamin D intake is inadequate, and (3) when patients are provided total parenteral nutrition (TPN) that is not supplemented with vitamin D. The major sources of vitamin D in the American diet are fortified milk, egg yolks, fatty fish, and fish liver oil.

Diagnosis
Clinical and Laboratory Manifestations

When obtaining the patient's history, the focus should be on the intake of vitamin D, amount of sunshine exposure, phosphorus and calcium in the diet, and circumstances in which these nutrients could have become deficient. Clinical findings commonly seen in patients with rickets include muscle weakness, bowing deformities of the long bones, and prominence of the costochondral junction (rachitic rosary). Patients may also develop kyphosis, lordosis, and a waddling gait. The most common complaint in patients with osteomalacia is diffuse bony pain; deformities of the pelvis and a waddling gait can also develop.

X-Rays

Radiographs show thinning of the cortex and disappearance of cartilaginous calcification. Stress fractures perpendicular to the bone shaft may be seen. DEXA shows diminished bone mass.

Biochemical Findings

The biochemical findings in patients with osteomalacia tend to be highly variable. Calcium and phosphorus levels may be normal or low, and alkaline phosphatase levels are frequently elevated. Serum 25-hydroxyvitamin D levels are low in patients with vitamin D deficiencies.

Treatment

Treatment is aimed at correction of the underlying cause. Calcium, phosphorus, and vitamin D should be supplemented as needed. Useful vitamin D preparations include ergocalciferol, cholecalciferol, calcifediol (25-hydroxyvitamin D_3, Calderol), and calcitriol (1,25-dihydroxycholecalciferol, Rocaltrol). Doses of vitamin D metabolites must be tailored to the cause of the deficiency. For example, a patient with renal disease who cannot hydroxylate 25-hydroxyvitamin D requires therapy with the 1,25-dihydroxy form (see Chapter 23). Patients with malabsorption require a higher dose of vitamin D than those with intact gastrointestinal tracts. Typical doses are the following: ergocalciferol (most often supplied as 50,000 IU capsules) and cholecalciferol, 25,000 to 100,000 IU daily or 3 times weekly; calcifediol, 20 to 50 µg daily or 3 times weekly (supplied in both doses); calcitriol, 0.25 to 1 µg once or twice daily (supplied as 0.25 and 0.50 µg capsules). Vitamin D, calcium, and phosphorus levels must be tracked to ensure they are in the normal range.

References

1. NIH Consensus Development Panel on Optimal Calcium Intake: Optimal calcium intake, *JAMA* 272:1942, 1994.
2. Devine A et al: A longitudinal study of the effect of sodium and calcium intakes on regional bone density in postmenopausal women, *Am J Clin Nutr* 62:740, 1995.

Suggested Readings

American Society for Bone and Mineral Research: *Primer on the metabolic bone diseases and disorders of mineral metabolism,* New York, 1993, Raven Press.

Cummings SR et al: Risk factors for hip fracture in white women, *N Engl J Med* 332:767, 1995.

Melton LJ: How many women have osteoporosis now? *J Bone Min Res* 10:175, 1995.

NIH Consensus Development Panel on Optimal Calcium Intake: Optimal calcium intake, *JAMA* 272:1942, 1994.

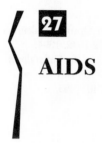

27
AIDS

NUTRITIONAL GOALS DURING HUMAN IMMUNODEFICIENCY VIRUS INFECTION

There are two principal goals of nutritional support during human immunodeficiency virus (HIV) infection. The first is to prevent the development of specific nutrient deficiencies because, among other reasons, such deficiencies can impair immune function. The second goal is to prevent loss of lean body mass, because when weight decreases to less than about 60% of ideal in patients with acquired immunodeficiency syndrome (AIDS) death becomes a near certainty. These nutritional goals should be pursued early in patients with HIV infection when signs and symptoms are few and later when AIDS has developed, because its opportunistic infections take a dramatic toll on nutritional status. Achieving these goals requires a systematic approach that involves periodic nutritional assessment, dietary evaluation, and dietary counseling. The benefits of specific interventions have not been conclusively documented, but results so far suggest that proper nutritional support can prolong survival and enhance quality of life in HIV patients.

NUTRITIONAL DEFICIENCIES AND IMMUNE FUNCTION
Protein-Energy Malnutrition

HIV infection impairs the cell-mediated immune response by specifically infecting and depleting lymphocytes called T helper cells (also known as CD4 cells). The result is an impaired immune response to pathogens that are normally eradicated by a T cell–mediated immune response, such as *Pneumocystis carinii* pneumonia, oral candidiasis, herpes infections, and tuberculosis. As HIV infection progresses to frank AIDS, peripheral blood CD4 numbers decrease to critical levels and infections develop. Protein-energy malnutrition (PEM) also affects T lymphocytes and can lower peripheral blood CD4 counts, impairing cell-mediated immunity in a similar fashion. In children with PEM, the T cell regions of the thymus and other lymphoid organs are specifically depleted, at least partly because of decreased production of hormones (e.g., thymulin) by thymic epithelial cells that promote T lymphocyte maturation. Thus fewer mature T lymphocytes are produced in the thymus and exported to peripheral blood and lymphoid tissue. Classic work done in the 1960s and 1970s among children with kwashiorkor and marasmus in developing countries showed that the types of infections from which they suffered were often the same as those found later to plague patients with AIDS in the United States.

The similar effects of PEM and AIDS on cell-mediated immunity suggest that the development of wasting malnutrition in patients with AIDS can exacerbate the already diminished T cell–mediated immune response. In children with acute PEM (kwashiorkor), provision of high-protein, high-energy food and treatment of intercurrent infections can restore cell-mediated immunity (as measured by the delayed-type hypersensitivity skin test response to recall antigens) within 1 week. Thus prevention and treatment of wasting in AIDS patients will hopefully benefit the maintenance of immune function.

Micronutrient Deficiencies

Micronutrient deficiencies can also impair the T lymphocyte–mediated immune response. In particular, deficiencies of vitamin A, zinc, and iron are detrimental, and replacing them can restore immune function. The mechanisms by which these nutrients affect immune function differ. Iron is a key component of cytochromes, which mediate cellular energy metabolism, as well as of enzymes that perform many important physiologic reactions. Thus the metabolism and proliferation of lymphocytes is impaired by iron deficiency. Zinc is important in the activity of many enzymes, DNA-binding proteins, and the thymic hormone thymulin; deficiencies impair lymphocyte function by a number of mechanisms. The active metabolite of vitamin A, retinoic acid, affects the production of immunologically significant cytokines such as interferon-γ and interleukin-4 and influences the ability of cells to respond to these cytokines. Vitamin A deficiency specifically impairs the ability of CD4 cells to respond to antigenic stimulation and thus can decrease the immune response to certain T cell–dependent antigens, particularly bacterial antigens. Deficiencies of other nutrients can also impair immune function. Depletion of antioxidant nutrients (e.g., vitamin E, vitamin C, and selenium) can impair the immune response, presumably by allowing greater oxidative damage to cells of the immune system than would normally occur. Deficiencies in B vitamins can also compromise immune function because of their roles as cofactors in many enzymes, including those involved in nucleic acid synthesis.

NUTRITIONAL DEFICIENCIES IN HIV PATIENTS

Body weight (particularly lean body mass) and biochemical indicators of nutritional status should be closely monitored during HIV infection. Weight loss, particularly if it is rapid, is often caused by an opportunistic infection and indicates a poor prognosis; but even when body weight is stable, care must be taken to maintain lean body mass and ensure that it is not being replaced by fat. This section will first discuss the problems associated with measuring micronutrient status during HIV infection and then consider the mechanisms by which infection can adversely affect nutritional status.

Biochemical Indicators of Nutritional Status

During the early stages of HIV infection, before AIDS has developed, active virus replication occurs in lymph nodes.

This apparently triggers an acute phase response that makes it difficult to interpret markers of nutritional status, such as serum levels of iron, zinc, copper, and retinol (vitamin A). Decreased serum levels of these micronutrients in otherwise healthy individuals indicate decreased body stores. However, the levels of iron, zinc, retinol, and retinol-binding protein decrease during the acute phase response, while serum copper levels rise. In addition, serum albumin and prealbumin are typically decreased during the acute phase response. In the early stages of HIV infection when opportunistic infections have not yet begun and weight is stable, albumin levels should not be affected by HIV infection, although prealbumin, iron, zinc, copper, and retinol serum concentrations may be altered. There is no accepted way to adjust for the effects of infection on these levels. However, when there is clinical evidence of infection and in particular when there are objective indicators of immune system activation (e.g., elevations in neopterin, $beta_2$-microglobulin) or the acute phase response ($alpha_1$-antitrypsin, C-reactive protein, interleukin-1 or interleukin-6, or tumor necrosis factor), serum nutrient levels should be interpreted with caution.

Energy Expenditure and Nutrient Intake

Resting energy expenditure (REE) in HIV patients appears to be slightly increased. At least one study indicated that food intake does not increase to compensate for the increase, but voluntary physical activity may decrease slightly, perhaps to maintain energy balance. The decrease in physical activity may contribute to depletion of lean body mass. Maintaining food intake early in HIV infection is usually not a problem because the patient often feels well and can maintain a normal, active life. By contrast, food intake decreases dramatically when patients have acute febrile illnesses and diarrhea and is not accompanied by the decrease in energy expenditure that normally occurs during fasting in otherwise healthy persons. Intake is especially a problem when individuals have oral and esophageal infections, such as candidiasis or herpes, and resulting lesions in the mouth and throat make eating painful. The "double-whammy" of increased REE and decreased intake is a major factor in the precipitous weight loss that develops in individuals with the opportunistic infections of AIDS.

Decreased Absorption

In the early stages of HIV infection, malabsorption of fat and carbohydrates may develop even if symptoms are absent. The malabsorption may be caused by HIV infection of cells in the intestinal epithelium and lamina propria. Opportunistic gastrointestinal infections and diarrhea also develop frequently in individuals infected with HIV. Decreased fat, carbohydrate, and micronutrient absorption are problems during and after these infections and to a lesser extent during nonenteric infections; both types of infection can contribute to weight loss. In addition to decreased intake, malabsorption appears to be a principal cause of "slim disease" in central African patients with AIDS.

Increased Excretion

Nitrogen excretion resulting from catabolism of lean body mass is part of the body's response to metabolic stress (Chapters 7 and 21). Loss of other nutrients due to increased excretion may also occur. For example, retinol and zinc are excreted in the urine during severe metabolic stress, such as major surgery or serious infection. Urinary losses of these nutrients may be significant during opportunistic infections, but appear not to be a problem in early HIV infection.

Increased Requirements

It is possible that the requirements for some micronutrients increase during HIV and other infections, but supporting data are sparse. For example, with the increase in REE, it is plausible that requirements for B vitamins and antioxidant nutrients such as vitamin C may be increased. This does not mean that nutritional supplements are required, but depending on the quality of the diet, Recommended Daily Allowance (RDA)-level multivitamin and mineral supplements may be advantageous. Slightly higher levels of some nutrients such as vitamins E and C may also be beneficial, but megadose supplements have no demonstrated value and are not recommended. Long-term ingestion of megadoses of vitamin A and zinc may be harmful and should be discouraged.

Altered Metabolism

Altered metabolism creates difficulties in assessing the micronutrient status of individuals with HIV and other infections, as discussed previously. Chronic inflammatory diseases that perturb the metabolism of these nutrients can affect nutritional status. For example, the anemia associated with chronic inflammatory diseases such as rheumatoid arthritis apparently results from iron being sequestered in reticuloendothelial cells rather than transported to erythropoietic tissue. This derangement is apparently beneficial in individuals with acute bacterial infections but detrimental in individuals with chronic inflammation. Other examples of altered nutrient metabolism are not so clearly beneficial (or detrimental). Changes in energy substrate utilization (e.g., increased glucose utilization) are prominent in individuals with opportunistic infections. Amino acid metabolism is also dramatically altered in patients with acute illnesses, with muscle tissue being catabolized and acute phase proteins synthesized in the liver. The resulting negative nitrogen balance depletes lean body mass. This serious and fundamental alteration in protein metabolism is a factor in individuals with acute infections but does not appear to be important in the early stages of HIV infection.

PREVENTING MALNUTRITION IN HIV PATIENTS
Preventing and Treating Opportunistic Infections

The best way to prevent weight loss in HIV patients is to prevent opportunistic infections from developing. Similarly, the key to minimizing weight loss from an ongoing infection is to treat the infection; this will also allow compensatory weight gain to begin as soon as the infection clears. The development of effective drug regimens to prevent and treat infections has been singularly important in prolonging the lives of AIDS patients. A contributing factor to enhanced survival is also maintenance of lean body mass. As discussed in Chapter 21, nutritional interventions can reduce the loss of lean body mass during metabolic stress, but no intervention can prevent it altogether.

Nutrition Education and Intervention

Nutrition education and appropriate nutrition interventions should be integral components of the preventive health care planning and medical treatment of patients with HIV infection. Care should begin immediately when HIV infection is diagnosed, with a complete assessment of nutritional status and identification of risk factors for malnutrition (see Chapter 8). The evaluation should include assessment of lean body mass as a benchmark against which to monitor subsequent changes in body weight and composition. The nutritionist should develop an individualized nutrition care plan to address dietary or other risk factors for developing malnutrition and to correct nutritional deficiencies. The plan should be implemented through periodic nutrition education sessions and counseling that address healthful eating principles and how to achieve them, risks from food-borne pathogens, alternative feeding methods (e.g., making foods more palatable or nutrient dense and using oral nutritional supplements), and guidelines for evaluating the nutritional value of foods. Counseling should also address unfounded food fads and nutritional "therapies" that are often attractive to patients with HIV infection.

Vigorous nutritional support strategies including enteral and parenteral feeding sometimes become necessary when frank AIDS develops. These interventions should be designed to minimize as much as possible the loss of lean body mass from opportunistic infections and recoup what has already been lost.

Appetite Stimulants

Megestrol acetate is a synthetic progestational agent that has been used in treating metastatic breast cancer and stimulates appetite and promotes weight gain in anorexic patients. In AIDS patients with weight loss and anorexia who have used this drug, weight gain, increased appetite, and an enhanced sense of well-being have been reported. Studies differ on the composition of the resulting weight gain, variously reporting increases in fat mass only or in both fat and lean body mass. Its efficacy in improving lean body mass and survival is still under investigation. In addition, a synthetic form of an ingredient in marijuana called dronabinol is a proven antiemetic and may increase appetite and decrease nausea in AIDS patients who have anorexia. The FDA has approved its use for this purpose.

Anabolic Hormones

Human growth hormone is being tested for its ability to maintain and recover lean body mass. Preliminary data indicate that protein catabolism can be reversed, thus promoting a gain of lean body mass. These effects have been seen in healthy subjects as well as HIV-infected individuals. The results of short-term studies are promising, but data are not yet available on the long-term use of human growth hormone in AIDS patients.

Suggested Readings

American Dietetic Association and Canadian Dietetic Association: Nutrition intervention in the care of persons with human immunodeficiency virus infection, *J Am Diet Assoc* 94:1042, 1994. (Published erratum appears in *J Am Diet Assoc* 94:1254, 1994.)

Grunfeld C: What causes wasting in AIDS? *N Engl J Med* 333:123, 1995.

Jewett JF, Hecht FM: Preventive health care for adults with HIV infection, *JAMA* 269:1144, 1993.

Keusch GT, Thea DM: Malnutrition in AIDS, *Med Clin N Am* 77:795, 1993.

Macallan DC, Noble C, Baldwin C: Energy expenditure and wasting in human immunodeficiency virus infection, *N Engl J Med* 333:83, 1995.

Myrvik QN: *Immunology and nutrition.* In Shils ME, Olson JA, Shike M, eds: *Modern nutrition in health and disease,* ed 8, Philadelphia, 1994, Lea & Febiger.

28

Organ Transplantation

Transplantations are performed of the kidney, pancreas, liver, heart, bone marrow, lung, and intestine at many clinical centers throughout the United States and other countries. Malnutrition is common in these patients before transplantation, and nutrition can play a major role in the outcome. The effects of nutrition on transplantation fall into three categories: preoperative nutrition, postoperative nutrition, and nutritional effects of pharmacologic agents. The specific nutritional issues in each of these categories may vary depending on the organ being transplanted. For example, patients undergoing liver transplantation tend to have problems with protein metabolism whereas those receiving bone marrow transplants may experience nutritional problems secondary to graft-vs.-host disease.

Although preoperative and postoperative nutritional support are extremely important, there is currently no evidence that providing parenteral nutrition during the transplant operation is beneficial, and doing so may predispose the patient to metabolic abnormalities that are difficult to manage. It is important to monitor blood glucose levels and provide solutions containing 5% dextrose during liver transplantation to minimize hypoglycemia, which may occur because of loss of hepatic gluconeogenesis. In addition, close monitoring of glucose levels is necessary during pancreas transplantation, as well as administration of 5% dextrose and insulin as needed to maintain the proper levels of glucose.

Immunosuppressive drugs can affect nutritional status in many ways. Although the effects of these agents are not organ specific, their interaction with the metabolic problems caused by each particular organ failure can produce different nutritional problems.

Energy expenditure and protein requirements vary among the different types of transplants. In most instances, energy expenditure can be calculated using the basal energy expenditure (BEE) estimated from the Harris-Benedict equation (see Chapter 9); details are outlined in the sections that follow. However, if complications occur, if long-term feeding is required, or if other factors arise that affect energy expenditure, it is prudent to measure the resting energy expenditure (REE) with indirect calorimetry. Although general estimates of protein requirements are provided in this chapter, protein balance should be monitored using the methods in Chapter 9.

All patients who are potential candidates for organ transplantation should undergo a preoperative nutritional assessment to address and treat preexisting nutritional problems. Improving preoperative nutritional status can reduce the morbidity and mortality associated with transplantation. This chapter will discuss some of the common nutritional problems associated with organ transplantation and immunosuppressive drugs. Nutritional issues in patients with hepatic and renal failure prior to transplantation are discussed in more detail in Chapters 20 and 23.

IMMUNOSUPPRESSIVE DRUGS

All transplant patients must receive immunosuppressive drugs to prevent rejection of the transplanted organ. In addition, patients undergoing bone marrow transplantation receive high-dose chemotherapy and sometimes radiation therapy. Common immunosuppressive agents include corticosteroids, cyclosporine, FK506, azathioprine, antilymphocyte globulin (ALG), and OKT3. These agents have different metabolic effects that may contribute to nutritional problems in transplant patients.

Corticosteroids are widely used in patients undergoing organ transplantation and often produce increased appetite, protein catabolism, sodium and fluid retention, hypertension, insulin resistance and hyperglycemia, hyperlipidemia, hypokalemia, and hypercalciuria. Large doses of corticosteroids are administered in the immediate postoperative period and tapered to a maintenance dose that must usually be maintained indefinitely, creating a substantial risk for osteoporosis. Patients receiving corticosteroids on a long-term basis should be advised to obtain adequate dietary calcium and perform weight-bearing exercises regularly if possible.

Cyclosporine is also used in most patients receiving transplants. Side effects include hypertension, nephrotoxicity (common), hepatotoxicity (uncommon), hyperlipidemia, glucose intolerance, hyperkalemia, and hypomagnesemia. FK506 is similar to cyclosporine in its mechanism of action although nausea, vomiting, and diarrhea may develop more frequently and hyperlipidemia and hypertension less frequently. ALG and OKT3 do not have many nutritional or metabolic complications but can lead to a flu-like syndrome during which nutrient intake may be depressed. Patients receiving azathioprine can develop nausea, vomiting, altered taste acuity, and liver dysfunction.

RENAL TRANSPLANTATION

As discussed in Chapter 23, malnutrition is common among patients with renal failure, in part because of the various dietary restrictions placed on patients with chronic renal failure, including sodium, potassium, phosphorus, magnesium, protein, and fluid restrictions. These restrictions in addition to the anorexia associated with renal failure commonly result in weight loss and micronutrient deficiencies. After transplantation, the return of adequate renal function allows many of the dietary restrictions to be removed. However, it may take some time before nutritional status improves, especially because immunosuppressive drugs administered to patients after a transplant can aggravate preexisting nutritional problems. Early in the posttransplant period, corticosteroids, cyclosporine, and FK506 may exacerbate hyperglycemia, protein catabolism, hypertension, and hyperlipidemia. The nutritional effects of immunosuppressive drugs may also be apparent during episodes of rejection when higher doses are administered.

In the early posttransplant period, the diet should be adequate (but not excessive) in energy and provide sources of high biologic-value protein such as egg whites and low-fat dairy products. Energy intake should be about 20% higher than the BEE value (estimated from the Harris-Benedict equation). Protein intake should be 1.3 to 2 g/kg per day. In addition, the diet should be low in salt, simple sugars (to help control hypertriglyceridemia), and saturated fat. Patients who develop complications or whose recovery from the transplant is delayed may need enteral or parenteral feeding to help meet their needs.

There are a number of long-term nutritional issues in renal transplant patients. Excessive weight gain can be a problem because of relaxed dietary restrictions, improved appetite and sense of well-being, and corticosteroid treatment. Avoiding excess calories and exercising regularly can help maintain an appropriate weight. There is a significant risk for cardiovascular disease in patients with diabetes mellitus and hypertension, so these conditions and hyperlipidemia must be controlled as well as possible using diet and pharmacologic treatment (if necessary). Some studies have suggested that a diet low in nucleotides (e.g., organ meats, meat extracts, anchovies, sardines) may augment the effect of cyclosporine and produce less rejection. There is also evidence that administration of fish oil containing omega-3 fatty acids has a beneficial effect on renal hemodynamics and blood pressure and is associated with significantly fewer rejection episodes. In addition, moderate protein restriction may decrease the progression of renal disease after transplantation.

PANCREAS TRANSPLANTATION

Transplantation of the pancreas is sometimes performed for patients with Type I diabetes mellitus and is usually done in conjunction with renal transplantation. Therefore many of the nutritional issues related to renal transplantation also apply to these patients. Side effects of diabetes, such as gastroparesis, are common in pancreas transplant patients. After successful transplantation, blood sugar levels return to normal.

LIVER TRANSPLANTATION

Preoperative malnutrition is common among patients with chronic liver failure who are candidates for transplantation. These patients may have decreased fat and lean-tissue stores, altered protein metabolism, sodium and water retention with ascites and edema, and vitamin and mineral deficiencies. Appropriate dietary treatment is necessary (see Chapter 20). In the preoperative period, selective bowel decontamination with antibiotics appears to reduce the incidence of infections in the early posttransplant period. Some centers using this treatment restrict foods including cheese, raw fruits, and raw vegetables that may contain certain bacteria. However, it is not clear to what extent the dietary restrictions add to the benefits of antibiotic treatment, and eliminating these foods could contribute to malnutrition.

In the early posttransplant period, energy expenditure does not appear to be substantially altered. However, there is an increase in protein catabolism, which gradually decreases but is not eliminated in most patients as clinical improvement occurs over the first month. This may be due to the perioperative stress, breakdown and use of endogenous amino acids as an energy source, and posttransplant corticosteroid therapy. Sodium and water retention and bicarbonate and potassium wasting can persist into the posttransplant period.

Some patients require parenteral nutrition in the preoperative period, and it is also used by many centers in the immediate posttransplant period. Approximately 1.2 g/kg per day of protein is usually provided. Although some centers use a formula enriched in branched-chain amino acids initially, its use is more appropriate in patients with hepatic encephalopathy. Barring complications, patients can often initiate oral feedings by the third postoperative day. Once oral intake is established, the administration of intravenous lipids can be discontinued. When the oral intake meets 50% of estimated requirements, parenteral nutrition can be decreased by 50% and discontinued as oral intake improves. Instead of using parenteral nutrition, some centers advocate starting enteral feeding within 18 hours of operation. Serum electrolyte and urea levels should be monitored periodically, and protein intake may need to be adjusted. If complications occur, nitrogen balance should be monitored with the goal of avoiding a negative balance but not necessarily achieving a positive balance because it is rarely possible until the metabolic stress subsides and clinical improvement occurs.

CARDIAC TRANSPLANTATION

Heart transplantations are most commonly performed in patients with cardiomyopathy resulting from ischemic heart disease. Candidates for heart transplantation commonly have cardiac cachexia caused by a combination of hypermetabolism, anorexia, and possibly malabsorption. Many patients also have diabetes mellitus, hypertension, or hyperlipidemia underlying their ischemic heart disease. Posttransplant dietary recommendations must take these factors into consideration.

As in patients receiving other organ transplants, parenteral nutrition may be required in the postoperative period, particularly if complications arise. Some studies have shown that depressed cardiac function is associated with high rates of lipid infusion, but this does not appear to be clinically significant at low infusion rates. Dietary prescriptions in the posttransplant period vary among centers, but most commonly a low-sodium, low-fat, low-cholesterol diet is prescribed to treat the salt and water retention, hypertension, and hyperlipidemia that often develop. In the immediate postoperative period, some centers liberalize calorie and protein intake to prevent weight loss and negative nitrogen balance. Patients commonly receive 1.2 to 1.5 g/kg per day of protein immediately postoperatively followed by 1 to 1.2 g/kg per day after 1 to 2 weeks. Drug therapy for hypercholesterolemia may be necessary in severe cases but should be used with extreme caution. Lovastatin has caused myositis in some patients, particularly when used with cyclosporine, gemfibrozil, or niacin.

BONE MARROW TRANSPLANTATION

Bone marrow transplantation has been used to treat a variety of malignant and benign hematologic disorders including leukemia, aplastic anemia, and thalassemia major. Treatment is intense, using chemotherapy and sometimes radiation therapy before transplantation, and complications are common. Thus many converging factors can predispose patients to nutritional problems. Patients receiving high-dose chemotherapy may experience nausea and vomiting and develop oropharyngeal mucositis, esophagitis, or altered taste perception. Liver disease may also occur.

Patients often receive parenteral nutrition before and after bone marrow transplantation. Enteral nutrition has advantages (see Chapter 12) but is often difficult to tolerate because of nausea, vomiting, and mucositis. The general recommendation for energy intake is 30% to 50% above the BEE as calculated by the Harris-Benedict equation. About 1.5 g/kg per day of protein is generally provided. Diarrhea secondary to chemotherapy and radiation therapy frequently develops after transplantation and may persist for weeks. However, diarrhea itself is not a contraindication to enteral feeding. If acute graft-vs.-host disease develops diarrhea can be severe. Vitamin and trace element deficiencies including vitamin K, thiamin, vitamin E, and zinc have developed in bone marrow transplant patients.

Nutritional problems remain highly prevalent during the first year after bone marrow transplantation, particularly if the individual has chronic graft-vs.-host disease, which can develop in up to two thirds of patients. Common symptoms include weight loss, oral sensitivity, xerostomia, stomatitis, anorexia, gastrointestinal reflux symptoms, and diarrhea. For these reasons, long-term monitoring of nutritional status is important.

LUNG TRANSPLANTATION

Lung transplants are performed for patients with cystic fibrosis, chronic obstructive pulmonary disease, idiopathic pulmonary fibrosis, primary pulmonary hypertension, and other conditions. Patients with cystic fibrosis and emphysema tend to be more malnourished before transplants than those with idiopathic pulmonary fibrosis and primary pulmonary hypertension. Lung transplant patients can experience prolonged ileus postoperatively because most procedures include omentopexy, in which the bronchial anastomosis is wrapped with omentum to enhance healing. Therefore most patients receive parenteral nutrition after the transplant.

Relatively little has been published about nutritional support in lung transplant patients. Energy and protein requirements have not been precisely defined, but overfeeding could potentially create problems in these patients. Excess energy intake can increase the metabolic rate, oxygen requirements, and carbon dioxide production (see Chapter 22), which creates an additional burden for patients whose pulmonary function is already inadequate (particularly for those being weaned from a ventilator) and requires a careful assessment of energy needs that includes indirect calorimetry.

INTESTINAL TRANSPLANTATION

Intestinal transplantation for intestinal failure is performed at only a few centers. Because most patients with intestinal failure can be maintained indefinitely with home parenteral nutrition, transplantation is usually done as a last resort when venous access has become impossible or hepatic failure develops (in which case the liver is also transplanted). Postoperatively, most patients require parenteral nutrition for a period of at least 1 to 2 months. Enteral tube feeding can be used once peristalsis of the transplanted bowel begins. Medium-chain triglycerides are used as a fat source because the lymphatic channels are severed during the transplant operation. Mortality is high after intestinal transplantation, but many patients who survive are able to discontinue home parenteral nutrition.

Suggested Readings

Nutrition and transplantation series, *Nutr Clin Pract* 8:3, 1993.

Appendixes

Normal Laboratory Values

	Normal values*
Hematology	
Hematocrit (Hct)	
Men	39%-49%
Women	34%-44%
Hemoglobin (Hgb)	
Men	14-17 g/dl
Women	12-15 g/dl
Children	12-14 g/dl
Newborn	14.5-24.5 g/dl
Mean cell volume (MCV)	83-99 fl
Mean cell hemoglobin (MCH)	27-32 pg
Mean cell hemoglobin concentration (MCHC)	32%-36%
Platelets	150,000-400,000/mm^3
Reticulocytes	0.5%-1.5%
White blood cells (WBC)	4,000-11,000/mm^3
Differential (Diff)	
Lymphocytes	15%-52% (higher in children)
Neutrophils	35%-73% (lower in children)
Monocytes	2%-10%

*Normal ranges vary among different laboratories.

Continued

	Normal values*
Hematology—cont'd	
Differential (Diff)—cont'd	
Eosinophils	0-5%
Basophils	0-2%
Serum iron (Fe)	60-180 µg/dl
Transferrin	212-405 mg/dl
Iron-binding capacity	
(total) (TIBC) %	250-450 µg/dl
saturation	15%-55%
Serum ferritin	
Males 18-30 years	30-233 ng/ml
Males 31-60 years	32-284 ng/ml
Premenopausal females	6-81 ng/ml
Postmenopausal females	14-186 ng/ml
Blood chemistry	
Alkaline phosphatase	
(Alk phos)	
1-3 mo	150-475 U/L
To 10 yr	120-320 U/L
Puberty	120-540 U/L
Adults	39-117 U/L
Ammonia (NH_3)	11-35 µmol/L
Bilirubin (Bili)	
Total	0-1 mg/dl
Direct	0.1-0.3 mg/dl
Calcium (Ca^{++})	8.4-10.2 mg/dl
Carbon dioxide content	23-29 mEq/L
(HCO_3^-)	
Carotene	79-233 µg/dl
Chloride (Cl^-)	96-108 mEq/L
Creatinine	0.4-1.2 mg/dl
GGT (gamma glutamyl	0-65 U/L
transpeptidase)	
GOT (AST, aspartate	0-31 U/L
aminotransferase)	
GPT (ALT, alanine	0-31 U/L
aminotransferase)	

*Normal ranges vary among different laboratories.

	Normal values*
Blood chemistry—cont'd	
Glucose, fasting	70-105 mg/dl
LDH (lactic dehydroge-nase)	120-240 U/L
Magnesium (Mg^{++})	1.7-2.2 mg/dl
Osmolality	280-305 mOsm/kg plasma
Phosphorus (Phos)	
Children	4.0-7.0 mg/dl
Adults	2.7-4.5 mg/dl
Potassium (K^+)	3.3-5.1 mEq/L
Proteins	
Total	6.5-8 g/dl
Albumin	3.5-5 g/dl
α_1 Globulin	0.15-0.4 g/dl
α_2 Globulin	0.5-0.9 g/dl
β Globulin	0.7-1.1 g/dl
γ Globulin	0.5-1.5 g/dl
Sodium (Na^+)	133-145 mEq/L
Urea nitrogen (BUN)	6-19 mg/dl
Nutrients	
(vitamins)	See Table 2-4
Urine tests (24-hour excretion; varies with intake)	
Calcium	100-240 mg (5-12 mEq)
Creatinine	See Tables 8-5 and 8-6
Magnesium	72-103 mg (6-8.6 mEq)
Phosphorus	0.7-1.5 g
Potassium	0.8-3.9 (20-100 mEq)
Sodium	3-8 g (130-360 mEq)
Urea nitrogen (UUN)	See Table 8-5
Stool tests	
Fat	
Total	<6 g/24 hr (with dietary fat intake >50 g/day); <30% of dry matter
Neutral	1%-5% of dry matter
Free fatty acids	1%-10% of dry matter

Continued

	Normal values*
Stool tests—cont'd	
Fat—cont'd	
Combined fatty acids (as soap)	1%-12% of dry matter
Nitrogen	<2 g/24 hr or 10% of urinary nitrogen
Function tests	
D-xylose absorption test: after overnight fast, 25 g xylose taken by mouth; urine collected for following 5 hr	Urine xylose 4-9 g/5 hr (or >20% of ingested dose); serum xylose 25-40 mg/dl 2 hr after oral dose
Schilling test: orally administered radio labeled vitamin B_{12} after "flushing" parenteral injection of B_{12}; intrinsic factor deficiency diagnosed with combination of pernicious anemia, gastric atrophy, and normalization of B_{12} excretion after exogenous intrinsic factor	Excretion in urine of >10% of oral dose/24 hr

*Normal ranges vary among different laboratories.

B

Commonly Used Equations

Equation	Reference chapter
Energy requirements	
Basal energy expenditure (Harris-Benedict equations), kcal/day	9

Men: BEE = 66.47 + 13.75W + 5.00H − 6.76A
Women: BEE = 655.10 + 9.56W + 1.85H − 4.68A

where

W = Weight (kg)
H = Height (cm)
A = Age (years)

FOR WEIGHT MAINTENANCE IN MOST PATIENTS   9

Energy requirement = BEE × 1.2-1.5

FOR WEIGHT GAIN IN STABLE PATIENTS   9

Energy goal = BEE × 2

Circulatory indirect calorimetry
(Fick equation for use in patients with
pulmonary artery catheters)

REE = CO × Hb(S_AO_2 − S_VO_2) × 95.18

Continued

where

REE = Resting energy expenditure, kcal/day
 CO = Cardiac output, L/min
 Hb = Hemoglobin, g/dl
S_AO_2 = Arterial oxygen saturation (decimal)
S_VO_2 = Mixed venous oxygen saturation (decimal)

FOR WEIGHT MAINTENANCE IN BURN PATIENTS   21
*Toronto formula** (probably most accurate)

Energy requirement $= -4343 + (10.5 \times \% \text{ TBSA}) +$
$(0.23 \times \text{CI}) + (0.84 \times \text{BEE}) + (114 \times \text{Temp}) - (4.5 \times \text{PBD})$

Modified Curreri formula (for TBSA ≤40%;
may overestimate requirements)

$= (20 \text{ kcal} \times \text{Wt}) + (40 \times \% \text{ TBSA})$

Traditional method (for TBSA > 40%; may
overestimate requirements)

$= \text{BEE} \times 2$

where

TBSA = Percent total body surface area burned
        (whole number, not decimal), estimated on
        admission and corrected where needed for
        amputation
   CI = Number of calories received in the
        previous 24 hours, including all dextrose,
        TPN, and tube feeding
 Temp = Average of hourly rectal temperature
        in the previous 24 hours (°C)
  PBD = Number of days postburn on the
        previous day
  BEE = Basal energy expenditure estimated by
        the Harris-Benedict equations
   Wt = Body weight in kilograms

*Allard JP, et al: Validation of a new formula for calculating the energy
 requirements of burn patients, *JPEN* 14:115, 1990.

Equation	Reference chapter

Protein loss

Urinary urea nitrogen

MOST PATIENTS ⟶ 8

Protein catabolic rate (g/day) =
$$[\text{24-hour UUN (g)} + 4] \times 6.25$$

BURN PATIENTS ⟶ 21

Protein catabolic rate (g/day) =
$$[\text{UUN} + (0.2\ \text{g} \times \%\ 3°) + (0.1\ \text{g} \times \%\ 2°)] \times 6.25$$

where
UUN = Measured urinary urea nitrogen in grams

% 3° = Percent body surface area with 3°
(full-thickness) burns (*whole number,
not decimal*)
% 2° = Percent body surface area with 2°
(partical-thickness) burns (*whole number,
not decimal*)

*Urea nitrogen appearance for patients with
changing BUN and/or body water* ⟶ 8

$$\text{UNA (g)} = \text{UUN (g)} + \frac{(\Delta\text{BUN} \times 10)(W_m)(BW) + (BUN_m \times 10)(\Delta W)}{1000}$$

where

ΔBUN = Change in BUN (mg/dl) during the urine
collection (Final BUN − Initial BUN)
BUN_m = Mean BUN (mg/dl) during the urine
collection [(Final BUN + Initial BUN)/2]
ΔW = Change in weight (kg) during the urine
collection (Final weight − Initial weight)
W_m = Mean weight (kg) during the urine
collection [(Final weight + initial weight)/2]
BW = Assumed body water as a proportion of
body weight (normal value = 0.5 for women and
0.6 for men; 0.05 subtracted for marked obesity or
dehydration; 0.05 added for leanness or edema)

Continued

Equation	Reference chapter
Protein balance	8
Protein balance (g/day) = Protein intake − Protein catabolic rate	
Midarm muscle circumference (MAMC)	8
MAMC (cm) = Upper arm circumference (cm) − [0.314 × triceps skinfold (mm)]	
Body mass index	15
$$BMI = \frac{Weight\ (kg)}{Height^2\ (m)}$$	
Total lymphocyte count (TLC)	8
TLC = Total white blood cell count × % lymphocytes	
Relative protein content of diet	9
Relative protein content (% of kcal) = $$\frac{Protein\ content\ (g) \times 4\ kcal/g \times 100}{Energy\ content}$$ Desired protein intake (g) = $$\frac{Energy\ requirement \times \%\ protein\ desired}{4\ kcal/g \times 100}$$	
Protein and energy content of parenteral nutrition formulas	13
Protein content = (ml aa)[aa conc (g/ml)] Energy content = (Protein content)(4 kcal/g) + (ml dex) [Dex conc (g/ml)](3.4 kcal/g) + (ml lipid)(1.1 or 2 kcal/ml)	

Equation	Reference chapter

where

Dex = Dextrose
  aa = Amino acids
conc = Concentration (e.g., 50% dextrose = 0.5
      g/ml and 8.5% amino acids = 0.085 g/ml
      1.1 kcal/ml applies to 10% lipid and 2 kcal/ml to
      20% lipid.

Respiratory quotient   9, 22

$$RQ = \frac{\text{Liters } CO_2 \text{ produced}}{\text{Liters } O_2 \text{ consumed}}$$

The RQ for oxidation of fat = 0.7;
for protein = 0.80; for carbohydrate = 1.

Stool osmotic gap   12

Stool osmotic gap = Stool osmolality −
          2 (Stool sodium + Stool potassium)
>140 = Osmotic diarrhea (likely due to
      medications or possibly tube feeding)
<100 = Secretory diarrhea (possibly due to
      pseudomembranous colitis or nonosmotic
      medications)

LDL cholesterol level   18

LDL cholesterol = Total cholesterol −
          (Triglycerides/5 + HDL cholesterol)
HDL cholesterol can be estimated as 40 to 45
  mg/dl if unknown.

Vitamin and Mineral Supplements

Because most vitamin supplements are classified by the U.S. Food and Drug Administration as foods rather than as drugs, they are not tightly regulated. However, vitamin preparations designated United States Pharmacopeia (USP) conform to established standards. It is important for clinicians to know the contents of the supplements they prescribe. A few generalizations can be made about multivitamin preparations:

1. There are no guidelines for the composition of multivitamins. Therefore amounts of specific micronutrients such as water-soluble vitamins and minerals vary widely from one manufacturer to another.
2. The fat-soluble vitamin content of most multivitamins is 100% to 200% of the Recommended Daily Allowance (RDA).
3. Multivitamins containing more than 400 μg of folic acid cannot be purchased without a prescription (see Chapter 24).
4. Few multivitamins contain vitamin K.
5. When supplied, the biotin content of multivitamins is between 5% and 15% of the recommended intake. (There is no RDA as such for biotin.)
6. The names of multivitamins can be deceiving. For instance, the term *stress vitamin* is a marketing tool and bears no relation to the physiologic stress referred to in this book. In fact, these preparations are marketed mainly to normal persons with "stressful" lifestyles, and yet there is no evidence that the normal stresses of

daily living increase vitamin requirements or that vitamin use aids in stress management.

Multivitamins are available with or without minerals. Both of these categories can be subdivided as follows according to the proportion of the RDA for most vitamins that they contain:

1. *Replacement vitamins* provide up to 100% of the RDA. Most pediatric multivitamins are in this category.
2. *Therapeutic vitamins* provide 100% to 200% of the RDA. Prenatal multivitamins fit in this category. There are no therapeutic multivitamins without minerals.
3. *Super-therapeutic vitamins* provide 200% to 1000% of the RDA. There are currently no multivitamins that strictly fit into this category, because most of the "stress" multivitamins have very large amounts of some individual vitamins, RDA amounts of others, and often omit some entirely. To consume these doses, individual vitamin supplements are often required. Levels of supplementation greater than 10 times the RDA are generally termed *megadose therapy*.

Vitamin supplementation is indicated in the following individuals. (Specific examples and recommended doses are listed in Tables 2-4 and 2-5.)

1. Pregnant and lactating women (chiefly calcium, iron, and folic acid; see Chapters 3 and 4); should consider folic acid supplementation for women of child-bearing potential also if their diets are not adequate
2. Newborns and infants (see Chapter 4)
3. Individuals in certain high-risk situations such as having a low socioeconomic status, having anorexia nervosa, participating in certain very-low calorie obesity regimens, and some persons who are elderly or vegans (strict vegetarians)
4. Individuals with documented deficiency states
5. Individuals with conditions or taking medications that interfere with micronutrient intake, digestion, absorption, metabolism, or excretion, such as malabsorptive gastrointestinal disorders, heavy menses, and renal dialysis
6. Individuals with vitamin-dependent genetic disorders

and diseases associated with defective vitamin transport
7. As an antidote in individuals who have ingested toxic antivitamins (e.g., folinic acid after high-dose methotrexate)
8. May add other indications periodically, if the results of research indicate that supplementation in addition to the RDA helps prevent or treat specific conditions (e.g., vitamin E supplementation in persons with CAD); many of these considered controversial

Pregnant or lactating women and infants should be given the appropriate multivitamins designed for them. Persons in the third group discussed should use a replacement multivitamin to achieve the RDA. Therapeutic vitamins are appropriate for treatment of deficiencies (fourth group), whereas doses in the super-therapeutic or megadose range are often needed for the individuals in the fifth, sixth, and seventh groups.

Multiple vitamin preparations

Name	Manufac-turer	Vitamin A (3333 IU)	Vitamin D (400 IU)	Vitamin E (10 IU)	Vitamin C (60 mg)	Thiamin B_1 (1.5 mg)	Ribo-flavin B_2 (1.8 mg)	Niacin B_3 (20 mg)	Pyridox-ine B_6 (2mg)
Replacement vitamins									
Adavite	Hudson	5000	400	30	90	3	3.4	30	3
Theravee	Vangard	5500	400	30	120	3	3.4	30	3
Thera-generix	Goldine	5000	400	30	90	3	3.4	20	
Thera-gran	Apothe-con	5000	400	30	90	3	3.4	20	3
Theravim	Nature's Bounty	5000	400	30	120	3	3.4	30	3
One-A-Day Essential	Miles Inc	5000	400	30	60	1.5	1.7	20	2
Dayalets	Abbott	5000	400	30	60	1.5	1.7	20	2
Family Tabs	Schein	5000	400	30	300	1.5	1.7	20	2
Unicap	Upjohn	5000	400	15	60	1.5	1.7	20	2
Centrum	Lederle	5000	400	30	60	1.5	1.7	20	2

Amounts of vitamins and minerals (RDA)

Continued

Multiple vitamin preparations—cont'd

Name	Manufacturer		Amounts of vitamins and minerals (RDA)								
		Folate (.2 mg)	B-12 (2 μg)	Beta carotene (IU)	Iron (15 mg)	Magnesium (400 mg)	Iodine (150 μg)	Zinc (15 mg)	Calcium (1200 mg)	Phosphorus (1200 mg)
Replacement vitamins—cont'd										
Adavite	Hudson	0.4	9	1250	—	—	—	—	—	—
Theravee	Vangard	0.4	3	—	—	—	—	—	—	—
Thera-generix	Goldline	0.4	9	—	—	—	—	—	—	—
Thera-gran	Apothecon	0.4	9	—	—	—	—	—	—	—
Theravim	Nature's Bounty	0.5	9	2500	—	—	—	—	—	—
One-A-Day Essential	Miles Inc	0.4	6	—	—	—	—	—	—	—
Dayalets	Abbott	0.4	6	—	—	—	—	—	—	—
Family Tabs	Schein	0.4	6	5000	—	—	—	—	—	—
Unicap	Upjohn	0.4	6	—	18	100	150	15	—	—
Centrum	Lederle	0.4	6	—	—	100	150	15	162	109

Multiple vitamin preparations—cont'd

Name	Manufacturer	Vitamin A (3333 IU) (per 5 ml)	Vitamin D (400 IU)	Vitamin E (10 IU)	Vitamin C (60 mg)	Thiamin B₁ (1.5 mg)	Riboflavin B₂ (1.8 mg)	Niacin B₃ (20 mg)	Pyridoxine B₆ (2mg)
Liquid replacement vitamins (per 5 ml)									
Syrite	Barre-National	2500	400	15	60	1.05	1.2	13.5	1.05
Daily Vitamins	Rugby	2500	400	15	60	1.05	1.2	13.5	1.05
Vi-Daylin Multi-vitamin	Ross	2500	400	11	60	1.05	1.2	13.5	1.05
Replacement vitamins with minerals									
Decagen	Goldeline	9000	400	30	90	10	10	20	5
Theravee-M	Vangard	5000	400	30	120	3	3.4	30	3
Adavite-M	Hudson	5000	400	30	90	3	3.4	20	3
Theravim-M	Nature's Bounty	5000	400	30	120	3	3.4	30	3

Continued

Multiple vitamin preparations—cont'd

Name	Manufacturer	Folate (.2 mg)	B-12 (2 µg)	Beta carotene (IU)	Iron (15 mg)	Magnesium (400 mg)	Iodine (150 µg)	Zinc (15 mg)	Calcium (1200 mg)	Phosphorus (1200 mg)
Liquid replacement vitamins (per 5 ml)										
Syrite	Barre-National	—	4.5	—	—	—	—	—	—	—
Daily Vitamins	Rugby	—	4.5	—	—	—	—	—	—	—
Vi-Daylin Multi-vitamin	Ross	—	4.5	—	—	—	—	—	—	—
Replacement vitamins with minerals										
Decagen	Goldeline	0.4	10	—	30	—	—	15	—	—
Theravee-M	Vangard	0.4	9	2500	27	—	—	15	—	—
Adavite-M	Hudson	0.4	9	—	27	—	—	15	—	—
Theravim-M	Nature's Bounty	0.4	9	2500	27	—	—	15	—	—

Amounts of vitamins and minerals (RDA)

Multiple vitamin preparations—cont'd

Name	Manufac-turer	Amounts of vitamins and minerals (RDA)								
		Vitamin A (3333 IU)	Vitamin D (400 IU)	Vitamin E (10 IU)	Vitamin C (60 mg)	Thiamin B₁ (1.5 mg)	Ribo-flavin B₂ (1.8 mg)	Niacin B₃ (20 mg)	Pyridox-ine B₆ (2mg)
Replacement vitamins with minerals—cont'd									
Optilets-M-500	Abbott	5000	400	30	500	15	10	100	5
Unicap T	Upjohn	5000	400	30	90	10	10	100	6
Avail	Menley and James	5000	400	30	90	2.25	2.55	203	3
Myadec	Parke Davis	5000	400	30	60	1.7	2	20	3
One-A-Day Maximum Formula	Miles	5000	400	30	60	1.5	1.7	20	2
Centrum Jr. + Iron	Lederle	5000	400	30	60	1.5	1.7	20	2
Unicap M	Upjohn	5000	400	30	60	1.5	1.7	20	2

Continued

Multiple vitamin preparations—cont'd

Name	Manufacturer	Amounts of vitamins and minerals (RDA)								
		Folate (.2 mg)	B-12 (2 μg)	Beta carotene (IU)	Iron (15 mg)	Magnesium (400 mg)	Iodine (150 μg)	Zinc (15 mg)	Calcium (1200	Phosphorus (1200 mg)
Replacement vitamins with minerals—cont'd										
Optilets-M-500	Abbott	—	12	—	18	80	150	1.5	20	—
Unicap T	Upjohn	0.4	18	—	18	—	150	15	—	—
Avail	Menley and James	0.4	9	—	18	100	150	22.5	400	—
Myadec	Parke Davis	0.4	6	—	18	100	150	15	162	125
One-A-Day Maximum Formula	Miles	0.4	6	—	18	100	150	15	129.6	100
Centrum Jr. + Iron	Lederle	0.4	6	—	18	40	150	15	108	50
Unicap M	Upjohn	0.4	6	—	18	—	150	15	—	—

Multiple vitamin preparations—cont'd

Name	Manufacturer	Amounts of vitamins and minerals (RDA)							
		Vitamin A (3333 IU)	Vitamin D (400 IU)	Vitamin E (10 IU)	Vitamin C (60 mg)	Thiamin B_1 (1.5 mg)	Riboflavin B_2 (1.8 mg)	Niacin B_3 (20 mg)	Pyridoxine B_6 (2mg)
Therapeutic vitamins with or without minerals									
Quintabs-M	Freeda	10,000	400	50	300	30	30	150	30
Generix T	Goldline	10,000	400	5.5	150	15	10	100	2
Total Formula	Vitaline	10,000	400	30	100	15	15	25	25
Nova-Dec	Rugby	9000	400	30	90	10	10	20	5
Centrum Silver	Lederle	6000	400	45	60	1.5	1.7	20	3
Theragran-M	Apothecon	6250	400	30	90	3	3.4	30	3
Liquid therapeutic vitamins (per 5 ml)									
Theragran	Apothecon	10,000	400	—	200	10	10	100	4.1
Theravite	Barre-National	10,000	400	—	200	10	10	100	4.1

Continued

Multiple vitamin preparations—cont'd

Name	Manufacturer	Folate (.2 mg)	B-12 (2 µg)	Beta carotene (IU)	Iron (15 mg)	Magnesium (400 mg)	Iodine (150 µg)	Zinc (15 mg)	Calcium (1200)	Phosphorus (1200 mg)
Therapeutic vitamins with or without minerals										
Quintabs-M	Freeda	0.4	30	—	15	—	—	30	—	—
Generix T	Goldline	—	7.5	—	15	—	—	1.5	—	—
Total Formula	Vitaline	0.4	25	—	20	—	—	30	—	—
Nova-Dec	Rugby	0.4	10	—	30	100	150	15	—	—
Centrum Silver	Lederle	0.2	25	—	9	100	150	15	200	48
Theragran-M	Apothecon	0.4	9	—	27	100	150	15	40	31
Liquid therapeutic vitamins (per 5 ml)										
Theragran	Apothecon	—	5	—	—	—	—	—	—	—
Theravite	Barre-National	—	5	—	—	—	—	—	—	—

Multiple vitamin preparations—cont'd

Name	Manufacturer	Amounts of vitamins and minerals (RDA)								
		Vitamin A (3333 IU)	Vitamin D (400 IU)	Vitamin E (10 IU)	Vitamin C (60 mg)	Thiamin B_1 (1.5 mg)	Ribo-flavin B_2 (1.8 mg)	Niacin B_3 (20 mg)	Pyridox-ine B_6 (2mg)
Prenatal vitamins									
Natafort Filmseals	Parke Davis	6000	400	30	120	3	2	20	15
Zenate	Solvay	4000	400	10	70	1.5	1.6	17	2.2
Filibon Forte	Lederle	8000	400	45	90	2	2.5	30	3
Prenate 90	Bock	4000	400	30	120	3	3.4	20	20
Materna	Lederle	5000	400	30	100	3	3.4	20	10
Secran	Scherer	8000	400	30	60	1.7	2	20	2.5
Niferex-PN Forte	Central	5000	400	30	80	3	3.4	20	4
Pramet FA	Ross	4000	400	—	100	3	2	10	5
Natalins RX	Mead Johnson	4000	400	15	80	1.5	1.6	17	4
Stuart-Natal 1 + 1	Wyeth Ayerst	4000	400	11	120	1.5	3	20	10

Continued

Multiple vitamin preparations—cont'd

Name	Manufacturer		Amounts of vitamins and minerals (RDA)								
		Folate (.2 mg)	B-12 (2 μg)	Beta carotene (IU)	Iron (15 mg)	Magnesium (400 mg)	Iodine (150 μg)	Zinc (15 mg)	Calcium (1200 mg)	Phosphorus (1200 mg)
Prenatal vitamins—cont'd										
Natafort Filmseals	Parke Davis	1	6	—	65	100	150	25	350	—
Zenate	Solvay	1	2.2	—	65	100	175	15	200	—
Filibon Forte	Lederle	1	12	—	45	100	200	—	300	—
Prenate 90	Bock	1	12	—	90	—	150	25	250	—
Materna	Lederle	1	12	—	60	25	150	25	250	—
Secran	Scherer	1	8	—	60	—	—	20	250	—
Niferex-PN Forte	Central	1	12	—	60	10	200	25	250	—
Pramet FA	Ross	1	3	—	60	—	100	—	250	—
Natalins RX	Mead Johnson	1	2.5	—	60	100	—	25	200	—
Stuart-Natal 1 + 1	Wyeth Ayerst	1	12	—	65	—	—	25	200	—

D

Conversion Factors for Various Minerals

SODIUM (Na$^+$)

Molecular weight = 23
1 mEq Na$^+$ = 23 mg
1 g Na$^+$ = 43 mEq (1000 mg/23 mg per mEq)
1 g NaCl = 0.4 g Na$^+$ (Na$^+$ = 40% of weight of NaCl)
1 g Na$^+$ = 2.5 g NaCl

POTASSIUM (K$^+$)

Molecular weight = 39
1 mEq K$^+$ = 39 mg

CALCIUM (Ca^{++})

Molecular weight = 40
1 mEq Ca^{++} = 20 mg (40/2)
For example, 15 mEq Ca^{++} in TPN = 300 mg

MAGNESIUM (Mg^{++})

Molecular weight = 24
1 mEq Mg^{++} = 12 mg (24/2)

PHOSPHORUS (P, phos)

Molecular weight = 31
1 mmol P = 31 mg

E

Intestinal Fluid

Volumes of fluid entering and leaving the intestinal tract daily

	Ingestion and secretion		Reabsorption		
Fluid*	Volume entering lumen (L)	Intestinal segment	Volume reabsorbed (L)	Approximate efficiency of reabsorption (%)	
Diet	2	Jejunum	4-5 of 9	50	
Saliva	1				
Gastric secretion	2	Ileum	3-4 of 4-5	75	
Bile	1				
Pancreatic secretion	2	Colon	1-2 of 1-2	>90	
Small intestinal secretion	1				
TOTAL	9	TOTAL	8-9		

*The stool normally contains 100 to 200 ml of fluid daily. If it contains >300 mg/day, diarrhea is usually present

Composition of abnormal external losses

Fluid	Na$^+$ (mEq/L)	K$^+$ (mEq/L)	Cl$^-$ (mEq/L)
Gastric	20-80	5-20	100-150
Pancreatic	120-140	5-15	90-120
Small intestine	100-140	5-15	90-130
Bile	120-140	5-15	80-120
Ileostomy	45-135	3-15	20-115
Diarrhea	10-90	10-80	10-110
Sweat			
Normal	10-30	3-10	10-35
Cystic fibrosis	50-135	5-25	50-110
Burns	140	5	110

Index

Page numbers in italics indicate illustrations; *t* indicates tables; *n* indicates notes.